Certified Ophthalmic Technician
Exam Review Manual
Third Edition

Certified Ophthalmic Technician
Exam Review Manual
Third Edition

Janice K. Ledford, COMT

EyeWrite Productions

Franklin, North Carolina

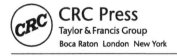

CRC Press
Taylor & Francis Group
Boca Raton London New York

CRC Press is an imprint of the
Taylor & Francis Group, an **Informa** business

Cover: Tinhouse Design

First published 2023 by SLACK Incorporated

Published 2024 by CRC Press
2385 NW Executive Center Drive, Suite 320, Boca Raton FL 33431

and by CRC Press
4 Park Square, Milton Park, Abingdon, Oxon, OX14 4RN

CRC Press is an imprint of Taylor & Francis Group, LLC

© 2023 Taylor & Francis Group, LLC

Janice K. Ledford and Aaron Shukla reported no financial or proprietary interest in the materials presented herein. Jane T. Shuman is President of Eyetechs, a consulting firm that trains technicians and encourages certification.

Library of Congress Control Number: 2023934504

ISBN: 9781630916442 (pbk)
ISBN: 9781003522973 (ebk)

DOI: 10.1201/9781003522973

Dedication

This one is for Cheryl.

Contents

Acknowledgments

This third edition would not, could not, have come into being without the assistance of Jane T. Shuman, MSM, COT, COE, OCS, OSC. Jane teaches a COT® review course and was willing to bring her much-valued opinion to this work; specifically, what may or may not constitute COT® material (vs COA® or COMT® level). In any case where I missed the mark, it is solely my error and not hers.

I am also grateful to many other colleagues, among whom are Al Lens, COMT (various graphics and advice on some questions about imaging devices); Aaron Shukla, PhD, COMT, (F)ATPO (reviewed/advised on some questions, submitted some questions for the optics chapter); and Rhonda G. Waldron, MMSc, COMT, CRA, ROUB, CDOS (advice on ultrasound). Others who gave an assist include Holly Hess Smith; Sergina M. Flaherty, COMT, OSC, CTC, (F)ATPO; and Monique Rinke, COMT.

I especially appreciate my fellow eye nerd pals in the Ophthalmic Techs on Facebook group, who have inspired and encouraged me, and kept me entertained.

Debbie Mason, Certification Manager at the IJCAHPO®, must certainly be glad that this book has finally gone to press. Her immeasurable patience with my many questions about the exam criteria is much appreciated.

Cheryl Pelham (to whom this edition is dedicated) simply would not let me give up. I cannot begin to tell you how many interruptions there have been to this work. I faced down COVID-19, bought a house and moved, lost my dear mother (for whom I was one of several caregivers), and other life challenges. Cheryl has been that steadying presence who encouraged me to let the work unfold its own way. (Every book I've ever written seems to have its own method of wanting to be composed.) Her favorite advice? "How does an ant eat an elephant? One bite at a time." True that.

SLACK Incorporated has also been patient. Tony Schiavo, Senior Vice President, deserves much credit in bringing this project to a satisfactory close. Thanks are also due to others at SLACK, including Jennifer Cahill, Joseph Magaletta, Erin O'Reilly, Megan Ritter, and Doris Zheku.

About the Author

She's been around forever. She loves her job and her patients. Her career mission statement is "Helping people see better, one person at a time." She loves to read and sing and play with her cat. She's a Judge Judy fan and a Trekkie. She's nuts over *The Hobbit* and *The Lord of the Rings*. She holds stubbornly (read: with a death grip) onto the Oxford comma. She thinks that eyes are the very coolest things *ever*. She thinks you should get certified. So get to work!

Foreword

For as many years that I have been in the field of ophthalmology, I have considered Jan Ledford, COMT, an invaluable asset to our industry. Although she has authored several texts, the ones she is most known for are the review manuals for each of the certification exams. Ophthalmic assistants and technicians have shared their copies with their coworkers but insist on getting them back for continual reference.

When an adult who has not been in school for many years takes an exam, they tend to be more stressed than they can recall being when they were in school. For some, it may mean an increase in pay, it might be a mandatory requirement of the job, or it may be for self-satisfaction (the best reason of all!). Whatever the motivation, Jan's review manuals have provided the test taker with a greater understanding of IJCAHPO's® knowledge areas.

If you referred to Jan Ledford's review manual for the COA® exam, you are familiar with the style and complexity of the questions. Not only does she provide the correct multiple-choice answer but teaches why. Furthermore, Jan takes the time to explain why the other answers are incorrect. In some cases, she includes responses that are outside the realm of possibility. If the reader remains confused, more self-study of that particular subject is needed.

In the years since the first editions were published, the field of ophthalmology has changed tremendously. There is more to learn about dry eye/ocular surface disease, new findings regarding glaucoma, and more diagnostic tests for our doctors to interpret. Although many of the review questions remained, Jan has tirelessly updated the material in *Certified Ophthalmic Technician Exam Review Manual* to acknowledge the changing workplace. I am honored that she chose me to validate the subject matter of the COT® questions and ensure it is appropriate for today's ophthalmic technician.

Like many others, we share a common passion for the field and a willingness to share our knowledge so others can advance as well. Each of our patients deserves a technician who is able to answer questions accurately and confidently. Each level of certification improves the depth of that knowledge and confidence.

Please use this book in the spirit with which it was written. Each chapter focuses on a different knowledge area of the exam. Begin with the sections with which you are least familiar, giving yourself ample time to return to them repeatedly. Reread chapters in your study book, ask your doctors questions when necessary. And most of all, go into your exam session feeling confident that you've got this.

—*Jane T. Shuman, MSM, COT, COE, OCS, OSC*
President
Eyetechs
Ashland, Massachusetts

Notes About the Book

SLACK is proud to feature the book *Principles and Practice in Ophthalmic Assisting: A Comprehensive Textbook* as a companion text to this exam review manual. Readings for study have been carefully selected and listed in each chapter.

- Ledford JK, Lens A, eds. *Principles and Practice in Ophthalmic Assisting: A Comprehensive Textbook*. SLACK Incorporated; 2018.

And here are a few disclaimers:

- Disclaimer #1: It is important (vital) to note that I didn't and don't have any inside info on the test, questions, or answers. My guide was the same criteria lists that you look at online or in the booklet from IJCAHPO®. Speaking of the criteria, I took great pains in attempting to interpret them at the appropriate (ie, COT®) level. I had help trying to do this, and they had no more inside info than myself.

- Disclaimer #2: As near as I could make it do so, at publication this book covered the COT® criteria as presented online. The criteria can change, however. Be sure you're using the latest criteria for your study efforts.

- Now for Disclaimer #3: Any opinions expressed herein are the author's and not those of any group, organization, clinic, or other entity with which she may be associated, including SLACK Incorporated and the Veterans Health Administration.

- Finally, Disclaimer #4: The information in this book is not intended for diagnosis or treatment of any disorder, medical or otherwise.

Chapter 1

History and Documentation*

* This topic comprises only 3% of the COT® exam. Since history taking is one of the most fundamental of COA® skills, if you desire more study questions, please see *Certified Ophthalmic Assistant Exam Review Manual, Third Edition*.

Ledford JK.
Certified Ophthalmic Technician Exam Review Manual, Third Edition (pp 1-10).
© 2023 Taylor & Francis Group.

ABBREVIATIONS USED IN THIS CHAPTER

- A/C   anterior chamber
- ACG   angle-closure glaucoma
- c/o   complains of
- E/M   evaluation and management
- OD   right eye
- OS   left eye
- OU   both eyes
- PFSH   past, family, and social history

Ocular

1. **Identify the elements in the following sample patient history. Some will be used more than once.**

    Pt presents complains of awakening with pain OD in middle of night X past 3 weeks. Does not happen every night, maybe 2 to 3 X a week. Pt states pain is +8 severe to the point of nausea. Vision cloudy and sees halos around bathroom light during this time. Tylenol helps some. Artificial tears no help. In the morning still somewhat achy and blurry but subsides after he's been up an hour or so. Pain is a throbbing, pressure sensation. Latest episode was last night.

    Elements:

    associated signs and symptoms _____

    chief complaint _____

    context _____

    duration _____

    location _____

    modifying factors _____

    quality _____

    severity _____

    timing _____

2. **Which of the following, if noted in the patient history, would *not* increase the E/M level of a patient presenting with a chief complaint of floaters?**

    a) no flashes

    b) no injury

    c) no tearing

    d) no "curtain" over vision

3. **A complete PFSH for a new patient must include which of the following elements?**

    a) past history

    b) family history

    c) social history

    d) all of the above

4. Your patient is returning to the clinic for an annual diabetic eye exam. In addition to carefully documenting their chief complaint, you have updated their systemic medications list. This is known as a:
    a) diabetic inquiry
    b) pertinent PFSH
    c) due diligence
    d) past history

5. Your patient is a 6-month-old infant where the mother states that the child's eyes do not seem to be straight. Which of the following questions is *most* pertinent?
    a) Has there been any discharge?
    b) Was the child born at term?
    c) Was the child delivered with forceps?
    d) Was this a Cesarean birth?

6. You have taken a phone call from an adult patient who splashed bleach in their eyes. What is the *most* important question?
    a) Have you rinsed with vinegar to counteract the bleach?
    b) One eye, or both?
    c) Have you been to our office before?
    d) Have you rinsed your eyes out?

7. Your adult patient presents with a metallic foreign body. From a *billing* standpoint, what is the *most* important question?
    a) Were you wearing eye protection?
    b) What were you doing when this happened?
    c) Did this happen on the job?
    d) When did this happen?

8. Of those listed, what is the *most* common cause of halos around lights?
    a) cataracts
    b) angle-closure glaucoma
    c) astigmatism
    d) migraine

9. Of those listed, which is the *most* emergent symptom?
    a) floaters
    b) flashes
    c) sudden painless loss of vision
    d) redness and photophobia

10. All of the following are symptoms *except*:
    a) intraocular pressure
    b) "curtain" over vision
    c) redness
    d) irritation

11. All of the following are signs *except*:
    a) phoria
    b) Marcus Gunn pupil
    c) diplopia
    d) cells in the anterior chamber

12. **Match the symptoms to the associated eye disorder. Symptoms may be used more than once.**

    Symptom | Disorder

    a) decreased vision   __ angle-closure glaucoma

    b) elevated intraocular pressure   __ cellulitis

    c) halos around lights   __ conjunctivitis

    d) mattering   __ endophthalmitis

    e) pain   __ foreign body

    f) photophobia   __ iritis

    g) redness   __ keratitis

    h) swelling   __ subconjunctival hemorrhage

    i) tearing

Medical

13. **Running through a check list of possible (nonocular) symptoms or inquiring after sets of systemic disorders is known as:**
    a) review of systems
    b) systematic evaluation
    c) mandatory review
    d) whole-body symptom review

14. **Your patient gives a history of asthma. This may be important if:**
    a) cataract surgery is necessary
    b) vitamin therapy is needed
    c) the patient is to be dilated
    d) a beta-blocker is prescribed for glaucoma

15. **You intend to check the patient's intraocular pressure with a Tono-Pen. Which of the following might be important?**
    a) photophobia
    b) claustrophobia
    c) high-frequency hearing loss
    d) latex allergy

16. **Your patient gives a history of sleep apnea. This could be important because:**
    a) the medication used in treatment can affect the eyes
    b) there is an increased risk of glaucoma
    c) the patient may fall asleep during the exam
    d) cataracts may worsen quickly

17. **Your patient gives a history of seizure disorder. This might affect which type of supplemental testing?**
    a) fluorescein angiogram
    b) A-scan ultrasound
    c) Schirmer's tear test
    d) potential acuity meter

18. **You notice that your patient's eyes seem to bulge a little. This should prompt you to ask about:**
     a) cancer treatments
     b) high blood pressure
     c) pituitary problems
     d) thyroid problems

Medication

19. **Match the disorder to the medication(s) commonly used to treat it. Disorders may be used more than once.**

Disorder

a) angina
b) asthma
c) blood clots
d) diabetes
e) erectile dysfunction
f) gastroesophageal reflux
g) high blood pressure
h) high cholesterol
i) inflammation
j) irregular heartbeat
k) pain
l) prostate problems
m) rheumatoid arthritis
n) risk of stroke
o) seizures
p) thyroid deficiency
q) urinary incontinence

Medication*

__ acetaminophen (Tylenol)
__ acetylsalicylic acid
__ albuterol (Proventil)
__ amiodarone (Cordone)
__ amlodipine (Norvasc)
__ atorvastatin (Lipitor)
__ gabapentin (Neurontin)
__ glucophage (Metformin)
__ hydrocodone (Lortab, Vicodin, Lorcet)
__ hydroxychloroquine (Plaquenil)
__ levothyroxine (Synthroid)
__ lisinopril (Prinivil, Zestril)
__ losartan (Cozaar)
__ omeprizol (Prilosec)
__ sildenafil (Viagra)
__ steroids
__ tamsulosin (Flomax)
__ warfarin (Coumadin)

20. **Match the systemic medication with the possible ocular complication. Medications may be used more than once.**

Medication

a) acetylsalicylic acid
b) amiodarone (Cordone)
c) hydroxychloroquine (Plaquenil)
d) sildenafil (Viagra)
e) steroids
f) tamsulosin (Flomax)
g) warfarin (Coumadin)

Possible Ocular Side Effect

__ "blue haze"
__ "red haze"
__ cataracts
__ corneal whorls
__ elevated intraocular pressure
__ excessive bleeding
__ intraoperative floppy iris
__ retinopathy/maculopathy

* Includes the top 10 most prescribed medications in the United States as of November 2021,[1] as well as medications of specific ophthalmic import.

Social

21. **Your patient is here for a refractive exam. Which of the following is *most* pertinent?**
    a) smoking
    b) occupation
    c) alcohol use
    d) marital status

22. **Your patient is here for a dry eye follow-up. Which of the following is *most* pertinent?**
    a) smoking
    b) illicit drug use
    c) social diseases
    d) alcohol use

23. **You ask the patient if they have been exposed to anyone who has had COVID-19. This is part of the patient's:**
    a) respiratory history
    b) risk factors
    c) ocular history
    d) social history

24. **Your patient asks to discuss their social history only with the practitioner. You should:**
    a) tell the patient that's your job, not the doctor's
    b) stop the exam and let the physician handle everything
    c) assure the patient of confidentiality then honor their wishes if they don't change their mind
    d) assure the patient of confidentiality and press them to answer

Family

25. **Which of the following is the *most* common genetically passed eye disorder?**
    a) refractive errors
    b) red-green color blindness
    c) strabismus
    d) retinitis pigmentosa

26. **Approximately what percentage of children with strabismus also have a family history of strabismus?**
    a) 1%
    b) 5%
    c) 40%
    d) 70%

27. **In some cases an ocular disorder is not itself inherited, but rather the propensity for developing it. This is known as:**
    a) genetic predetermination
    b) genetic inevitability
    c) genetic predisposition
    d) recessive inheritance

28. **Which of the following is *not* a potentially inherited ocular disorder?**
    a) acquired color vision defect
    b) aniridia
    c) corneal dystrophy
    d) albinism

29. **Which of the following is *not* likely to be inherited?**
    a) ptosis
    b) corneal scar
    c) epicanthal folds
    d) eye color

30. **Which of the following is a genetic disorder that is sometimes associated with dislocation of the crystalline lens?**
    a) Marfan syndrome
    b) Brown syndrome
    c) Violet syndrome
    d) retinitis pigmentosa

Study Notes

Suggested reading in *Principles and Practice in Ophthalmic Assisting: A Comprehensive Textbook:*
　　Chapter 7: History Taking (pp 77-91)
　　Chapter 9: Basic Eye Exam (*History Taking* p 119)
　　Chapter 10: Ocular Motility, Strabismus, and Amblyopia (*History Taking* p 156)
　　Chapter 21: Contact Lenses (*Patient Selection* pp 396-397)
　　Chapter 22: Pharmacology (*Identification of Ophthalmic Drugs* pp 420-421, *Ocular Effects of Systemic Drugs* pp 434-435)
　　Chapter 24: Genetics (*Genetics of Ophthalmic Diseases* pp 464-467)
　　Chapter 25: Neuro-Ophthalmology (*History* p 481)
　　Chapter 29: Glaucoma (*History Taking* pp 529 and 531)
　　Chapter 32: Ocular Trauma (*History Taking* pp 568-569)
　　Chapter 33: Non-Traumatic Ocular Emergent and Urgent Situations (*History Taking* pp 587-588)
　　Chapter 35: Low Vision (*History Taking* p 613)
　　Chapter 38: Refractive Surgery (*History Taking Considerations* p 650)
　　Chapter 43: The Basics of Coding in an Outpatient Setting (*Elements of the Eye Exam* p 698)

Explanatory Answers

1. associated signs and symptoms: nausea, vision cloudy, sees halos
    chief complaint: pain in OD
    context: wakens with
    duration: X past 3 weeks; maybe 2-3 X a week; in the morning still somewhat achy and blurry, but subsides after he's been up an hour or so
    location: OD
    modifying factors: Tylenol helps some, artificial tears no help
    quality: throbbing, pressure sensation
    severity: pain is +8 severe
    timing: in middle of night, last episode was last night

2. c) Negative answers only "count" if related to the chief complaint. Since tearing is not classically associated with floaters, it would not bump the history up to the next level of E/M.

3. d) For a new patient, the PFSH must include all 3 history types.

4. b) Since this is an established patient, while a complete PFSH is not required, you should document at least one of them. In this case it is appropriate to update the medications. Since they are diabetic, their medications are pertinent to the exam.

5. b) Premature infants have a higher rate of strabismus than those born at term.

6. d) *Triage* is taking a history and figuring out where the patient/incident falls in the continuum of emergent vs urgent vs routine. But the need for immediate first aid trumps history; ask the patient if they have irrigated their eyes yet and if not, send them to do so for at least 15 minutes.

7. c) For *billing*, you need to know if this will be a Worker's Compensation case. From a medical standpoint, you will also want to know if any treatment was attempted as well as the information requested in Answers a), b), and d).

8. a) The disruption of a cataract in the path of vision will often diffract light, causing halos around lights. Corneal edema caused by angle-closure glaucoma (ACG) may also be accompanied by halos, but ACG is not common. Astigmatism usually has a "starburst" effect on lights. Migraine is sometimes associated with a shimmering, colored aura, but not specifically around lights.

9. c) A sudden, painless loss of vision is usually at the top of everyone's ocular triage list because it portends several serious eye problems: retinal vein or artery occlusion, hemorrhage, giant cell arteritis, and retinal detachment.

10. a) Symptoms are what the patient is experiencing. You may or may not be able to see it for yourself (eg, you can see the redness but you cannot feel the patient's irritation or see the "curtain").

11. c) Signs are things that you, as an observer, can discover, usually with testing. In the examples, a phoria is not seen until you do a cover test, the Marcus Gunn pupil is revealed when you do a swinging flashlight test, and cells in the A/C are seen only under the slit lamp. Diplopia, however, is something you cannot observe—double vision is a symptom that the patient tells you about that you cannot see for yourself.

12. **Matching**:
    angle-closure glaucoma: a), b), c), e), g)
    cellulitis: e), h)
    conjunctivitis*: d), g), h), i)
    endophthalmitis: a), e), f), g)
    foreign body: e), g), i)
    iritis: a), e), f), g)
    keratitis: a), e), f), g), i)
    subconjunctival hemorrhage: g)

---

* *Conjunctivitis* is a term that encompasses allergic, bacterial, and viral forms, among others. Symptoms vary according to the cause

13. a) Review of systems involves evaluating the patient for systemic disorders. This can be done by asking about specific symptoms (Do you have shortness of breath?) and/or about specific organ systems (Do you have any problems with your lungs?). For the visit to "qualify" as comprehensive, a review of systems must be included. If the exam is at the "lower" levels, then review of systems is not needed as far as coding/billing is concerned.

14. d) A beta-blocker (as used for treating glaucoma) can exacerbate bronchospasms in a patient with asthma.

15. d) The disposable tip covers for the Tono-Pen contain latex. While it is unlikely that such brief contact would elicit an allergic reaction, it is still a good idea to use an alternate method of checking this patient's intraocular pressure.

16. b) Studies have found an increased risk of glaucoma in patients with obstructive sleep apnea. This is theorized to be due to damage to the optic nerve caused by hypoxia (lack of oxygen).[2]

17. a) Some seizure disorders can be triggered by flashing/strobe-like lights, so any photographic procedure could be problematic.

18. d) Exophthalmia (bulging eyes) can be related to thyroid problems.

19. **Matching**:
    angina: amlodipine (Norvasc)
    asthma: albuterol (Proventil)
    blood clots: acetylsalicylic acid, warfarin (Coumadin)
    diabetes: glucophage (Metformin)
    erectile dysfunction: sildenafil (Viagra)
    gastroesophogeal reflux: omeprizol (Prilosec)
    high blood pressure: amlodipine (Norvasc), lisinopril (Prinivil, Zestril), losartan (Cozaar)
    high cholesterol: atorvastatin (Lipitor)
    inflammation: acetaminophen (Tylenol), acetylsalicylic acid, steroids
    irregular heartbeat: amiodarone (Cordone)
    pain: acetaminophen (Tylenol), acetylsalicylic acid (aspirin), hydrocodone (Lortab, Vicodin)*
    prostate problems: tamsulosin (Flomax)
    rheumatoid arthritis: hydroxychloroquine (Plaquenil)
    risk of stroke: acetylsalicylic acid (aspirin), losartan (Cozaar), warfarin (Coumadin)
    seizures: gabapentin (Neurontin)
    thyroid deficiency: levothyroxine (Synthroid)
    urinary incontinence: tamsulosin (Flomax)

20. **Matching**:
    acetylsalicylic acid: excessive bleeding
    amiodarone (Cordone): corneal whorls
    hydroxychloroquine (Plaquenil): retinopathy/maculopathy
    sildenafil (Viagra): "blue haze," "red haze" if exceeding recommended dose
    steroids: elevated intraocular pressure, cataracts
    tamsulosin (Flomax): intraoperative floppy iris
    warfarin (Coumadin): excessive bleeding

21. b) Although each element listed is part of the patient's social history, the important one in this case is occupation. You need to know the patient's visual activities and working distances to provide the best information for the prescriber.

22. a) Again, each element is a part of the social history. Smoking can be a key factor in dry eye.

23. d) Asking about exposure to contagious disorders would be part of the social history.

---

* If you listed gabapentin here, that's okay: it's used for nerve pain in addition to seizures.

24.   c) The patient has the right to discuss matters with only the practitioner if desired. You might say, "Okay, we don't have any problem with that! But I can assure you that anything you tell me is strictly confidential." If the patient is not reassured, then defer the discussion to the doctor.

25.   a) Refractive errors are the most common genetically inherited eye disorder. Surprised?

26.   c) About 40% of children with strabismus have someone in the family who had it as well.[3] *The point here isn't to actually memorize this statistic, but to emphasize how important family history is to the overall patient history.*

27.   c) Genetic predisposition means that conditions were inherited that makes a person more likely to develop a specific ocular disorder. A simple example would be high hyperopia, which might make a person more likely to have narrow angles, and therefore more likely to develop ACG. It's more complicated, of course.

28.   a) The word "acquired" should have tipped you off that this one is not genetic. It is, rather, developed as a side effect, usually of medication.

29.   b) A corneal scar would be caused by an injury, not by heredity.

30.   a) Marfan syndrome is a genetic disorder where the affected person has elongated limbs (including fingers and toes). Dislocation of the lens is a common ocular disorder associated with it. It is believed that Abraham Lincoln had Marfan syndrome. Brown syndrome involves the extraocular muscles; Violet syndrome is made up; retinitis pigmentosa is genetic but does not involve the lens.

References

1.   The GoodRx Top 10. GoodRx Website. November 2021 Accessed March 12, 2023. https://www.goodrx.com/drug-guide

2.   Chaitanya A, Pai VH, Mohapatra AK, VeRs. Glaucoma and its association with obstructive sleep apnea: a narrative review. *Oman J Ophthalmol.* 2016;9(3);125-134. doi:10.4103/0974-620X.192261

3.   Hereditary eye conditions and diseases. Auckland Eye Blog. March 6, 2019. Accessed March 12, 2023. https://www.aucklandeye.co.nz/about/blog/hereditary-eye-conditions-and-diseases

Chapter 2

Visual Assessment*

* For questions on stereo acuity, near point of accommodation, and near point of convergence, see Chapter 7: Ocular Motility Testing.

Ledford JK.
Certified Ophthalmic Technician Exam Review Manual, Third Edition (pp 11-23).
© 2023 Taylor & Francis Group.

```
┌─────────────────────────────────────────────────────┐
│        ABBREVIATIONS USED IN THIS CHAPTER             │
│   •  CF          count fingers                        │
│   •  ETDRS       Early Treatment Diabetic Retinopathy │
│                  Study                                │
│   •  ft          foot/feet                            │
└─────────────────────────────────────────────────────┘
```

Visual Acuity: Test and Record

1. **Your patient can correctly count fingers at 10 ft. This roughly translates to:**
   a) 20/100 acuity
   b) 20/200 acuity
   c) 20/400 acuity
   d) 20/600 acuity

2. **Count fingers acuity is less acceptable to some practitioners because:**
   a) results are dependent on size of examiner's hand
   b) it is not standard of care
   c) it cannot be performed in dim light
   d) a 20-foot test distance is required

3. **All of the following are disadvantages to hand motion acuity testing *except*:**
   a) lack of uniformity of background contrast
   b) varying hand size of different examiners
   c) varying illumination
   d) difficult for patient to understand

4. **When comparing count fingers to hand motion, it is generally accepted that hand motion is:**
   a) 2 X worse than counting fingers at the same distance
   b) 10 X worse than counting fingers at the same distance
   c) 20 X worse than counting fingers at the same distance
   d) more accurate

5. **The difference between light perception and light projection is:**
   a) light perception is the ability to locate the light; light projection is the ability to see the light
   b) light perception vision is better than light projection
   c) light perception is the ability to see light; light projection is the ability to locate the light
   d) light perception can be done with children; light projection is done in adults

6. **Your patient cannot detect direction or presence of light as tested with a pen light/transillumi-nator. Your next step is to:**
   a) record vision as no light perception
   b) try a pinhole vision
   c) check again with the indirect ophthalmoscope light
   d) check pupils for Marcus Gunn

7. **At what age would we expect an infant to have developed some binocular vision?**
    a) 1 month
    b) 3 months
    c) 12 months
    d) 24 months

8. **You are evaluating vision in a 4-month-old with your pen light. The light reflex falls slightly nasal on the right eye. This is noted as:**
    a) central fixation
    b) noncentral fixation
    c) eccentric fixation
    d) exotropia

9. **In evaluating an infant, the term** *steady fixation* **means that:**
    a) the infant remains still during evaluation
    b) the baby easily reaches for the target
    c) the infant keeps looking at the target
    d) the baby refuses to look at the target

10. **You are examining a 3-month-old. She looks directly at your pen light and keeps her eye on it as you move it slowly to the left and right. This would be documented as:**
    a) responds to light
    b) fix and follow
    c) orthophoria
    d) normal versions/ductions

11. **You are examining a 6-month-old. Vision is central and steady with each eye. With both eyes together, vision is still central and steady. This is referred to as:**
    a) binocular vision
    b) light perception
    c) light projection
    d) maintained

Optotypes*

12. **A vision of 15/20 is tested how far from the target?**
    a) 0.5 ft
    b) 10 ft
    c) 15 ft
    d) 20 ft

13. **The figures on an eye chart or acuity card—whether letters, numbers, symbols, or pictures— are known as:**
    a) Snellens
    b) optotypes
    c) points
    d) Allens

* Since testing patients who are preliterate, illiterate, aphasic, and foreign-speaking is largely a matter of choosing an appropriate optotype, the material regarding these are mixed in with the rest of the visual acuity questions.

14. **The generally accepted standard optotype is:**
    a) Snellen letters
    b) Allen pictures
    c) Landolt chart
    d) Jaeger chart

15. **Snellen letters are calibrated so that each letter falls within a 5 x 5 grid. Each block of the grid:**
    a) subtends 5 minutes of arc
    b) subtends 1 minute of arc
    c) subtends 5 degrees of arc
    d) subtends 1 degree of arc

16. **Which of the following is *not* a recognition-type acuity test?**
    a) ETDRS chart
    b) Sloan letters
    c) Lea symbols
    d) Tumbling Es

17. **Tumbling Es and Landolt broken ring optotypes are examples of:**
    a) recognition tests
    b) resolution tests
    c) contrast tests
    d) glare tests

18. **Assessing a person's acuity using optotypes on a chart is an example of:**
    a) kinetic vision
    b) static vision
    c) dynamic vision
    d) control testing

19. **You cannot speak your patient's language. Which of the following acuity tests is most appropriate?**
    a) count fingers
    b) light perception
    c) E-game
    d) pictures

20. **Which of the following acuity tests are *most* appropriate for an illiterate patient?**
    a) Snellen letters, numbers, and pictures
    b) Snellen letters, Sheridan Gardner test, and numbers
    c) Snellen letters, E-game, and numbers
    d) E-game, Landolt C, and sometimes numbers

21. **Which of the following are commonly used letter optotypes for children?**
    a) HOTV
    b) ABC
    c) XYZ
    d) KAJSV

22. In checking visual acuity of children, the most important information is:
     a) whether or not the vision is 20/40 or better
     b) the patient's vision with both eyes opened
     c) any difference between the acuity of the 2 eyes
     d) whether or not the vision in each eye is 20/20

23. Crowding bars are used on some vision charts especially for testing patients with:
     a) cataracts
     b) strabismus
     c) amblyopia
     d) agoraphobia

24. When testing vision using hand-held optotype cards, it is important to:
     a) use only Allen picture cards
     b) test the patient first for hand motion
     c) properly record the testing distance
     d) test in a dark room

25. A *disadvantage* of the Landolt C and Tumbling E tests is that:
     a) there is a 25% guess rate
     b) they are not easily recognized by children
     c) they are more time-consuming to use
     d) they are not accepted for low vision testing

26. The standard Snellen chart may not be adequate for evaluating how a patient really sees because:
     a) it cannot be used in varying light conditions
     b) it does not measure macular function
     c) it is high contrast
     d) it is easy to memorize

27. If the metric system is used, at what distance is visual acuity checked?
     a) 2 meters
     b) 6 meters
     c) 10 meters
     d) 20 meters

28. Which of the following would indicate that the patient has low vision?
     a) 20/10
     b) 20/400
     c) 10/10
     d) 400/20

29. You are going to check a patient's near acuity. The near card should be held:
     a) wherever the patient can see it most clearly
     b) 10 inches
     c) 14 inches
     d) 20 ft

30. **One key feature of the ETDRS acuity chart is that:**
    a) only numbers are used
    b) only easily recognized pictures are used
    c) every line has the same number of optotypes
    d) every line is 20/100

31. **The ETDRS chart would be *most* useful in which testing situation?**
    a) children
    b) low vision patients
    c) literate adults
    d) non–English-speaking patients

32. **Which of the following is *not* true regarding a distance visual acuity chart designed specifically for testing low vision patients?**
    a) it can be used with a variety of low vision aids
    b) it provides larger optotypes than traditional charts
    c) it provides more graded lines in the larger sizes
    d) it provides continuous reading text

33. **When testing near vision in the low vision patient, the best type of card to use is the:**
    a) continuous text
    b) same chart used for distance
    c) contrast sensitivity card
    d) any near chart may be used

34. **In order to *best* assess the functional vision at near of a patient who is legally blind, one should:**
    a) encourage the patient to guess at the letters on the acuity chart
    b) simply ask if the patient can see that there are letters on the chart; reading them is not necessary
    c) have the patient read only the smallest text that can be read easily and comfortably
    d) try all available low vision aids until finding the one that gives the best acuity

35. **Visual acuity in a patient with nystagmus should be tested using the following tips *except*:**
    a) use a +6.00 diopter trial lens as an occluder and have them keep both eyes opened
    b) allow the patient to tilt their head if they normally do so
    c) occlude the eye not being tested with an occluder as usual
    d) allow the patient to wear their usual distance correction

Pinhole

36. **An intelligent, literate patient sees 20/400 without correction, 20/200 with the pinhole, and 20/200 with correction. The most reasonable assumption is:**
    a) they need a change of glasses
    b) they are malingering
    c) they are uncooperative
    d) they have some type of ocular pathology

37. **Your healthy patient has clear media, although you have not looked at the retina. Your best refraction yields only 20/40 vision. What should you do next?**
    a) record the measurement as final
    b) label that eye as amblyopic
    c) get a pinhole vision
    d) perform a stereo test

38. **The pinhole improves vision by:**
    a) eliminating polarized light
    b) correcting color vision
    c) eliminating scattered (indirect) light rays
    d) eliminating blur from pathology

39. **Potential vision of a person with uncorrected aphakia may *best* be evaluated by using:**
    a) a pinhole disk
    b) a +10.00 or +12.00 diopter trial lens
    c) a +10.00 or +12.00 diopter trial lens and a pinhole
    d) count fingers

Low Vision Definitions

40. **The term *low vision* means that the patient:**
    a) has difficulty with everyday tasks due to impairment
    b) will not benefit from low vision aids
    c) has no functional vision
    d) is eligible for government assistance

41. **In the United States, the term *legal blindness* refers to which best corrected acuity (in the better eye)?**
    a) 20/40
    b) 20/100
    c) 20/200
    d) 20/400

42. **The term *legal blindness* refers to which limitation of peripheral vision?**
    a) 20 degrees
    b) 40 degrees
    c) 60 degrees
    d) 80 degrees

43. **Your patient's best corrected acuity in the better eye is 20/100. Because they do not qualify as legally blind:**
    a) they are not eligible for any type of assistance
    b) they cannot be referred to a low vision clinic
    c) they may be disabled and eligible for some type of compensation
    d) no optical low vision aids will be helpful

44. **The largest group of individuals who are legally blind are:**
    a) preschool children (infants to age 5 years)
    b) school-aged children (ages 5 to 18 years)
    c) young adults (ages 20 to 60 years)
    d) older persons (ages 65+ years)

45. **The leading cause of blindness in adults living in the Western world is:**
    a) cataracts
    b) glaucoma
    c) retinal disease
    d) trachoma

46. **Of those who are legally blind:**
    a) most have some residual vision
    b) most are totally blind
    c) most have developed nystagmus
    d) most have tunnel vision

Low Vision Aids

47. **The 2 basic divisions of low vision aids are:**
    a) optical and nonoptical
    b) tactile and auditory
    c) low and high magnification
    d) magnifiers and telescopes

48. **Examples of optical low vision aids include:**
    a) magnifiers, telescopes, and high-powered bifocals
    b) reading glasses, large print, and yellow filter
    c) stand magnifier, Braille, and high-intensity lamp
    d) closed-circuit television and books on tape

49. **Examples of nonoptical low vision aids include:**
    a) high-powered reading glasses and magnifying glass
    b) writing guide, high illumination lighting, and large print
    c) magnifiers, telescopes, and closed-circuit television
    d) magnifying page, Braille, and reading guide

50. **Patients with reduced visual fields would be expected to benefit most from:**
    a) optical magnification
    b) optical minification
    c) increased illumination
    d) infrared rejection lens

51. **Magnification functions as a low vision aid by:**
    a) shortening the viewing distance
    b) shortening the working distance
    c) increasing the size of the retinal image
    d) using only one lens

52. **Advantages of telescopes modified for near vs a regular magnifier include:**
    a) increased working distance
    b) comparative lightness and reduced size
    c) relatively wide field
    d) all of the above

53. **An older person with hand tremors might do well with any of these low vision aids *except*:**
    a) stand magnifier
    b) hand magnifier
    c) page magnifier
    d) reading stand with light

54. **A college law student with low vision might benefit most from using:**
    a) a reading telescope
    b) a stand magnifier
    c) a hand magnifier
    d) a computerized low vision scanner

Study Note

Suggested reading in *Principles and Practice in Ophthalmic Assisting: A Comprehensive Textbook*:
   Chapter 8: Vision Testing (pp 93-116)

Explanatory Answers

1. c) "CF at a given distance is usually converted to a Snellen equivalent by assuming that the fingers are approximately the size of the elements of a '200 letter."[1] So if you are at a 10-foot testing distance, that would be 10/200. To convert that to the traditional 20 ft (ie, to make the numerator 20), multiply by 2/2 (which equals one) = 20/400. (If following standard protocol, you would have already tried the eye chart before resorting to count fingers; but try again with the 20/400 letter and encourage them a bit.)
2. a) Some practitioners do not want a count fingers acuity notation for several reasons. For one thing, it is somewhat subjective, depending on the examiner's interpretation of the patient's replies (which often vary), background contrast, and size of the examiner's hand and fingers. It is more useful (and comparable) to bring an optotype to the patient until it is recognized and then converting the answer to a 20-foot format.
3. d) The hand motion test is easily understood. When checking acuity with optotypes, the illumination, background, and optotype size are controlled. This is not the case with either counting fingers or detecting hand motion.
4. b) Hand motion is roughly considered to be 10 times worse than count fingers at same distance.[2] Hand motion at 2 ft is approximately equivalent to 20/20,000. (If count fingers at 2 ft = 20/2000, then hand motion at 2 ft would be around 20/20,000.)
5. c) Light perception means the patient can perceive the presence of light. In light projection, the patient can also detect from which direction the light projects, which is considered a higher level of vision than light perception alone.
6. c) Once it's determined that the patient cannot detect the pen light, your final step before declaring no light perception is to check with "noxious" light. Hold the indirect headset in your hand, turn the light on full blast, and check for light perception again. *Note:* be sure that the fellow eye is well occluded. I usually use my own hand, using my palm to create a "seal" around the fellow eye.

7.   b) At 1 month, an infant should be able to follow a slow-moving target. Binocular vision is expected by 3 months. By 6 months the child should be reaching for toys, by 12 months looking for hidden toys, and at 24 months may actually be able to match pictures.

8.   a) In evaluating vision in infants, one thing you're looking for is the eye to fixate on the object (your pen light in this case) using the fovea. This is indicated when the corneal reflex falls slightly nasal to center. If it does, then vision is documented as central for that eye. If not, then fixation is noted as being noncentral (you may also see the term *uncentral*). Eccentric fixation means that an area other than the fovea is used for fixation; this would also be termed noncentral. Each eye is evaluated separately. It is normal for the fixation reflex to be slightly nasal; this does not indicate exotropia.

9.   c) An eye that "finds" the target and locks onto it most likely has at least some visual function. If fixation is not steady, you may see movement of the eye as if the baby is searching for the target. Fixation would also be not steady if nystagmus was present.

10.   b) Most infants with vision will look at (fix) and smoothly follow a slowly moving target at 1 to 2 months of age. The test is done for each eye. Remember, this should be a silent target. An infant following a noisy squeaky toy (or your talking face) could be simply responding to sound.

11.   d) Central and steady are first evaluated for each eye alone. Then you look for any shift in fixation when you uncover one eye and then the other. (Yes, this is like a cover test for strabismus.) If neither eye shifts during cover/uncover, then fixation is considered *maintained*, and it is likely that vision is equal in each eye.

12.   c) The numerator indicates the test distance; thus, the patient was 15 ft from the target or chart.

13.   b) Visual acuity testing figures are called optotypes. Snellen and Allen are variations of optotypes. *Point* is a print size.

14.   a) Snellen letters are generally accepted as the industry standard. Allen pictures feature common objects (eg, car, horse, house, hand) and are generally used for testing children. The Landolt chart has "C" or "broken rings," where the patient must identify if the opening is right, left, up, or down. The Jaeger system is used for near testing, but the size of the letters is not standardized.

15.   b) Each part of the 5 x 5 grid subtends 1 minute of arc; the total subtends 5 minutes of arc (ie, each part of the letter is 1/5 of the whole). This actually corresponds to the arrangement of cone cells in a healthy macula. A single degree, as in Answers c) and d), is made up of 60 minutes of arc. "To say that an object 'subtends XX minutes of arc' means that the rays emanating from an object of a specific size and a specific distance away eventually converge to a specific point, creating a specific angle."[3] In vision testing, that specific point is the macula.

16.   d) In recognition acuity tests, the question is, "Can the patient successfully identify smaller and smaller optotypes?" The tests in a), b), and c) are all recognition tests, requiring the patient to be familiar with the optotypes themselves. In the Tumbling E test, the patient does not have to know that the optotype is an E in order to discern the orientation of smaller and smaller optotypes.

17.   b) Resolution-based acuity tests require that the patient be able to discern (and identify) the orientation of smaller and smaller details on the same optotype. See Answer 16 for information on recognition tests. The contrast and glare tests are not considered visual acuity tests per se.

18.   b) Static vision means that the target is stationary (ie, not moving). Kinetic (also called dynamic) vision refers to how well you perceive moving objects such as a tennis ball. *Control testing* is a bogus term.

19.   c) The E-game is most appropriate if there is a language barrier. The patient can easily be taught the procedure using pantomime. If desired, the patient can be given a hand-held E-card that they can turn to match each optotype, giving the most accurate measurement possible. Count fingers and light perception are not appropriate, nor are pictures (also problematic because of the language difference).

20. d) An illiterate patient might be tested with the E-game or Landolt C. Many illiterate patients also recognize numbers. (Of course, pictures might be used, too, but did not appear in a proper answer combination. Be sure to read all items in an answer.) The "functionally literate" can usually recognize letters, but this situation was not identified in the question.

21. a) HOTV are symmetrical (ie, the left and right sides of the letters are identical) and are often easily recognized by children.

22. c) It is most crucial to find amblyopia at as early an age as possible, while it is still correctable. So, finding a difference between the 2 eyes is more important than the actual vision. (An exception might be the child with low vision, but that was not offered as a response.)

23. c) Crowding bars are used to "frame" each optotype in order to prevent the crowding phenomenon, in which a child with amblyopia seems to have better acuity when presented a single optotype vs a row of them.

24. c) Remember, the numerator (top number) of the visual acuity fraction is the testing distance, which varies if you're using hand-held cards. If you are using a card with a 20/200 E on it, and the farthest away the patient can correctly identify the orientation of that E is 10 ft, then vision is 10/200. This can be algebraically converted to a standard acuity of 20/400.

But you must also be sure you're using the proper denominator. Allen cards, for example, have a denominator of /30 (so be sure to read instructions that come with any test). The top number, then, is the farthest distance at which the patient can correctly identify the optotypes. Suppose that the farthest distance at which the patient can correctly identify the pictures is 10 ft. The vision is 10/30. Again, this can be converted to standard format: 20/60.

25. a) Because there are only 4 options (right, left, up, or down), these tests have a 25% guess rate. Because of this they are not as accurate as other tests. They are ideal for young children because the patient does not have to know that the optotype is a "C" or an "E," but simply to identify the orientation of the opening or "legs." The test is not particularly time consuming and can be used with low vision patients (although the ETDRS chart is *much* better for low vision).

26. c) The standard Snellen chart employs black letters on a bright, white background. In other words, it has high contrast. How much of our world is of such high contrast? Most of what we look at is shades and shadows. Therefore, the Snellen chart may give an exaggerated sense of the patient's acuity. Low contrast situations that are difficult for a person with normal contrast sensitivity may be virtually debilitating to a person with low contrast sensitivity.

27. b) In countries where the metric system is used, the standard distance for testing distant acuity is 6 meters.

28. b) In patients with low vision, the numerator (top number) still indicates the distance from the patient to the chart. The denominator (bottom number) indicates the smallest optotype that patient can identify from the indicated distance. Thus, a) and c) represent vision that is normal or better than normal. Answer b) means that the person identifies, at 20 ft, an optotype that a person with normal vision could identify from 400 ft away: the correct answer. Answer d) would be an impossible situation where a person could identify from 400 ft what a person with normal vision could see at 20 ft.

29. c) The standard near card is held at 14 to 16 inches.

30. c) Because the ETDRS chart has the same number of letters in each row, it is a more accurate representation of the patient's acuity. Standard acuity charts, for example, often have only 2 letters on the 20/100 line but 6 on the 20/20 line. This can skew the testing results.

31. b) The ETDRS system was developed in 1982 for use in scientific study, which requires that multiple examiners use the same standards and are able to obtain the same results over and over. The ETDRS chart meets those requirements, at least to a better degree than the standard Snellen charts. Some feel that the system is too time consuming for use in the average eye clinic. The same features that make the ETDRS system so useful for research also make it the preferred system for low vision patients (see Answer 30). It can be used for other groups, of course, but of those listed the best answer is low vision.

32.   d) The charts for *near* testing of low vision provide continuous text, not the distance charts. The "normal" Snellen distance charts usually jump from 20/100 to 20/200 to 20/400. A distance chart for low vision patients provides several rows of letters (or test objects) that fall between these gradations.

33.   a) See Answer 32.

34.   c) The low vision patient is not usually encouraged to guess at the letters because we are concerned with functional vision. (Some may feel, however, that guessing is useful in order to know the patient's visual threshold, so opinions vary.) Use a near card of continuous text rather than single letters or numbers. The acuity to record is the last line that the patient can read with ease.

35.   c) In patients with nystagmus, covering one eye may cause the amplitude/speed of the nystagmus to increase, blurring the vision. For conventional visual acuity testing, allow the patient to wear their own glasses, assume any habitual head posture (which likely decreases the amplitude/speed of the jerking), and occlude the eye not being tested with a high plus lens such as +6. Both eyes should be kept open; the +6 lens effectively acts as occlusion without increasing the nystagmus.

36.   d) The patient sees no better with correction than with the pinhole, so changing the glasses will not help. The residual poor acuity would be due to pathology.

37.   c) Anytime a healthy-looking eye does not refract to 20/20, do a pinhole vision. If the pinhole improves the vision, you should be able to improve acuity with the correct lenses. If the pinhole does not improve the vision, your refraction is probably the best you can do, and the doctor will look for pathology.

38.   c) The pinhole improves vision by eliminating light rays that are not central, focused, and coming straight into the eye, temporarily eliminating the visual effects of a refractive error. If pinhole vision is less than 20/20, one must suspect a pathological reason for less than optimal vision.

39.   c) While a pinhole disk alone may be used, the person with aphakia needs a large amount of plus to correct for the lack of a crystalline lens. Put a +10 or +12 lens in the trial frames and put the pinhole disk over that to get your best evaluation.

40.   a) "Low vision" is not a legally regulated term. It usually refers to those who are visually impaired because of problems that cannot be permanently corrected (optically or otherwise), where the loss interferes with the person's activities of daily life. Low vision aids may be of immense benefit.

41.   c) In the United States, legal blindness is defined as having vision of no better than 20/200 as the best corrected vision in the best eye. (This is with traditional correction, without the use of any low vision aids.) Remember, "low vision" is not defined by laws and regulations; "legal blindness" is. Also remember that "legal blindness" includes *both* the partially sighted and the totally blind.

42.   a) Legal blindness also exists if the patient's visual field is restricted to 20 degrees or less.

43.   c) While being legally blind is necessary to receive free government assistance, the federal registry still recognizes the fact that, while a person may not be legally blind, they may still be visually impaired and thus disabled to some degree. Such a person may qualify for some type of insurance, social services, or Social Security compensation.

44.   d) Unfortunately, many causes of legal blindness are age related. More older adults fall into the category of legal blindness than the other groups listed.

45.   c) Retinal disorders (including diabetic retinopathy and macular degeneration) are the leading cause of blindness in adults in the Western world.

46.   a) Stein, Stein, and Freeman report that of legally blind persons, most (approximately 66%) have some residual vision. In the United States and Canada, not quite 10% of those legally blind are actually totally blind (ie, have no light perception).[4]

47.   a) The 2 main types of low vision aids are optical and nonoptical. Items in answer b) are nonoptical aids, and items in answers c) and d) are optical aids.

48.   a) Examples of optical aids include magnifiers, telescopes, high-powered bifocals, and stand magnifiers. Large print, yellow filters, Braille, high-intensity lamps, CCTV, and books on tape are nonoptical. Answer a) was the only option that offered *only* optical aids.

49. b) Nonoptical aids include those mentioned in Answer 48, plus writing and reading guides. Answer b) is the only list of nonoptical aids without any optical aids thrown in.
50. b) Minifying the distant scene for a visual field–impaired person helps shrink the view to within their available field.
51. c) Any type of magnifying system enlarges the image that falls on the retina.
52. a) A telescope that has been modified for near work allows the user to have a greater working distance than with magnifiers.
53. b) A person with a hand tremor would have trouble holding a hand magnifier still. The other 3 options don't require the user to hold anything.
54. d) A computerized low vision scanner (closed-circuit TV) allows a wide range of magnification capabilities combined with being able to save the reading material on disk.

References

1. Schulze-Bonsel K, Feltgen N, Burau H, Hansen L, Bach M. Visual acuities "hand motion" and "counting fingers" can be quantified with the Freiburg visual acuity test. *Investig Ophthalmol Vis Sci.* 2006;47:1236-1240. doi:https://doi.org/10.1167/iovs.05-0981
2. Holladay JT. Proper method for calculating average visual acuity. *J Refract Surg.* 1997;13:388-391. doi:https://doi.org/10.3928/1081-597X-19970701-16
3. Ledford JK. Vision testing. In: *Principles and Practice in Ophthalmic Assisting: A Comprehensive Textbook.* SLACK Incorporated; 2018.
4. Stein HA, Stein RM, Freeman MI. *The Ophthalmic Assistant: A Text for Allied and Associated Ophthalmic Personnel.* 10th ed. Elsevier: 2018.

Chapter 3

Visual Field Testing

Ledford JK.
*Certified Ophthalmic Technician Exam
Review Manual, Third Edition* (pp 25-74).
© 2023 Taylor & Francis Group.

> ## ABBREVIATIONS USED IN THIS CHAPTER
>
> - cm   centimeter
> - D   diopter
> - m   meter
> - mm   millimeter
> - OD   right eye
> - OS   left eye
> - OU   both eyes
> - Rx   prescription (for glasses)
> - SITA   Swedish Interactive Thresholding
>   Algorithm

Part I*

Anatomy and Physiology of Peripheral Vision**

1. The extent of vision beyond the fixation point is known as the:
    a) binocular field
    b) visual field
    c) neurological field
    d) visual pathway

2. The normal extent of human peripheral vision of is:
    a) 60 degrees temporal, 60 degrees inferior, 75 degrees nasal, and 95 degrees superior
    b) 75 degrees temporal, 60 degrees inferior, 95 degrees nasal, and 60 degrees superior
    c) 95 degrees temporal, 60 degrees inferior, 75 degrees nasal, and 60 degrees superior
    d) 95 degrees temporal, 75 degrees inferior, 60 degrees nasal, and 60 degrees superior

3. The configuration of the normal visual field is limited by:
    a) the ear and nasal bridge
    b) the brow and nose
    c) the location of the fovea
    d) the size of the optic nerve

4. In the island of vision analogy, vision exists in:
    a) a sea of blindness
    b) a sea of vision
    c) an expanse of vision
    d) a time-space continuum

---

* Sections have been inserted into this lengthy chapter for ease of study, to allow for a logical "break" point.
** In order to understand the basis of all visual field testing, I determined it prudent to include some ocular anatomy here, as well as questions on the visual pathway.

5. **The blind spot would be represented on the island of vision profile as:**
    a) a bottomless hole
    b) a peak
    c) a shallow dip
    d) a deep pit

6. **The peak of the island of vision profile corresponds to the:**
    a) optic nerve
    b) center of the crystalline lens
    c) nerve fiber layer
    d) fovea

7. **In the island of vision analogy, peripheral vision that gradually decreases as it extends outward would be represented by a:**
    a) bottomless hole
    b) gentle slope
    c) sharp drop-off
    d) flat area

8. **The retinal nerve fibers are axon extensions of the:**
    a) rods and cones
    b) ganglion cells
    c) bipolar layer
    d) Mueller cells

9. **Label the following drawing of the retinal nerve fibers (Figure 3-1):**
    __ horizontal raphe
    __ optic disc
    __ radiating nasal fibers
    __ temporal fibers

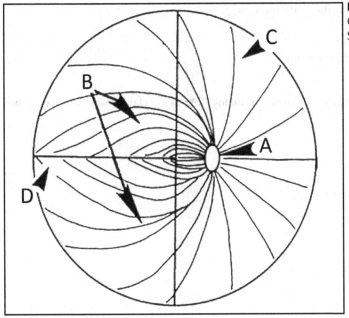

Figure 3-1. Right eye. (Adapted from Garber N. *Visual Field Examination.* SLACK Incorporated; 1998.)

10. **A visual field defect involving the inferior nasal radiating fibers would appear:**
    a) as a scotoma near the central fixation point
    b) as an arch that stops at the vertical
    c) as an arch over the central vision
    d) as an arch under the central vision

11. **At the chiasm:**
    a) nerve impulses are magnified before traveling on to the brain
    b) nerve impulses are sorted before traveling on to the brain
    c) nasal nerve fibers from each eye cross over to the opposite side
    d) temporal nerve fibers from each eye cross over to the opposite side

12. **The gland that lies in the chiasmal region and can have a direct impact on the visual field is the:**
    a) thyroid
    b) pituitary
    c) adrenal cortex
    d) hypothalamus

13. **The characteristic visual field defect due to a lesion at the chiasm is:**
    a) bitemporal hemianopsia
    b) binasal hemianopsia
    c) left hemianopsia
    d) right hemianopsia

14. **After nerve fibers cross at the chiasm, they pass next through the:**
    a) lamina cribrosa
    b) optic tract
    c) optic radiations
    d) optic nerve

15. **As the nerve fibers pass through the optic tract, they:**
    a) intensify the light impulses
    b) rotate, thus changing position
    c) cross over to the other side of the brain
    d) pass under the pituitary gland

16. **After leaving the optic tract, the nerve fibers bundle together at a "relay station" known as the:**
    a) optic radiations
    b) optic disk
    c) visual cortex
    d) lateral geniculate body

17. **Visual nerve fibers terminate at the:**
    a) brainstem
    b) occipital cortex
    c) thalamus
    d) Meyer's loop

18. **The anatomic pattern of the nerve fibers throughout the visual pathway produces visual field defects:**
     a) that are total blind spots
     b) that correspond to the location of the rods and cones
     c) that correspond to the location of the nerve fibers
     d) that respond well to treatment

19. **Sensory input (light impulses) on the patient's left is transmitted to the:**
     a) temporal retina OS and nasal retina OD
     b) left side of each retina
     c) left optic tract
     d) right side of the brain

20. **Visual field defects become more similar:**
     a) if both optic nerves are affected
     b) if the intraocular pressure in both eyes is elevated
     c) if the lesion is in one eye only
     d) the closer the lesion is to the occipital cortex

21. **Match the term to the correct definition.**

Term	Definition
__ absolute	a) central dot on the visual field chart
__ altitudinal	b) rings around the center point designated in degrees on the visual field chart
__ Bjerrum's area	c) diameter lines designated in degrees on the visual field chart
__ congruous	d) point where a stimulus is seen 50% of the time
__ constricted	e) a stimulus that is too small or too dim to be seen
__ depression	f) a stimulus that exceeds threshold and is seen over 50% of the time
__ eccentricities	g) boundary of points with the same sensitivity
__ fixation	h) area within an isopter where threshold is not seen
__ hemianopsia	i) scotoma that is blind to every stimulus
__ heteronymous	j) scotoma that is sensitive to suprathreshold stimuli
__ homonymous	k) an entire isopter that is moved inward from expected normal
__ incongruous	l) a portion of an isopter that is moved inward from expected normal
__ infrathreshold	m) constriction of the isopter along the 180-degree meridian
__ isopter	n) area between the 10-degree and 18-degree eccentricities
__ meridians	o) defect involving the superior or inferior field
__ quadrantanopsia	p) defect involving half of the field
__ relative	q) defect involving one fourth of the field
__ scotoma	r) defect involving opposite sides of each eye
__ step	s) defect involving the same side of each eye
__ suprathreshold	t) defect that looks the same in both eyes
__ threshold	u) defect that looks different in each eye

22.   **Label the following visual field defects (Figure 3-2):**
___ Bjerrum's scotoma
___ cecocentral scotoma
___ central scotoma
___ nasal step
___ paracentral scotoma
___ physiologic blind spot
___ Seidel scotoma

Figure 3-2. Types of visual field defects. (Reproduced with permission from Al Lens, COMT.)

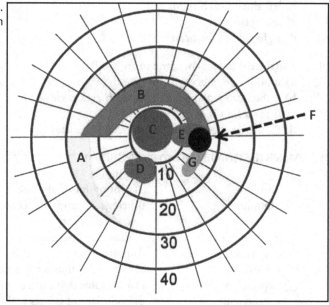

Amsler Grid

23.   **The blind spot *cannot* be plotted by which of the following methods?**
a) bowl perimeter
b) automated perimeter
c) Amsler grid
d) tangent screen

24.   **The patient in your exam chair complains of a "black dot" in the right eye, just barely to the left of center. It doesn't seem to swish around like a normal floater. Which of the following is *most* appropriate?**
a) Amsler grid
b) Maddox rod test
c) confrontation fields
d) red glass test

25.   **When testing a patient with the Amsler grid, they should:**
a) wear habitual reading correction
b) hold the material at the habitual reading distance
c) focus on the central dot
d) all of the above

Confrontation Fields

26. **What is the given assumption in confrontation field testing?**
     a) The patient has 20/20 vision.
     b) The fields are tested in the central area.
     c) The examiner's field is normal.
     d) The procedure is fully qualitative.

27. **The confrontation field:**
     a) requires the use of elaborate equipment
     b) will not pick up gross visual field defects
     c) can be performed on a patient in any position
     d) cannot be performed on children

28. **Which of the following is *not* true regarding the confrontation visual field test?**
     a) Ideally, the examiner's back should be toward a blank wall.
     b) Only the examiner's fingers should be used as a target.
     c) The eye not being tested is occluded.
     d) A defect can be either described in words or drawn out in the chart.

Tangent Screen*

29. **The tangent screen and Autoplot are used to map:**
     a) the central 20 degrees
     b) the central 30 degrees
     c) the central 40 degrees
     d) the peripheral field outside 20 degrees

30. **If you are using a felt-type tangent screen, patient responses should be marked using:**
     a) a chalk marker
     b) standard sewing pins
     c) black-head pins
     d) a pencil

31. **During a tangent screen test the patient should:**
     a) wear their distant correction
     b) wear their near correction
     c) remove all correction
     d) wear a contact lens if the refractive error is over 3.00 diopters

32. **If you are performing a tangent screen and the patient wears bifocal lenses, the patient should:**
     a) remove the glasses when you test the inferior field
     b) tuck the chin so the screen is viewed with the distance portion of the lens
     c) look through the bifocal when you test the inferior field
     d) remove the glasses for the entire test

---

* Although the tangent screen is not listed per se, IJCAHPO® suggests that "candidates be familiar with a variety of methods."

33. **When plotting the patient's left field using a tangent screen, the examiner should stand:**
    a) on the patient's left, facing the patient
    b) on the patient's right, facing the patient
    c) on the patient's left, facing the screen
    d) in the center

34. **The correct speed for moving a tangent screen target is approximately:**
    a) 1 degree per second
    b) 5 degrees per second
    c) 10 degrees per second
    d) it doesn't matter as long as the motion is smooth

35. **You look at a patient's previous tangent screen test and see the notation "2/1000 green." This means that:**
    a) a 2-mm green target was used at 1 m
    b) the patient's vision is 2/1000 and their eyes are green
    c) a 2-mm target was used at 1 m and the patient's eyes are green
    d) a 2-mm green target was used at 1000 cm

36. **For a tangent screen test on a 2 x 2 m screen, the patient is usually seated:**
    a) 1000 cm from the screen
    b) 1 m from the screen
    c) 2 m from the screen
    d) 4 m from the screen

37. **Using the tangent screen to confirm a severely constricted field of 5 degrees in a patient suspected of malingering, the patient first is tested with a 3-mm target at 1 m. Then the test is repeated at 2 m using a:**
    a) 1-mm target
    b) 2-mm target
    c) 3-mm target
    d) 6-mm target

Perimetry/General*

38. **The validity of all visual field testing depends on:**
    a) the technical skill of the operator
    b) the patient's ability to maintain fixation
    c) the complexity of the program
    d) the illumination capabilities of the instrument used

39. **The boundary of an area that responds to the same stimulus intensity is called a(n):**
    a) isopter
    b) scotoma
    c) decibel
    d) homonymous

---

* This is general information that applies to both Goldmann and automated visual field testing. It's not listed as a specific criteria item.

40. An area inside a visual field isopter that does *not* respond to any of the targets available on that particular instrument is termed a:
    a) contortion
    b) constriction
    c) Bjerrum's
    d) scotoma

41. On the visual field, the average blind spot is located:
    a) 25 degrees temporal to fixation
    b) 5 degrees nasal to fixation
    c) 15 degrees nasal to fixation
    d) 15 degrees temporal to fixation

42. The size of the average blind spot is:
    a) 5.5 degrees wide and 7.5 degrees high
    b) 7.5 degrees wide and 5.5 degrees high
    c) 3.5 degrees wide and 5.5 degrees high
    d) 7.5 degrees wide and 10.5 degrees high

43. If you increase the visual field testing distance, the blind spot will:
    a) stay the same in both cm and degrees
    b) get larger in both cm and degrees
    c) get larger in cm but remain the same in degrees
    d) stay the same in cm but get larger in degrees

44. Which of the following is *true* regarding visual field *screening* techniques?
    a) They are difficult for patients because of the time required.
    b) They are not practical for evaluating large groups.
    c) Their main purpose is to rule out pathology.
    d) They cannot be used to confirm changes in prior fields.

45. Which of the following is *not* true regarding visual field screening techniques?
    a) Always plot the blind spot if the chosen technique permits.
    b) A defect should be verified by more in-depth testing.
    c) Limited information is generated.
    d) The same screening protocol is used for every patient.

46. The main challenge in testing the visual fields of low vision patients is:
    a) their inability to understand the test
    b) their inability to see the fixation area
    c) finding the appropriate threshold
    d) finding the appropriate correcting lens

47. The visual field in a patient with high hyperopia will be:
    a) compressed, with a blind spot closer to fixation than normal
    b) expanded, with a blind spot farther from fixation than normal
    c) compressed, with a smaller blind spot than normal
    d) expanded, with a larger blind spot than usual

48. **A patient with high myopia will have a field that is:**
   a) compressed, with a blind spot closer to fixation than normal
   b) expanded, with a blind spot farther from fixation than normal
   c) compressed, with a smaller blind spot than normal
   d) expanded, with a larger blind spot than usual

49. **The smallest size pupil diameter allowable for adequate mapping of the periphery is:**
   a) 1 mm
   b) 3 mm
   c) 5 mm
   d) 7 mm

50. **Regarding visual field testing with a perimeter, the term *calibration* refers to:**
   a) proper selection of the target size
   b) checking the light intensity and adjusting if needed
   c) checking and installing the recording paper
   d) installing the proper bulbs prior to use

51. **Moving a target across a screen or other surface from a point where it is not seen to a point where the patient responds is known as:**
   a) static perimetry
   b) kinetic perimetry
   c) threshold perimetry
   d) formal perimetry

52. **Using stationary targets to measure a retinal receptor's ability to detect the stimulus is known as:**
   a) static perimetry
   b) kinetic perimetry
   c) automated perimetry
   d) threshold perimetry

53. **Which of the following involves finding the dimmest and smallest target that the corresponding point of the retina can detect?**
   a) mapping the blind spot
   b) binocular testing
   c) threshold testing
   d) gaze tracking

54. **The threshold level in kinetic perimetry is affected by:**
   a) the fact that a larger target is necessary
   b) the fact that the target is moving
   c) the fact that the target is stationary
   d) computer or operator error

55. **Before starting Goldmann or automated fields, it is a good idea to perform a confrontation field on the patient. In addition to providing the examiner general information about possible gross defects, this serves to:**
   a) indicate a possible starting threshold setting
   b) educate the patient about fixation and response
   c) quantify possible defects
   d) evaluate the patient's visual acuity

56. **Occlusion of the eye not being tested on visual fields is best done with:**
     a) any eye patch that is comfortable
     b) the patient's hand
     c) a piece of tape running from upper to lower lid
     d) a white patch

57. **The visual field patient should be told all of the following *except*:**
     a) you won't see every light
     b) some of the lights will be dimmer or smaller than others
     c) be sure to look at the light once you see it
     d) press the button as soon as you're aware of the light

58. **The visual field patient should be positioned so that they:**
     a) are not leaning forward at all
     b) are on an eye level with the fixation area
     c) have their chin jutted forward as far as possible
     d) have their forehead tilted forward as far as possible

59. **What is the best way for a visual field patient who is physically unable to push the buzzer button with the thumb to indicate their response?**
     a) The test cannot be done.
     b) Have them push the upside-down buzzer against their leg or tabletop.
     c) Have them give a verbal response.
     d) Have them nod when they see the stimulus.

60. **If the visual field patient's head is tucked into a chin-down position:**
     a) the brow may obstruct the upper field
     b) the cheek bone may obstruct the lower field
     c) the eye cannot be aligned properly
     d) fixation will be impossible

61. **If a visual field patient has a beard:**
     a) tape the facial hair back out of the way
     b) request that they shave before the test
     c) position them so there is as little hair as possible in the chin rest
     d) no special modifications are necessary

62. **Which of the following is more comfortable during the visual field exam?**
     a) The feet should not touch the floor.
     b) The back should be curved gently.
     c) The patient should not have to lean forward at all.
     d) The back should be straight, with feet flat on floor.

63. **Adaptations that might allow a patient who is wheelchair-bound to be positioned at the perimeter include all of the following *except*:**
     a) placing a sturdy board across the wheelchair armrests and having the patient sit on the board
     b) raising the table so the chair will fit under it, and using pillows to help prop the patient
     c) removing the wheelchair armrests so that the chair will slide under the table
     d) removing the footrests so the chair will fit closer to the table

64. **In general, the longer the test time:**
    a) the less reliable the patient becomes
    b) the more reproducible the test
    c) the more accurate the test because more data are provided
    d) the more reliable the patient becomes

65. **You are halfway through the field when your patient begins to complain that their eye is stinging and watering. This might indicate that you forgot to instruct the patient to:**
    a) maintain fixation
    b) use artificial tears before the test
    c) blink often during the test
    d) take their allergy medication before the test

66. **A correcting lens is required to test:**
    a) presbyopic patients
    b) every patient
    c) hyperopic patients only
    d) on a patient-by-patient basis

67. **The area of the field that is tested by using a near add is:**
    a) the central 20 degrees
    b) the central 30 degrees
    c) the foveal area
    d) the blind spot

68. **The best type of lens to use for the near add is:**
    a) the patient's glasses
    b) a lens from any trial lens set
    c) spheres only
    d) a lens with a thin rim

69. **If the patient's distance correction is over + 10.00 D:**
    a) a contact lens is required to do the test
    b) typical field landmarks will be displaced
    c) a trial lens is required for the entire test
    d) there is no difference from any other field test

70. **In a fully dilated, emmetropic patient, which near add correction is required to test the central field?**
    a) none
    b) +1.25 D
    c) +2.00 D
    d) +3.25 D

71. **The trial lens(es) should be placed:**
    a) with the sphere closest to the eye, and as close to the eye as possible
    b) with the cylinder closest to the eye, and as close to the eye as possible
    c) with the sphere closest to the eye at the patient's habitual vertex distance
    d) with the cylinder closest to the eye at the patient's habitual vertex distance

72. **The chances of producing a correcting lens artifact on visual field testing can be reduced by:**
    a) using only wide-rimmed trial lenses
    b) using spherical correction and placing it as close to the eye as possible
    c) using the proper lens and placing it as close to the eye as possible
    d) using the proper lens to test the field beyond the central 30 degrees

73. **Selecting a correcting lens of improper power may result in:**
    a) apparent field depression
    b) artificial enlargement of the blind spot
    c) misplacement of the blind spot
    d) spiral fields

Part II

Automated Perimetry

Note: Questions 74-128 refer to automated perimetry.

74. **At the beginning of each day before using an automated perimeter:**
    a) the background reflectance must be calibrated
    b) the stimulus illumination must be calibrated
    c) the technician should run a diagnostic test
    d) ensure that all patient-contact points have been sanitized

75. **Decreased bulb brightness in an automated visual field machine may be indicated by:**
    a) the instrument's failure to power up
    b) threshold values other than < 0
    c) failure to find the blind spot
    d) unexplained field contraction

76. **Maintenance measures for automated perimeters include all of the following *except*:**
    a) a surge protector for the electrical outlet
    b) initializing (formatting) the hard drive once a week
    c) using antistatic spray on carpeted surfaces around the instrument
    d) covering the instrument when not in use

Terms/Techniques

77. **For the most part, the basic mapping technique used by automated perimeters is:**
    a) static perimetry
    b) kinetic perimetry
    c) confrontation perimetry
    d) Amsler technique

78. **In automated perimetry, stimuli are presented at specific locations. Which of the following is *not* true?**
    a) Test accuracy depends on the density of the test points and the retina's sensitivity at those points.
    b) If tested points are spaced 6 degrees apart, a scotoma the size of the blind spot could be missed.
    c) All tests are based on a 120-point system.
    d) Tested locations are usually placed on meridians and eccentricities.

79. **Target exposure time on an automated perimeter is usually:**
    a) 0.1 to 0.4 seconds
    b) 0.5 to 0.7 seconds
    c) 0.9 to 1.0 seconds
    d) 1.0 to 1.5 seconds

80. **The most commonly used automated visual field programs test points that are:**
    a) 2 degrees apart
    b) 6 degrees apart
    c) 20 degrees apart
    d) 30 degrees apart

81. **The SITA involves the use of:**
    a) artificial intelligence
    b) comparisons to normals in Sweden
    c) advanced catch trials
    d) more sensitive gaze monitoring

82. **The term *catch trials* refers to:**
    a) methods used in automated perimetry to ensure reproducible fields
    b) methods used in manual/Goldmann perimetry to ensure reliable fields
    c) methods used in automated perimetry to rate patient reliability
    d) the trial lens used during the central part of a field test

83. **In automated visual fields, the monitoring of fixation loss, false positives, and false negatives are collectively known as:**
    a) reliability indicators
    b) field losses
    c) malingering identifiers
    d) hysteria identifiers

84. **Match the automated field terms with the definitions. Definitions may be used more than once.**

    Term

    __ false negative

    __ false positive

    __ fixation loss

    __ fluctuation

    Definition
    a) evaluates the patient's understanding of the test
    b) the patient does not respond to the brightest target available in an area where they previously responded to a dimmer light
    c) the patient responds to a target that appears within the previously designated blind spot
    d) the patient responds to the sound of the perimeter when no stimulus was presented
    e) a measure of the patient's consistency
    f) evaluates the patient's alertness

g) some perimeters will retest the points that were evaluated just before this occurred

h) this factor can be affected by certain eye diseases

i) a higher number indicates that the patient is giving varying responses to the same point

j) may be detected continually by a photoelectric sensor

Understanding Threshold

85. **The differences between a screening program and a threshold program include the fact that:**
    a) threshold is faster
    b) screening gives more data
    c) threshold is more appropriate for glaucoma suspects
    d) screening is more accurate

86. **"At threshold" means that the patient responds to a given stimulus in the same area:**
    a) 25% of the time
    b) 50% of the time
    c) 75% of the time
    d) 100% of the time

87. **Threshold is dependent on all of the following *except*:**
    a) background and stimulus intensity
    b) the patient's age
    c) the patient's level of stereopsis
    d) distance of stimulus from the fovea

88. **Automated threshold testing:**
    a) basically gives a yes/no response
    b) measures sensitivity at each tested point
    c) tests each point with a suprathreshold stimulus
    d) tests each point with a standardized stimulus

89. **Accurately determining threshold requires:**
    a) using a "normal" threshold as a starting point
    b) moving from seeing to nonseeing
    c) a single testing of a point
    d) multiple testing of the same point

90. **In order for a threshold point to be considered abnormal:**
    a) it must fall outside the 95th percentile for normal patients
    b) it must be consistently measured as > 50 dB
    c) it must be consistently measured as < 10 dB
    d) it must be seen 50% of the time

91. **A patient might not respond to a suprathreshold stimuli:**
    a) by chance
    b) because it is too dim
    c) because it is too small
    d) because it is too large

92. **Automated threshold tests generally start with a suprathreshold stimulus, then:**
     a) test all points at that illumination
     b) increase illumination until the stimulus is not seen, then gradually decrease illumination until the stimulus is seen again
     c) decrease illumination until the stimulus is not seen and record this as threshold
     d) decrease illumination until the stimulus is not seen, then gradually increase illumination until the stimulus is seen again

93. **The starting point to determine threshold in an automated perimeter program might come from all of the following *except*:**
     a) information from the patient's last test
     b) the patient's threshold at several predetermined points
     c) the threshold at the patient's optic nerve
     d) using age-related normal values

Strategies/Programs

94. **The term that describes the selection of points that are tested in any particular program is:**
     a) point array
     b) kinetic array
     c) central baseline array
     d) peripheral baseline array

95. **A full-field suprathreshold test would be appropriate for:**
     a) the glaucoma suspect
     b) the patient with known glaucoma
     c) the patient with 2.0-mm pupils
     d) general screening

96. **Which of the following automated strategies is most appropriate in screening for suspected glaucoma?**
     a) full field 120
     b) central threshold 24-2
     c) superior 64
     d) central 10-2

97. **An automated array suited for glaucoma testing might not be appropriate in other optic nerve disease because:**
     a) the blind spot is not checked as thoroughly
     b) the central 30 degrees is not checked as thoroughly
     c) the array designed for glaucoma may de-emphasize temporal points
     d) the array designed for glaucoma may de-emphasize nasal points

98. **If a defect includes or is close to fixation, it would be best to choose an automated test array that:**
     a) checks points that are 2 degrees apart for the entire field
     b) checks points that are 2 degrees apart in the central 10 degrees
     c) provides a wider variety of stimuli
     d) utilizes a red test object

99. **Which of the following automated threshold strategies would be most appropriate for a patient with optic neuritis?**
a) Using results of a previous test.
b) Determining threshold at a point in each quadrant.
c) Full field at a higher intensity than a previous test.
d) Using age-related normals.

Test Prep

100. **Regarding data entry on an automated perimeter:**
a) one may use all the data from a previous test
b) the computer automatically makes changes from one test to another
c) you should override the instrument's data fields
d) it must be entered in the prescribed manner or the computer will not find it later

101. **When testing a return patient for an annual automated field exam, it is important to:**
a) use the same test parameters as the previous test
b) use the same correcting lens as before
c) not fatigue the patient with test instructions
d) have the same tech run the test

102. **Calculation of the add for automated perimetry includes the factors of:**
a) full distance correction and age-related add
b) full distance correction and habitual add
c) full distance correction, age-related add, and bowl depth
d) full distance correction and a 30-cm bowl depth

103. **New technology that takes the place of conventional trial lenses in Humphrey automated field testing is a(n):**
a) adjustable contact lens
b) liquid lens
c) focal lens
d) accommodating trial lens

104. **To provide for patient comfort and rest during an automated visual field, the patient should be:**
a) told to hold down the button to pause the test after every couple of stimuli
b) told to close their eye whenever needed
c) encouraged periodically to continue, then allowed to rest between testing eyes
d) allowed to take a break every 5 minutes

Modifications to Parameters

105. **In automated perimetry there are a number of features that can be modified according to patient need. These types of features are called:**
a) standards
b) programs
c) isopters
d) parameters

106. **If the patient has poor vision and cannot see the fixation target in the center of the automated perimeter:**
    a) activate an alternate fixation pattern
    b) turn off the fixation monitoring option
    c) increase the size of the stimulus
    d) use a +3.00 correcting lens to provide magnification

107. **Your patient appears alert and capable, but seems to have a delayed response to the stimuli. In such a case you might:**
    a) recheck the blind spot
    b) switch to a different program
    c) discontinue the test
    d) slow down stimulus presentation

Conducting the Test

108. **Once the automated visual field test has begun, the perimetrist should:**
    a) encourage the patient frequently
    b) be totally quiet
    c) leave the room
    d) speak only if the patient repeatedly loses fixation

109. **In automated instruments that use an infrared monitor to evaluate fixation:**
    a) a fixation loss in a patient with blue eyes will register more easily than in a patient with brown eyes
    b) a fixation loss in a patient with brown eyes will register more easily than in a patient with blue eyes
    c) having the patient wear a soft contact lens will increase the sensitivity of the monitor
    d) a correcting lens cannot be used because it will interfere with the monitor

110. **During automated visual fields, if the patient repeatedly responds to the blind spot check, yet seems to be maintaining fixation:**
    a) encourage the patient to continue to fixate
    b) relocate the blind spot or reduce the fixation stimulus
    c) pause the test and allow the patient to rest
    d) turn off the fixation check

111. **Your physician-employer has sent a patient to you for automated full threshold visual field testing. Five minutes into the test it is obvious that the patient is physically unable to cope with threshold testing. You should:**
    a) increase stimulus speed
    b) switch to a screening strategy
    c) stop the test and inform the physician it is impossible
    d) stop the test and re-educate the patient

112. **You check the gaze-tracking graph on the bottom of the patient's field and see a relatively flat line above the base line. This means that:**
    a) the patient almost never blinked
    b) the patient was not paying attention
    c) the patient neglected to punch the button
    d) the patient had little eye movement

113. **There are numerous points greater than 40 dB on the patient's decibel graph. This probably means that:**
    a) the patient is "trigger happy"
    b) the stimulus is too bright
    c) the bulb is about to burn out
    d) there is significant field loss

Results

114. **A "normal" screening test means that:**
    a) the patient has no visual field defect
    b) the patient has no field defect detectable by this instrument
    c) confrontation visual fields are adequate for future testing
    d) the patient does not have glaucoma

115. **Which of the following is *not* true regarding test results found with an automated perimeter?**
    a) The data can be rearranged into a variety of printouts.
    b) It is valid only if the same person performs the test each time.
    c) The data can be compared with the patient's previous test(s).
    d) The data can be compared to normal age-related values.

116. **In order for an automated field test to be considered reliable, the false positives and/or false negatives must be *less* than:**
    a) 33%
    b) 45%
    c) 52%
    d) 68%

117. **In order for an automated field test to be considered reliable, the fixation losses must be *less* than:**
    a) 5%
    b) 10%
    c) 20%
    d) 40%

Analysis

118. **Which of the following is *not* displayed on the single field analysis printout?**
    a) patient demographics and reliability data
    b) numeric sensitivities and grayscale
    c) total and pattern deviation plots
    d) defect depth and change analysis

119. **The threshold sensitivity display for an automated field:**
    a) displays a threshold using symbols on a grid that corresponds to the test points
    b) displays probability on a grid that corresponds to the test points
    c) displays the decibel threshold on a grid that corresponds to the test points
    d) displays the decibel threshold on a table that corresponds to the test points

120. **On the threshold sensitivity (numeric) printout of an automated field, the number zero indicates that:**
    a) the stimulus was seen 100% of the time
    b) the stimulus was infrathreshold
    c) the dimmest stimulus was used
    d) the brightest stimulus was not seen

121. **A grayscale printout for automated fields:**
    a) displays the threshold decibel measurements as a graphic display of varying shades
    b) displays an "x" if the target was seen and an "o" if the target was not seen
    c) displays the probability of a normal person seeing that point as a graphic display of varying shades
    d) displays the differences of the patient's current test to a previous test using a graphic display of varying shades

122. **A point that is not seen is represented on a grayscale printout by:**
    a) a white area
    b) a dot
    c) a black area
    d) an x

123. **The display that compares the patient's results to age-corrected normals and then calculates the probability that any deviation occurred by chance is the:**
    a) total deprivation display
    b) partial deviation display
    c) total deviation display
    d) total corrected display

124. **A black block on a patient's total deviation display indicates that:**
    a) the probability that the deviation occurred by chance is low
    b) the patient had a false positive
    c) the patient had a false negative
    d) the patient did not respond

125. **The analysis that may reveal scotomas that are "hidden" by a generalized field depression is the:**
    a) total deviation
    b) pattern deviation
    c) island of vision
    d) catch trials

126. **Conversion of the visual field map into a three-dimensional representation results in:**
    a) isopters
    b) the island of vision profile
    c) a comparison analysis
    d) a graytone analysis

127. **The comparison printout on an automated perimeter is designed to:**
    a) compare the patient's results to normal
    b) compare the patient's test with and without a correcting lens
    c) compare the patient's current results to a previous test
    d) compare the patient's responses to one stimulus with another

128. **A notation of –2 on a point from a comparison printout means:**
    a) the previous test was 2 dB lower than the present test
    b) a loss of 2 dB from the previous test to the present
    c) that particular point has a threshold less than 2 dB
    d) the patient had 2 varying responses for that point

Part III

Goldmann Perimetry

Note: Questions 129-163 refer to Goldmann perimetry.

129. **Manual perimetry involves testing the visual field:**
    a) at preset points
    b) using stationary stimuli
    c) using moving stimuli
    d) using both stationary and moving stimuli

130. **An advantage to manual perimetry over automated is that manual perimetry:**
    a) permits testing of preselected points
    b) permits testing of the entire visual field
    c) is more accurate with static threshold testing
    d) is more reproducible

131. **One disadvantage of manual perimetry is that:**
    a) the entire visual field cannot be tested
    b) it is difficult to locate scotomas
    c) it requires a higher degree of technical skill
    d) isopters cannot be accurately plotted

132. **Advantages of the Goldmann perimeter include all of the following *except*:**
    a) fixation can be monitored easily
    b) its portability
    c) its versatility in kinetic testing
    d) the target can be projected and the chart marked simultaneously

133. **In general, mapping out isopters and scotomas with the Goldmann perimeter is accomplished by:**
    a) moving the stimulus from seeing to non-seeing
    b) moving the stimulus from non-seeing to seeing
    c) presenting a stationary stimulus for a yes/no response
    d) moving the stimulus from left to right

134. **In Goldmann perimetry, a static target is used for each of the following *except*:**
    a) determining threshold at a particular point
    b) determining the target to use for plotting an isopter
    c) spot-checking specific areas
    d) mapping an isopter

135. **In Goldmann perimetry, a kinetic target is used to:**
    a) plot isopters
    b) determine suprathreshold
    c) determine infrathreshold
    d) spot-check the blind spot

136. **For kinetic perimetry, the Goldmann stimulus should be moved:**
    a) smoothly at 5 degrees per second
    b) in an oscillatory motion at 5 degrees per second
    c) in a straight line at 1 degree per second
    d) around the eccentricities at 10 degrees per second

Calibration

137. **The Roman numeral designations on the Goldmann filter levers refer to stimulus:**
    a) brightness
    b) grayness
    c) size
    d) speed

138. **Regarding the Arabic number and alphabetic levers on the Goldmann perimeter:**
    a) the Arabic numbers designate stimulus size and the alphabet designates stimulus intensity
    b) both control the stimulus intensity
    c) the Arabic numbers designate brightness and the alphabet designates shape
    d) the Arabic numbers designate intensity and the alphabet designates duration of presentation

139. **Regarding calibration of the Goldmann perimeter:**
    a) the bulb and background reflectance should be calibrated daily prior to use
    b) the bulb and background reflectance should be calibrated and adjusted for each patient
    c) the bulb should be calibrated daily and the background reflectance adjusted for each patient
    d) the bulb should be calibrated weekly and the background reflectance should be adjusted daily

140. **An apostilb is a measurement of:**
    a) target size
    b) target value
    c) light intensity
    d) target color wavelength

141. **Decreasing the illumination of the Goldmann perimeter background:**
    a) increases the visibility of the target
    b) decreases the visibility of the target
    c) means that a smaller target can be used
    d) decreases contrast

142. **The Goldmann visual field chart is traditionally:**
    a) marked with checks and x's in lead pencil
    b) color coded to indicate the size and intensity of the stimulus
    c) grayscale coded to indicate the size and intensity of the stimulus
    d) automatically created by the pantograph

Set-Up

143. **Fixation monitoring on the Goldmann perimeter:**
     a) can be done continuously through the viewer port
     b) can be done even with the fixation mirror in place
     c) is done only when testing the blind spot
     d) is adequate if checked once every 5 minutes

144. **Fixation losses in Goldmann perimetry may be minimized by:**
     a) telling the patient where the next kinetic stimulus is going to come from
     b) telling the patient that you can see their eye during testing
     c) use of the correct near add
     d) enlarging the fixation point for every patient

145. **If the patient has poor vision and is having trouble seeing the fixation area in the Goldmann bowl:**
     a) the mirror inside the viewing port should be put in place
     b) use a +3.00 add for the entire test
     c) have the patient wear their glasses
     d) put a cross of black tape over the fixation area to enlarge it

146. **When calculating the near add for Goldmann visual field testing:**
     a) cylinder amounts under 1.00 D can be ignored
     b) cylinder amounts over 1.00 D are incorporated as a spherical equivalent
     c) cylinder amounts are incorporated as a spherical equivalent regardless of amount
     d) cylinder amounts under 1.00 D are incorporated as a spherical equivalent

147. **An emmetropic patient who is 35 years old:**
     a) requires no near add for central fields
     b) requires a -0.50 D add for central fields
     c) requires a +1.00 add for central fields
     d) requires an add only if dilated

148. **Calculation of the correcting lens for Goldmann perimetry in an ametropic patient:**
     a) uses the distance Rx plus the power of the patient's habitual add
     b) uses the distance Rx without any add
     c) starts with the distance Rx, then uses an add related to the patient's age
     d) uses the power of the patient's add without regard to any distance correction

149. **The patient should be warned not to sit back suddenly during a Goldmann visual field test because:**
     a) this will make the test take longer
     b) this will interrupt fixation and invalidate the test
     c) it is difficult to realign the patient
     d) they might come into contact with the projector arm

Techniques

150. **Once the Goldmann perimeter is calibrated, and the patient is educated and positioned, one should:**
    a) map the blind spot to ensure fixation
    b) determine threshold to find a starting place
    c) begin testing immediately to reduce patient fatigue
    d) show a few static stimuli to acquaint them with the procedure

151. **Begin the Goldmann visual field by:**
    a) plotting the blind spot
    b) plotting the outer isopter with the I4e
    c) finding a static threshold starting point
    d) statically spot-checking several points outside the central 30 degrees

152. **In Goldmann perimetry, the central field is tested and mapped inside which eccentricity?**
    a) 5 degrees
    b) 15 degrees
    c) 30 degrees
    d) 90 degrees

153. **In Goldmann perimetry, to find a suitable stimulus for mapping the central field, determine the threshold:**
    a) of central fixation
    b) 15 degrees temporal to fixation
    c) 25 degrees temporal to fixation
    d) use 2 "notches" dimmer than that for the outermost isopter

154. **To find threshold for the central field, use a static target at 25 degrees temporal and set the instrument to which setting?**
    a) I2e
    b) I1a
    c) II4e
    d) IV2d

155. **If the patient is having a follow-up Goldmann visual field:**
    a) use threshold stimuli as determined on this date
    b) use the same stimuli as the last test
    c) use a stimulus 1 degree brighter or larger than the last test
    d) use a stimulus 1 degree dimmer or smaller than the last test

156. **Maximum illumination of the smallest stimulus is achieved at the I4e setting. If the patient does *not* respond to this stimulus anywhere in the central 5 to 10 degrees:**
    a) one cannot perform a Goldmann on this patient
    b) use a +3.00 add for the entire test
    c) have the patient sit 1 m back from the bowl and try again
    d) increase the target size

157. **Difficulty in finding the blind spot with the Goldmann perimeter may be due to all of the following *except*:**
    a) failure to patch the opposite eye
    b) enlarged blind spot due to glaucoma
    c) a stimulus that is too large or moved too fast
    d) fixation loss

158. **When using the Goldmann perimeter, the outer isopter should be mapped with the threshold stimulus found:**
    a) at central fixation
    b) within the central 30 degrees
    c) 15 degrees temporal to fixation
    d) 50 degrees temporal to fixation

159. **You are mapping the central isopter, and the patient sees the stimulus before you get to the 30-degree eccentricity. This means that:**
    a) you are moving the stimulus too slowly
    b) you forgot to patch the other eye
    c) the stimulus you are using is too bright/large
    d) you are using the wrong correcting lens

160. **In Goldmann perimetry, if the patient's vision is hand motion or finger counting, it makes the most sense first to try mapping the outermost isopter using which target?**
    a) I4e
    b) I2e
    c) V4e
    d) VI6f

161. **When plotting the isopter with the Goldmann perimeter at 90 degrees, 0 degrees, and 180 degrees:**
    a) plot the isopter at 30-degree intervals
    b) plot the isopter directly at 90, 0, and 180, plus 15 degrees on either side
    c) plot the isopter at 5 and 15 degrees to either side
    d) plot the isopter every 5 degrees for 30 degrees on either side

162. **If a constriction or scotoma is detected with the Goldmann perimeter:**
    a) continue using only standard examination technique
    b) map the defect with at least 2 different targets
    c) map the defect only with the stimulus with which it was detected
    d) introduce a +3.00 add and see how the size changes

163. **If the patient's responses are inconsistent in a certain area, this can be indicated on the Goldmann perimeter chart by:**
    a) plotting as a definite isopter or border using your best judgment
    b) moving the target faster and plotting as a definite isopter labeled "faster"
    c) drawing a crosshatch in that area and labeling it as "in and out"
    d) such an area should not be plotted or reported

Part IV

Perimetry Errors*

164. The most common areas for artifacts in the visual field are:
a) superior nasal or inferior nasal
b) superior temporal or inferior temporal
c) temporal nasal or superior nasal
d) nasal temporal or inferior temporal

165. Common errors in testing the central 30 degrees include all of the following *except*:
a) forgetting to remove the correcting lens
b) presenting static targets in a steady rhythm
c) using a stimulus that stretches the isopter beyond 30 degrees
d) moving the stimulus too quickly, creating a falsely enlarged blind spot

166. Match the following visual fields to the artifacts (Figures 3-3 through 3-6):

Visual Field	Artifact
__ decentered correcting len	a) Figure 3-3
__ hysteria or malingering	b) Figure 3-4
__ ptotic upper eyelid	c) Figure 3-5
__ thick rim on correcting lens	d) Figure 3-6

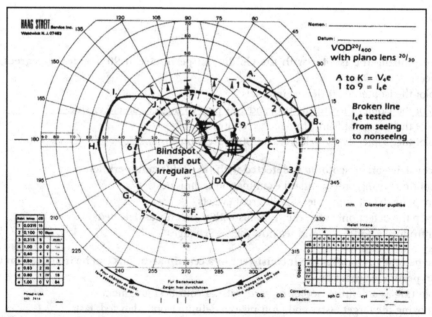

Figure 3-3. (Reproduced with permission from Garber N. *Visual Field Examination.* SLACK Incorporated; 1998.)

* Questions 164-166 refer to both automated and Goldmann perimetry unless otherwise noted.

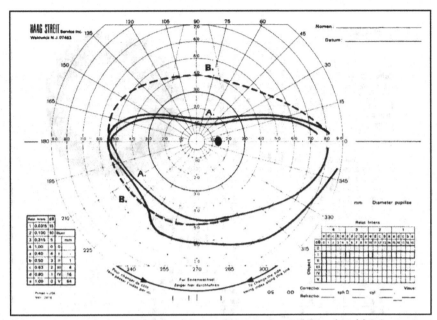

Figure 3-4. (Reproduced with permission from Garber N. *Visual Field Examination*. SLACK Incorporated; 1998.)

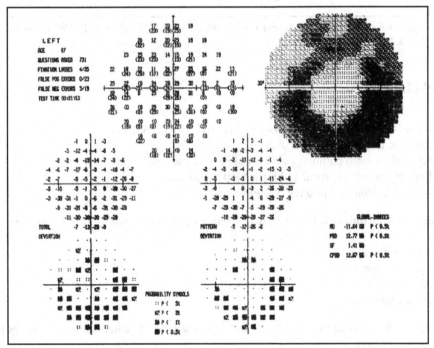

Figure 3-5. (Reproduced with permission from Choplin N, Edwards R. *Visual Fields*. SLACK Incorporated; 1998.)

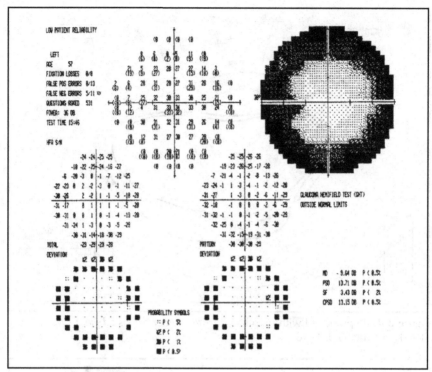

Figure 3-6. (Reproduced with permission from Choplin N, Edwards R. *Visual Fields*. SLACK Incorporated; 1998.)

Visual Field Defects*

167. **All of the following are characteristics of retinal area defects *except*:**
    a) defects at this level are binocular
    b) most field-related pathology also is visible with the ophthalmoscope
    c) they can cross the vertical and horizontal meridians
    d) defects are projected into the opposite quadrant

168. **If a retinal detachment is found in the superior nasal retina, where is the corresponding field loss?**
    a) superior nasal
    b) superior temporal
    c) inferior nasal
    d) inferior temporal

169. **The retinal field defect that results in the highest degree of visual limitation occurs in the:**
    a) Bjerrum's fibers
    b) periphery
    c) macula
    d) disc

* For more on field defects, see also Answers 8-22 regarding the visual pathway.

170. **Damage in the nerve fiber layer commonly produces which of the following field defects?**
    a) hemianopsia
    b) quadrantanopsia
    c) congruous
    d) Bjerrum's scotoma

171. **In the case where nerve fiber layer damage has caused a constriction in the isopter, the isopter will:**
    a) progress toward the horizontal meridian
    b) progress toward the disc
    c) progress toward the vertical meridian
    d) show no particular pattern of progression

172. **Common characteristics of nerve fiber layer defects include all of the following *except*:**
    a) arc-shaped constrictions or contractions
    b) nasal step
    c) enlarged blind spot
    d) left homonymous hemianopsia

173. **Which of the following has *no* resulting field loss?**
    a) optic neuritis
    b) macular hole
    c) ocular hypertension
    d) central retinal artery occlusion

174. **Enlargement of the blind spot might typically be expected to occur in all of the following conditions *except*:**
    a) glaucoma
    b) retinal detachment
    c) papilledema (papillitis)
    d) optic nerve coloboma

175. **Except in glaucoma, enlargement of the blind spot caused by optic nerve damage generally is:**
    a) oriented vertically
    b) oriented horizontally
    c) rounded or concentric
    d) tapered at the top

176. **The most common visual field defect found in optic nerve damage is:**
    a) nasal step
    b) enlarged blind spot
    c) central scotoma
    d) Bjerrum's scotoma

177. **Optic nerve damage that causes a visual field defect in both eyes cannot occur anterior to:**
    a) the junction of the optic nerve and the chiasm
    b) the chiasm
    c) where the fibers leave the chiasm
    d) the optic tract

178. **All of the following regarding field loss in optic neuritis are true *except*:**
    a) field loss is permanent
    b) the most common defect is a central scotoma
    c) it can cause a defect anywhere in the nerve fiber bundle
    d) centrocecal defects can also occur

179. **Optic disc drusen can cause field defects that mimic:**
    a) retinal detachment
    b) glaucoma
    c) pituitary tumor
    d) hysteria

180. **The most common field defect in optic disc drusen is:**
    a) progressive contractions
    b) localized depressions
    c) scotomas
    d) inferior nasal step

181. **A patient taking Plaquenil (hydroxychloroquine) should have periodic visual field examinations to check for:**
    a) bitemporal hemianopsia
    b) temporal wedge
    c) nasal step
    d) paracentral scotoma

182. **Which areas are most important when evaluating for glaucomatous defects?**
    a) fovea, superior, and temporal
    b) central 30 degrees
    c) outer 30 degrees
    d) nasal, central 20 degrees, and blind spot

183. **Changes in the visual field of the glaucoma patient correspond to:**
    a) intraocular pressure readings
    b) choroidal blood supply to the retina
    c) the progression of nerve fiber bundle damage at the rim of the optic disc
    d) how far posteriorly into the visual pathway the damage has progressed

184. **The nasal contraction seen in the glaucomatous field is:**
    a) an inferior nasal step
    b) a superior nasal step
    c) a vertical nasal step
    d) attached to the blind spot

185. **The most common initial field loss(es) seen in open-angle glaucoma is/are:**
    a) central scotoma and vertical step
    b) nasal step
    c) paracentral scotoma and nasal step
    d) temporal wedge and arcuate scotoma

186. The Bjerrum's scotoma seen in open-angle glaucoma occurs in which eccentricity?
    a) 7.5 degrees
    b) 15 degrees
    c) 30 degrees
    d) 45 degrees

187. Which of the following field defects extends superiorly from the blind spot, arcs over the central vision, and stops at the horizontal/nasal midline?
    a) Bjerrum's scotoma
    b) enlarged blind spot
    c) nasal step
    d) hysterical field

188. The very last area of the visual field remaining in end-stage glaucoma is the:
    a) nasal step
    b) blind spot
    c) central 5 degrees
    d) temporal crescent

189. In general, the more congruous the defect, the more likely that the problem site is:
    a) prechiasmal
    b) related to the optic nerve
    c) more posteriorly located
    d) more anteriorly located

190. About half of your patient's field is gone, but the central area around 8 degrees is clear. This is known as:
    a) arcuate scotoma
    b) nasal step
    c) cecocentral scotoma
    d) macular sparing

191. Macular sparing is most often seen in problems of the:
    a) occipital cortex
    b) optic nerve head
    c) optic radiations
    d) chiasm

192. One hallmark of the neurological field is:
    a) respect for the vertical meridian
    b) respect for the horizontal meridian
    c) the macula is never affected
    d) the blind spot is never affected

193. Which location should be screened when ruling out a neurological defect?
    a) the horizontal meridian
    b) the vertical meridian
    c) the central 20 degrees
    d) the nasal area

194. **A total homonymous hemianopsia can result from a defect in all of the following** *except*:
   a) the optic nerve
   b) the optic tract
   c) the temporal lobe
   d) the occipital lobe

195. **Bitemporal field defects can occur** *only* **in the:**
   a) retina
   b) optic nerve
   c) chiasm
   d) temporal lobe

196. **"Pie-in-the-sky" and "pie-on-the-floor" defects are indications of damage in the:**
   a) optic tract
   b) lateral geniculate body
   c) optic radiations
   d) visual cortex

197. **Your patient's visual field result shows an overall decrease but no specific areas of loss. This is likely due to:**
   a) pituitary tumor
   b) optic nerve disease
   c) ocular hypertension
   d) media opacity

198. **Which of the following patterns often indicates fatigue or poor concentration?**
   a) clover leaf
   b) overall depression
   c) enlarged blind spot
   d) ring scotoma

199. **Field patterns typical of a hysterical patient include all of the following** *except*:
   a) spiral
   b) star-shaped
   c) tubular
   d) square

200. **Hysterical visual field loss is usually a product of:**
   a) the patient's desire to fool the examiner
   b) elevated intraocular pressure
   c) mental conflict
   d) pseudotumor cerebri

201. **Which technique is more useful in determining that a visual field loss is** *not* **due to an injury or disorder?**
   a) automated full-field threshold
   b) confrontation fields
   c) Amsler grid
   d) Goldmann fields

202. **In automated testing, one clue that field loss might *not* be caused by a physical injury or disorder is:**
    a) a field loss pattern that is not later reproduced
    b) high rate of fixation loss
    c) presence of grayscale artifacts
    d) generalized constriction

203. **Match the visual field to the most likely diagnosis (Figures 3-7 through 3-13).**

Diagnosis	Visual Field
__ chiasmal defect	a) Figure 3-7
__ glaucoma	b) Figure 3-8
__ nerve fiber layer defect	c) Figure 3-9
__ nonorganic defect	d) Figure 3-10
__ optic disc drusen	e) Figure 3-11
__ post-chiasmal defect	f) Figure 3-12
__ retinal detachment	g) Figure 3-13

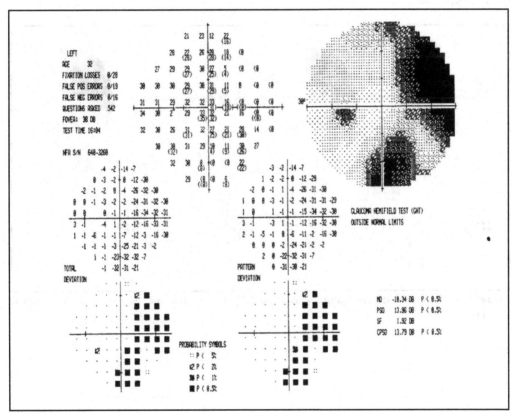

Figure 3-7. (Reproduced with permission from Choplin N, Edwards R. *Visual Fields*. SLACK Incorporated; 1998.)

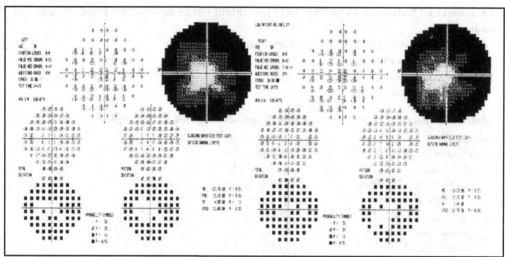

Figure 3-8. (Reproduced with permission from Choplin N, Edwards R. *Visual Fields*. SLACK Incorporated; 1998.)

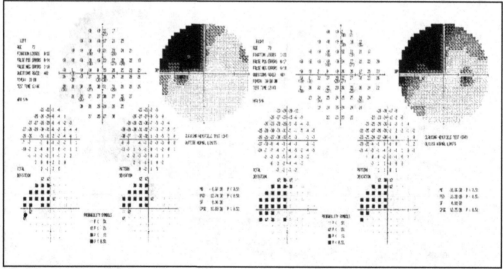

Figure 3-9. (Reproduced with permission from Choplin N, Edwards R. *Visual Fields*. SLACK Incorporated; 1998.)

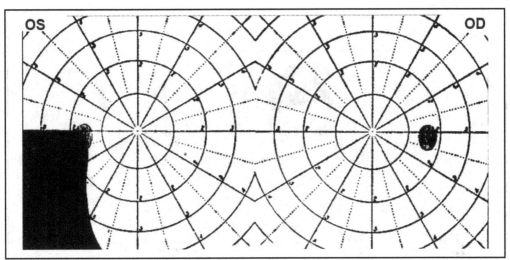

Figure 3-10. (Reproduced with permission from Garber N. *Visual Field Examination*. SLACK Incorporated; 1998.)

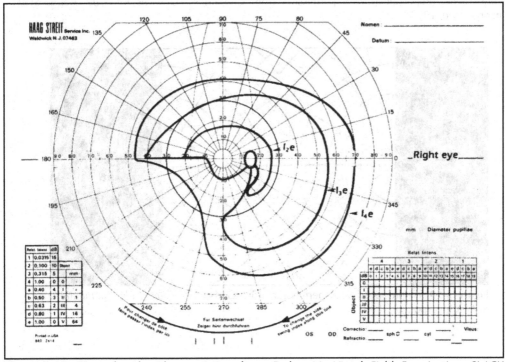

Figure 3-11. (Reproduced with permission from Garber N. *Visual Field Examination*. SLACK Incorporated; 1998.)

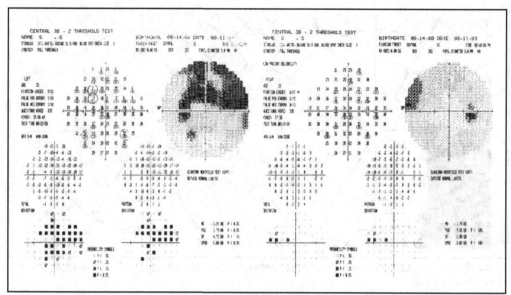

Figure 3-12. (Reproduced with permission from Choplin N, Edwards R. *Visual Fields*. SLACK Incorporated; 1998.)

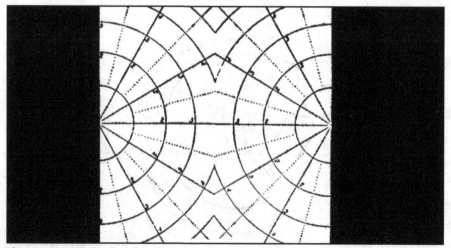

Figure 3-13. (Reproduced with permission from Garber N. *Visual Field Examination*. SLACK Incorporated; 1998.)

Study Notes

Suggested reading in *Principles and Practice in Ophthalmic Assisting: A Comprehensive Textbook*:
> Chapter 2: Ocular Anatomy (*Optic Nerve* pp 22-23)
> Chapter 9: Basic Eye Exam (*Confrontation Visual Fields* pp 120-122)
> Chapter 14: Visual Fields (pp 253-274)

TEXT CORRECTION: If studying from *Principles and Practice in Ophthalmic Assisting: A Comprehensive Textbook*, please note that the caption for Figure 9-3 should read: "Drawing results of confrontation visual field testing, showing an inferior nasal constriction of **the left eye from the patient's point of view** (N = nasal, T = temporal)."

Explanatory Answers

Part I

1.   b) Vision beyond fixation is the visual field. Binocular field is the visual field with both eyes. A neurological field is a particular method of testing. The visual pathway refers to the ocular structures responsible for sight.
2.   d) The normal visual field is approximately 95 degrees temporal, 75 degrees inferior, 60 degrees nasal, and 60 degrees superior. You could pick this out even if the numbers were slightly different, if you remember that the temporal field is the largest and the nasal and superior fields are the smallest. Remember, though, that if a large, very bright target was used the field would be larger; if a small, dim target was used the field would be smaller. The figures given are "standard."
3.   b) The superior and nasal fields are limited by the anatomical boundaries of the brow and nose. (The superior field also is limited by the lids, which are not mentioned in this question.)
4.   a) The island of vision is afloat in a sea of blindness, because anything that is not seen is in a blind area. (The time-space continuum is a term I borrowed from *Star Trek*.)
5.   a) The blind spot is devoid of light receptor cells and would be represented by a bottomless hole. A peak is the point of highest sensitivity. A dip and a pit have a bottom, indicating that a stimulus could be found to which that area would respond.
6.   d) The peak of the island represents the area of highest visual sensitivity, the fovea.
7.   b) Gradually decreasing vision would be represented by a gradually decreasing slope. A bottomless hole is a place of absolutely no vision. A sharp drop-off would be produced by an area where seeing suddenly becomes nonseeing. A flat area would be the same throughout, no increase or decrease.
8.   b) The nerve fibers are actually the axons of the ganglion cells.
9.   **Labeling (Figure 3-1):**

horizontal raphe	D
optic disc	A
radiating nasal fibers	B
temporal fibers	C

10.   c) Look back at Figure 3-1. The nasal retinal nerve fibers move in an arch over the central fixation point. Such a defect does cross the vertical meridian, but not the nasal.
11.   c) At the chiasm, the nasal nerve fibers from each eye cross over to the other side. The temporal nerve fibers do not cross but remain on the same side.
12.   b) The pituitary gland lies just under the chiasm where the nasal fibers cross. If the pituitary swells, it can put pressure on the chiasm. This affects the crossing nasal fibers that receive impulses from the temporal field, producing a bitemporal field defect.

13.   a) See Answer 12. The fibers that cross at the chiasm are more likely to be damaged in this scenario, thus the bitemporal hemianopsia is the most common. This type of loss affects the right field of vision in the right eye and the left field of vision in the left eye. *Note*: The terms *hemianopsia* and *hemianopia* are interchangeable.

14.   b) After the chiasm, the nerve fibers continue on through the optic tract.

15.   b) The nerve fibers rotate or twist as they pass through the optic tract.

16.   d) The optic tract ends in the lateral geniculate body, which acts as a gathering place and relay station for the nerve fibers.

17.   b) The visual nerve fibers terminate into the occipital cortex of the brain. The eye-related fibers that terminate in the brain stem (only 10% of all the fibers) are concerned with pupillary action and are not visual.

18.   c) Because the nerve fibers fan out in a specific anatomic pattern, visual field defects occurring in the nerve fibers also follow the same pattern. This makes diagnosis easier because the patterns are identifiable.

19.   d) An object on the patient's left will stimulate the nasal retina OS and temporal retina OD. The nasal fibers from OS will cross over to the right at the chiasm, while the temporal fibers from OD will remain on the right. These fibers then stay on the right as they pass through the right optic tract, right lateral geniculate body, right optic radiations, and right occipital cortex.

20.   d) The closer a lesion is to the occipital cortex, the more similar (*congruous*) the visual field defects. This means that the field defect in one eye is more similar to the defect in the other. This phenomenon occurs because the fibers that correspond to neighboring visual spaces get closer and closer together as they course back to the occipital lobe.

21.   **Matching:**

absolute	i)
altitudinal	o)
Bjerrum's area	n)
congruous	t)
constricted	k)
depression	l)
eccentricities	b)
fixation	a)
hemianopsia	p)
heteronymous	r)
homonymous	s)
incongruous	u)
infrathreshold	e)
isopter	g)
meridians	c)
quadrantanopsia	q)
relative	j)
scotoma	h)
step	m)
suprathreshold	f)
threshold	d)

22.   **Labeling (Figure 3-2):**

Bjerrum's scotoma	B)
cecocentral scotoma	E)
central scotoma	C)
nasal step	A)
paracentral scotoma	D)
physiologic blind spot	F)
Seidel scotoma	G)

23. c) The blind spot cannot be plotted on the Amsler grid because it falls outside of the grid's testing range of the central 20 degrees.

24. a) Because the Amsler grid evaluates the central 20 degrees of vision, it could be quite informative. Consider performing the test on the unaffected eye first, so the patient gets the idea. Then do the affected eye, asking the patient to draw in the "black dot." Include this drawing with the information presented to the physician. Confrontation fields is not a bad answer, but Amsler grid is better. Maddox rod and red glass tests evaluate extraocular muscles.

25. d) The patient should wear any reading correction they normally use. I usually tell the patient to hold the Amsler grid "where you would hold a magazine." (I once had a patient who refused to use the grid at home to monitor macular degeneration, because he complained that "the whole grid is blurry." I found out he was holding the grid at 12 inches. His habitual reading distance was 18 inches.) The patient is to focus on the central dot and evaluate the grid for completeness/no parts missing or "grayed-out," all 4 corners visible, and all lines straight and square.

26. c) In confrontation visual field testing, the examiner is comparing the patient's field to their own. Therefore, the assumption is that the examiner's visual field is normal. The patient need not have 20/20 vision. The peripheral area, rather than the central area, is tested. The test is not qualitative.

27. c) The advantage of the confrontation field is that it requires no equipment and can be performed on a patient in any position (ie, sitting or lying down). Properly done, the test will pick up gross defects. Most school-aged children can cooperate for a confrontation field test.

28. b) While the examiner's fingers most often are used as the target, one also may use objects such as a dropper bottle lid. The other statements are true.

29. b) The central 30 degrees are mapped on the tangent screen or Autoplot.

30. c) The patient's responses should be marked with black-headed pins if using a felt screen. The nap would be ruined when trying to erase chalk or pencil marks. Shiny sewing pin heads could distract the patient.

31. a) The patient should wear their habitual distance correction when taking the tangent screen test.

32. b) The patient should tuck their head to lower the bifocal add out of the way when testing the lower portion of the field. Make sure the patient maintains fixation, however. Using the bifocal for the inferior field would invalidate the test, since the upper half would be tested with one correction and the lower half in another.

33. a) Stand on the patient's left when plotting the left and on the right when plotting the right. Don't reach across the screen with the wand and target.

34. b) Move the target smoothly at about 5 degrees per second.

35. a) "2/1000 green" refers to a 2-mm test object, a test distance of 1000 mm (which equals 1 m), and a green test object.

36. b) Most tangent screens are 2 x 2 m, and the usual test distance is 1 m. In some situations (such as suspected malingering or hysteria), the patient might be moved back to a test distance of 2 m. There is a 4 x 4 m screen with a test distance of 2 m.

37. d) If doubling the test distance to catch a malingerer, you also should double the object size (in this case, to 6 mm). If, with this combination, the patient still plots the exact same isopter, you should strongly suspect malingering or hysteria.

38. b) The validity of any type of field testing depends on the patient's ability and willingness to maintain fixation. Automated perimetry requires minimal technical skill as compared to the manual Goldmann. Other factors involved (but not listed as responses) are the patient's response time, vision, and mental capabilities.

39. a) An isopter is a boundary created around an area of the visual field that responds to the same stimulus.

40. d) A scotoma is an area within an isopter where vision is impaired or absent. The definition given (ie, no response to *any* stimulus on that particular machine) actually refers to an absolute scotoma. Bjerrum's is a particular type of scotoma that extends from the blind spot/optic nerve.

41.   d) The average blind spot is located 15 degrees temporal to fixation. (The optic disc is anatomically located in the nasal part of the retina, which picks up the temporal field.)

42.   a) The average blind spot is 5.5 degrees wide and 7.5 degrees high.

43.   c) If you increase the test distance, the size of the blind spot increases in cm, but not in degrees. The size of the average blind spot is 5.5 x 7.5 degrees, regardless of test distance. However, at 1 m the blind spot is 9 x 13 cm; at 2 m the blind spot is 18 x 26 cm. This occurs because the size of the spot expands as you get farther away, but the degree stays the same (like a cone).

44.   c) The main purpose of screening techniques is to give a yes/no answer to the question: Is this patient's peripheral vision grossly normal? In general, screening techniques are quicker, and practical for evaluating large groups of people (not all at once, of course!). They also are useful in comparing a patient's screening results from one test to the next.

45.   d) The screening protocol should vary according to the patient's presumed diagnosis. By the nature of the screening, the information obtained is not thorough; some defects will be missed.

46.   b) Because of poor vision, many low vision patients have difficulty seeing the fixation area and maintaining fixation on it. For tangent screen testing, a large X of white tape can be placed over the fixation button. Many automated perimeters have an alternate fixation area made up of several lights instead of just one, that may be used in low vision testing situations.

47.   a) A patient with high hyperopia will exhibit a compressed field with a blind spot displaced closer to fixation than normal.

48.   b) By contrast, a patient with high myopia will have an expanded field with a blind spot farther away from fixation than normal.

49.   b) If the pupil is smaller than 3 mm, consider dilating the patient before proceeding with the test.

50.   b) In Goldmann visual field testing, calibration is done prior to testing by checking and adjusting the projector light. Automated field instruments are generally self-calibrating, performing this task when first turned on.

51.   b) Bringing a target from nonseeing into seeing until the patient responds is kinetic perimetry. The word *kinetic* refers to motion or movement. Static perimetry involves a stationary target, as does threshold. Formal perimetry usually refers to Goldmann or computer-generated visual fields (as opposed to confrontation, for example).

52.   a) See Answer 51. Automated perimetry means that the test was computerized, not necessarily how the test was done. While threshold perimetry does use stationary targets, the term generally refers to finding the smallest, dimmest target that a receptor can detect. (That qualification was not mentioned in this question.)

53.   c) In threshold testing, you are trying to find the smallest and dimmest stimulus that the patient reliably responds to, at that particular point or area. The blind spot (theoretically) will not respond to even the largest, brightest target on most perimeters. Perimetry for mapping the peripheral vision is a monocular test. Gaze tracking is used in automated perimetry to monitor the patient's eye movement.

54.   b) Since kinetic perimetry involves a moving target, the patient is responding to movement as well as size and intensity.

55.   b) Performing a confrontation field on the patient prior to formal perimetry serves to reinforce the idea that "you will not be looking directly at the stimulus" and "you need to look straight ahead during the entire test." Confrontation fields will not give you a threshold, quantitate defects, or visual acuity.

56.   d) Ideally, an opaque white patch is used because it not only covers the untested eye but keeps the eye light adapted. A black patch allows the eye to become dark adapted. (A person can be dark adapted in one eye and light adapted in the other.) There are now single-use press-on patches available.

57.   c) Patients should be told *not* to look at the stimulus. Telling patients that they won't see every light reduces a lot of stress, because normally they think, "I must be doing terribly because I don't see anything." Tell them that they may go for a while without seeing anything. They also should know that they are to respond regardless of the size or brightness of the stimulus. Patients should respond as soon as they are aware of the light, and not wait for it to get crystal clear.

58.   b) The eye should be level with the fixation area. It is okay if the patient has to lean forward a little as long as the back is straight and not hyper-extended. The plane of the face should be parallel to the plane of the back of the bowl or screen. If the chin is jutted forward, this will minimize the lower field. If the forehead is jutted out, the size of the superior field is reduced.

59.   b) Patients who cannot press the buzzer may turn the buzzer upside down and press the button into their knee, leg, armrest, or tabletop. Giving a verbal response or a nod will interfere with fixation and positioning.

60.   a) A patient with the chin tucked down has a reduction of the superior field because of interference by the brow. You must visually check the head position because it still is possible to align the eye and for the patient to fixate even if the head is malpositioned.

61.   c) If a person has a full beard, have them put their chin beyond the chin rest, then slide back into the chin cup. Then the hair can be parted to either side of the chin cup so as not to interfere with the inferior field. A beard can cushion the chin in the cup, making it difficult to maintain alignment.

62.   d) The patient's back should be straight, not hyper-extended, even if they have to lean forward a little. Feet should be flat on the floor, thighs parallel to the floor.

63.   a) Perching the wheelchair (or any) patient on a board for the test would be uncomfortable and probably dangerous. Remove parts of the wheelchair, if possible, in order to accommodate. If you remove the armrests, be sure the patient isn't going to fall out of the chair. Propping with pillows may help with comfort and positioning.

64.   a) The longer the test continues, the greater the patient's fatigue, boredom, and "hypnosis." These all lower reliability. The test may stretch on because the program does not find that the data are reliable.

65.   c) Burning, watery eyes are symptoms of dryness. In the case of a visual field exam, dryness usually is caused by staring. Before starting the test and sometime during the test, remind the patient to blink periodically. You can stop the test and instill artificial tear drops if necessary.

66.   d) The need for a correcting lens is determined on a patient-by-patient basis. A 50-year-old who is −2.50 sphere will probably not require a near add. A 20-year-old who wears +6.00 sphere will need an add. The words "every" and "only" should have clued you in that Answers b) and c) were wrong.

67.   b) The central 30 degrees is the testing area where a near add is required. True, the fovea and blind spot are within this area, but Answer b) is the best because it includes both.

68.   d) A lens with a thin rim is the best type of trial lens to use. The patient's glasses or a trial lens with a thick rim most likely will cause artificial field losses because the edge of the lens or the rim will block off part of the patient's side vision. Cylinder power cannot be ignored, either (see Answer 146).

69.   b) Visual field landmarks will be displaced in this case, where the distance correction is over +10.00. (*Note:* A patient with high hyperopia will exhibit a compressed field with a blind spot displaced closer to fixation than normal. By contrast, a patient with high myopia will have an expanded field with a blind spot farther away from fixation than normal.) The use of a contact lens is desirable, but not required. A trial lens never is used for the entire test as long as some stimulus can be detected outside the central 30 degrees.

70.   d) A +3.25 add is required for a fully dilated patient, regardless of age.

71.   a) The near add should be placed with the sphere closest to the patient's eye (if cylinder is also required) and as close to the patient's eye as possible. Vertex distance is not usually considered when going from glasses or phoropter to trial lens.

72.   c) Using the wrong power lens can wreak havoc on the field, giving you some truly strange results. For one thing, minification or magnification might be a factor. Blurred vision might be another. In addition, placing the lens as close to the eye as possible reduces any interference by the lens rim (even a thin lens rim, which is the only type that should be used anyway). Using spherical correction is not proper if the patient has astigmatism over 1.00 diopter. The lens is used to test the field within the central 30 degrees, not beyond it.

73.   a) The wrong correcting lens power may cause a generalized depression of the field.

Part II

74.   d) Automated perimeters are self-calibrating and run their own internal diagnostic without any prompting, so a) to c) aren't necessary. But you should be sure that all points of patient contact are properly sanitized.

75.   b) If you see threshold values other than < 0, it is time to change the bulb. The instrument can still be turned on, and it can still find the blind spot. Unexplained field contraction is not related to the bulb.

76.   b) Initializing or formatting a disk erases *all* of the information on it. You never will initialize the hard drive. This would erase not only data files but potentially program files as well.

77.   a) Automated perimeters most often use static perimetry, presenting a single non-moving target. There is no such thing as "Amsler technique."

78.   c) Automated tests may include any number of points.

79.   a) Most automated perimeters present the target for 0.1 to 0.4 seconds.

80.   b) Most automated field programs test points that are 6 degrees apart. Certain macular evaluations might test points that are 2 degrees apart, but they are not the most commonly used programs.

81.   a) The Swedish Interactive Thresholding Algorithm applies a complex set of data analyses to guide the visual field of each person. Released in the late 1990s, it is basically the application of artificial intelligence to automated field testing.

82.   c) "Catch trials" refers to the methods used by automated perimetry programs to evaluate patient cooperation and performance. These include monitoring fixation losses, false positives, and false negatives.

83.   See Answer 82.

84.   **Matching:**
       false negative   b), f)
       false positive   a), d)
       fixation loss   c), g), j)
       fluctuation   e), h), i)

85.   c) The threshold test gives more data, is more accurate, takes longer, and is more appropriate for glaucoma suspects. It is also more appropriate for following glaucoma patients. The screening test is faster but not as accurate, nor does it provide more data. Screening is adequate in most cases for simple detection (ie, is there a defect?).

86.   b) Threshold refers to a response to a stimulus, in a given area, 50% of the time.

87.   c) Stereopsis is a binocular phenomenon. Visual fields testing is monocular. The intensity of the background and stimulus affects threshold, in that a dimmer background increases contrast and a brighter stimulus is easier to see. Threshold decreases with age and with distance from the fovea.

88.   b) While automated screening gives a yes/no response, automated *threshold testing* gives a value of threshold to each point that is tested. The illumination of the stimulus is individualized to each patient's responses.

89.   d) In determining threshold (whether manual or automated), a point is tested numerous times. Starting with expected normal for a particular point is all right but is not required.

90. a) The automated field machine compares the patient's responses to that of normal individuals. If the patient's response falls outside the 95th percentile, it is considered abnormal.

91. a) A suprathreshold stimulus is not seen 100% of the time, but rather is considered to be seen only 95% of the time. It is extrapolated that suprathreshold could be missed 5% of the time, in part by chance alone.

92. d) Automated threshold tests usually start with suprathreshold, decrease intensity until the light is not seen, then increase again to confirm the reading. In manual threshold, it is customary to start infrathreshold and increase intensity until the target is seen.

93. c) The optic nerve has no threshold because it cannot perceive any light stimulus.

94. a) The testing programs are generally preloaded into the automated perimeter. Each program will have its own point array, which defines which points are tested during that particular program. The point array and program are specific to the type of information desired. The other answers are made up.

95. d) Suprathreshold testing is a screening tool, not intended for glaucoma evaluation. Nor does the size of the pupil matter in this scenario.

96. b) The central 24 degrees of the visual field includes the blind spot, one of several key points in glaucoma field loss. Most glaucoma defects occur within the central 24 degrees. A full field 120 tests out in the periphery as well, which is generally not necessary for glaucoma. The superior 64 array is used to evaluate upper lid position (eg, ptosis, dermatochalasis). The central 10-2 might be used in advanced glaucoma but is not appropriate for screening as it does not plot the blind spot.

97. c) An array that is intended for glaucoma screening will emphasize Bjerrum's area, the blind spot, and the nasal meridian. Other optic nerve diseases may show up in the temporal area, which is not tested as closely on a glaucoma test.

98. b) If a defect is close to fixation (such as a defect found on an Amsler grid), choose an array that will test the central 10 degrees with more concentration, 2 degrees apart. Testing the entire field at 2-degree intervals would be very time-consuming. A red stimulus usually is used in neurological testing.

99. b) Running a threshold test that used starting points determined by a threshold point in each quadrant would be most appropriate in evaluating optic neuritis. This is because the field loss in optic neuritis can change rapidly. Thus, the results of a previous test may be drastically different from the current situation. The test would take longer as the program fumbles around trying to find threshold. The same is true of using age-related normals. A field performed at 2 dB higher than a previous test assumes that improvement greater than this is not possible; thus, this test isn't suitable either.

100. d) Data must be entered the same way every time. If you enter *Aaron Jacob* for one test and *Jacob Aaron* for the next, the computer will not know they are the same patient. Data from a previous test need to be updated. For example, pupil size or near add Rx might have changed. The computer only knows what you tell it. Trying to override an instrument's pre-set data fields is counter productive.

101. a) In order for tests to be comparable, they must be run with the same parameters. Otherwise, you are trying to compare apples and stones. The correcting lens used for one test may not be appropriate for the next. The patient always should be instructed, even if they have done numerous field tests. One of the beauties of automated testing is that it is fairly repeatable, regardless of who runs the test (barring some sort of human error).

102. c) In automated perimetry, the near add calculation must include the patient's full distance correction, an age-related add, and the bowl depth. Bowl depth can range from 30 cm (equal to a Goldmann perimeter) to 50 cm. Most computerized perimeters calculate the add for you once you input the distance Rx and patient age. This is why it is key to enter the correct patient data.

103. b) New technology called a liquid lens combines water and oil (between 2 pieces of glass) to which an electric current is applied. Because of the charge of the molecules in the water, the voltage changes the shape of the water-lens, moving the focal point. Once the patient's refractive error is entered into the automated visual field machine, the appropriate charge is applied, and the lens automatically corrects for near. *Note:* at least one source suggests that if the astigmatic correction is over 2 diopters, a conventional trial lens is better.[1]

104. c) Give patients verbal encouragement. This helps them stay alert and motivated. For example, tell them they're doing well, or that they're halfway through, etc. Answer a) might be considered correct by some. My opinion is that if you tell patients to hold down the button and pause whenever they want to, it will lengthen the test and add to the stress, instead of helping the patient. It is better to let pauses remain in the control of the perimetrist. Patients should not be allowed to sit at the machine with their eyes closed during the test. Resting every 5 minutes might be allowed in extreme cases, but not as a general rule.

105. d) There are several test features that can be changed in order to better test a particular patient. These are known as parameters. In automated visual fields, these parameters can include alternate fixation points, speed at which stimuli are presented, stimulus color, and other features (which may be dependent on which program is chosen).

106. a) Most automated perimeters have an alternate fixation pattern that can be used for low vision patients. This pattern is offset from normal fixation, and if activated, the instrument automatically adjusts the blind spot and other points to coincide. Turning off the fixation monitor won't help the patient see the fixation point any better, nor will using a larger target. The correcting lens must be calculated for each patient; a +3.00 lens used across the board is unacceptable.

107. d) There are generally 2 presentation speeds: normal and slow. If you notice that the patient has a delayed response time, go to the parameters menu and select slow; hopefully this will help.

108. a) Communication during an automated field is almost constant. The droning of the machine and rhythm of responses can be tiring for even the most alert patients. Automated fields are taxing; therefore, reinforce the patient often. Leaving the room is not a good idea. Even the best patient can slip out of alignment.

109. a) An infrared monitor evaluates fixation via the corneal reflex in front of the pupil. The change from a black pupil to a blue iris is more pronounced than the change from a black pupil to a brown iris, hence fixation losses in a blue eye are registered more easily.

110. b) If the patient seems to be fixating, yet the instrument is registering fixation losses, tell the program to relocate the blind spot. If the blind spot is not placed accurately, the patient will respond when the light is flashed in that area. Reducing the intensity of the stimulus may help, as well.

111. b) If, during threshold testing, it becomes obvious that the patient cannot physically cope with the testing time required, switch to a screening strategy. This will provide *some* information and won't take as long. Increasing the stimulus speed won't help. And education is not the problem here; endurance is.

112. d) Blips above the baseline on the gaze-tracking graph indicate eye movement. The more blips, the more eye movement there was during the test. Spikes below the baseline represent blinks, so there should be some of these. (If, during the test, you are seeing no blips below baseline, remind the patient to blink periodically.)

113. a) The decibel graph is what you see on the screen during testing. The numbers that pop up are a representation of the patient's ability to see stimuli and can range from 0 (no points seen at any intensity) and 50 (can see the very dimmest of dim stimuli). Normal is around 30 dB, so if you see a bunch of 40s, it is likely that the patient is trigger happy.

114. b) Normal for a screening test does not necessarily mean that there is no field loss. It means that there is no field loss detected at this time by this particular instrument and this particular test. Screening programs can miss the shallow defects that indicate the early stages of disease. The need for future formal visual field tests depends on the patient's diagnosis and complaints. Screening tests are not adequate in glaucoma evaluation. Diagnosis of glaucoma requires elevated pressures and nerve damage, in addition to field loss.

115. b) One of the beauties of automated perimetry is that it is largely independent of operator bias and expertise.
116. a) If there are over 33% of either false positives or false negatives, the test is considered unreliable.
117. b) If fixation losses are greater than 10%, the test is considered unreliable.
118. d) The single field analysis printout is the most commonly used. It displays all the data in Answers a), b), and c). The defect depth and change analysis is a separate printout (also called the 3-in-1) and not used as often.
119. c) The decibel values corresponding to the point where the number is printed on the chart is characteristic of the threshold sensitivity (also called the numeric pattern or value table) printout. The numbers represent actual retinal sensitivity. A "0" means that the brightest stimulus was shown and not seen. Lower numbers indicate brighter lights and are more commonly elicited in the periphery. The higher numbers around the fovea represent dimmer lights and greater retinal sensitivity. Numbers are used, not symbols. The numbers are the actual, raw values, not statistically altered in any way.
120. d) A "0" on the decibel graph/numeric print out indicates that the brightest stimulus available on that instrument was not seen. On a normal field, the only 0 will be the physiologic blind spot (optic nerve head).
121. a) The grayscale printout gives each decibel measurement a graphic symbol, then prints the field using the symbols. The symbols used are varying shades of gray. The darker the symbol, the higher the decibel and the less sensitive the receptors. *Note:* You may also see the spellings *gray-scale* and *grey-scale*.
122. c) A point that is not seen would appear as a black area on the grayscale printout.
123. c) The total deviation display shows a numeric field on top, which shows any differences between the patient's test and the tests of other patients of the same age with normal fields. Beneath this is a graphic representation (blocks of varying shades of gray) that shows the probability that the patient's deviations occurred simply by chance.
124. a) The darker the block in the graphic display of the total deviation indicates that there is a very low probability that the patient's deviation was due to chance alone. See Answer 123.
125. b) The pattern deviation analysis "corrects" a field's island of vision, thus (possibly) revealing scotomas that may be hiding under a field that is depressed overall. Regarding total deviation analysis, see Answer 123; island of vision, see Answer 126; catch trials, see Answer 82.
126. b) The island of vision profile is a 3-dimensional representation of the visual field. An isopter is a boundary. Comparison and graytone analyses are other ways of representing the field (see Answers 127 and 121-122, respectively).
127. c) The comparison printout is designed to compare a patient's previous test to the current test.
128. b) A –2 on a comparison printout means that the patient has lost 2 decibels (at that particular point) since the previous test.

Part III

129. d) Manual perimetry, from confrontation to Goldmann, involves moving and stationary targets. Theoretically, any and every point could be tested with the Goldmann, not merely preselected ones (as in automated perimetry).
130. b) See Answer 129. *Automated* perimetry uses preselected points, is more accurate with static threshold testing, and is more reproducible.
131. c) It is a disadvantage that manual visual field testing, as with the Goldmann perimeter, requires more technical skill than automated.
132. b) The Goldmann perimeter is very bulky and not portable at all.

133. b) Isopters and scotomas are mapped by moving the stimulus from an area where it is not seen to an area where it is seen (and the patient responds). A stationary stimulus is not used to plot borders. Moving the stimulus from left to right is useful only when plotting the 180-degree meridian.

134. d) Mapping an isopter involves kinetic testing, where the target is moved from nonseeing to seeing. A static stimulus is used to determine threshold at a particular point, which gives you information as to what brightness/size target to use to plot an isopter. Static testing is also used to spot-check specific areas, such as the nasal area in glaucoma (searching for nasal step) or the vertical area in neurological fields.

135. a) Isopters are plotted by moving the stimulus from an area where it is not seen toward an area where it might be seen. A mark is made on the chart when the patient responds, to indicate the isopter's boundary.

136. a) Move the stimulus at a steady pace about 5 degrees per second. If you oscillate the target, it effectively becomes larger (which makes it easier to see) and gives a false representation of the field. Isopters are measured along meridians (the straight lines), not eccentricities (the circular lines).

137. c) The Roman numeral levers control the size of the stimulus.

138 b) The Arabic number and alphabetic levers both control the intensity of the stimulus. Each number designates a 0.5 step (4 being the brightest), and each letter designates a 0.1 step (e being the brightest).

139. c) The bulb of the Goldmann perimeter should be calibrated once every day. The background should (ideally) be adjusted for every patient with the patient seated at the instrument, because various clothing materials and colors reflect and absorb light in differing amounts.

140. c) An apostilb is a measurement of light intensity. It is not related to size (a large or small target may have the same brightness or intensity).

141. a) A dimmer background means that the stimulus will show up more because contrast is increased. This would result in a falsely expanded field. It is important to calibrate the bowl's background illumination to maintain comparability between a patient's tests.

142. b) The Goldmann field chart traditionally is hand-marked with colored pencils. Each color corresponds to a different stimulus size and intensity and is coded to the chart at the lower right corner of the chart. Checks and x's in lead pencil would be hard to decode. Grayscale printouts are products of automated fields. There is no automated pantograph.

143. a) Monitoring fixation on the Goldmann perimeter can be done constantly by looking through the viewer port. Unfortunately, the fixation mirror obstructs the view. If you need to use the mirror you can flash it by hand or move it every now and then to check the patient's position. Many automated perimeters check fixation by flashing a light on the blind spot. If the patient responds, it is recorded as a fixation loss. A manual field on a cooperative patient takes about 12 minutes; checking fixation once every 5 minutes is not enough.

144. b) Just knowing that you are watching will make the patient more motivated to hold fixation. Some Goldmann perimetrists advocate telling the patient where the next kinetic stimulus is coming from, but most do not feel this is a good idea. Using the near add may clear the fixation target but cannot be used to plot the outer isopter. The fixation point need be enlarged only for low vision patients.

145. a) If the patient has trouble seeing the central fixation area, use the mirror in the viewing port. You can either flash it manually during testing, or just flip it down and leave it in place (after determining that fixation will be adequate, since the eye no longer can be seen through the telescope). An add for the whole test will not give an accurate outer field, nor will the patient's glasses. Never tape anything to the inside of the bowl, as this will mar the paint finish.

146. d) Cylinder is translated to a spherical equivalent if the amount is under 1.00 diopter. If over 1.00 diopter, the full correction is used.

147. c) An emmetropic patient between 30 and 40 years old is given a near correcting lens (+1.00 sphere).

148. c) The near add calculation starts with the patient's distance refraction and then incorporates an add related to the patient's age. The habitual near add cannot be used because it may not be set to the 300-mm test distance of the Goldmann (and some automated instruments).

149. d) The projector arm of the Goldmann swings around the patient. If a patient sits back unannounced, they could get clobbered. True, sitting back means the test takes longer, fixation is lost, and the patient must be repositioned. But d) is the best answer because the test is not invalidated, nor is repositioning difficult (even if it is bothersome; *Note:* been there, done that!).

150. d) It is helpful to show the patient a few test points to give them an idea of what the test is like before you begin plotting anything.

151. c) Before proceeding with the field, determine a static threshold point at about 25 degrees temporal to fixation. (Since usually you are evaluating for glaucoma, start with the near portion of the field, as most early glaucoma defects occur in the central 30 degrees.)

152. c) Central fields are within 30 degrees.

153. c) To map the central field, use a stimulus that is threshold at 25 degrees temporal to fixation. The threshold stimulus at central fixation would be too dim to test the central field. The blind spot is at the 15 degrees temporal point. It may be that the proper stimulus *is* 2 notches dimmer than that used for the outer isopter, but you must test to find out.

154. a) The Roman numerals are target size, I being the smallest in common use (there is a 0, which is generally not used); always start with the instrument at I. The e intensity is also almost always used. The Arabic numbers are the first ones you should change when determining threshold. Start at the setting I2e, at 25 degrees temporal. Turn on the stimulus and see if the patient responds. If they do respond, then use this setting as threshold. If they do not respond, turn the levers to I3e and try again. If the target is *not* seen, continue to increase brightness using the Arabic numbers until the target is seen. The first stimulus the patient responds to is your threshold. (This applies both to threshold for central field and peripheral field where a brighter light must be used because sensitivity decreases the farther out you go.)

155. b) When performing a follow-up test, use the same stimuli as the original test. This provides better comparisons. If changes have occurred, you may have to plot additional isopters/points using other stimuli as well.

156. d) See Answer 154. 4e is the brightest target, so if the patient doesn't respond to it, the target *size* must be increased, adjusting the Roman numeral lever.

157. b) Enlargement of the blind spot should make it *easier* to find, not more difficult. The other answers are common errors.

158. d) The normal field extends to 95 degrees temporally. Central is 30 degrees. To map the outer isopter, use a target that is threshold between 30 and 95, or around 50 degrees temporal to fixation. A target that is threshold at fixation or 30 degrees would be too dim to map the outer periphery. At 15 degrees temporal, you run into the blind spot.

159. c) You want the widest part of the central field isopter to fall just *inside* the 30-degree eccentricity. If the patient is seeing the stimulus prior to 30 degrees, you need to first make it smaller (until you're on the I setting, if you're not already there) or dimmer (decreasing the Arabic number lever downward).

160. c) In the case of extreme low vision, try starting with the V4e, which is the largest and brightest stimulus. (There is no such thing as a VI6f setting.)

161. c) To map at 90 and 180 degrees, plot meridians 5 and 15 degrees to either side. Plotting exactly at 90 or 180 might cause you to miss a step defect. In addition, the Goldmann bowl itself has a gap at 180 and 0 degrees, so the patient's true response might be missed because the stimulus is not actually being projected.

162. b) A defect should be mapped with at least 2 different stimuli. A test strategy is necessary, but the strategy must be modified as you accommodate every patient. An add is not used for fields beyond the central 30 degrees, and a +3.00 is not right for every patient.

163. c) Areas of inconsistency can be marked with crosshatching and labeled "in and out" or "variable." Such an area cannot be plotted as if it had definite borders. Moving the target faster would make the area map as smaller (or even cause it to disappear), but it would be a false response. The same speed should be used throughout the test. Ignoring such a finding is likewise incorrect.

Part IV

164. a) The most common areas for visual field artifacts are superior nasal (because of brows and lids) and inferior nasal (because of the nose).
165. a) The correcting lens should be in place when you are testing the central 30 degrees.
166. **Matching:**
     decentered correcting lens   c) Figure 3-5
     hysteria or malingering   a) Figure 3-3
     ptotic upper eyelid   b) Figure 3-4
     thick rim on correcting lens   d) Figure 3-6
167. a) Retinal defects are monocular. The remaining statements are true.
168. d) Retinal defects are projected to the opposite quadrant. Thus, superior is projected to inferior and nasal to temporal.
169. c) Since the macula is the area of fine central vision, any defect involving the macula will be more debilitating than a defect in any other location.
170. d) Nerve fiber layer damage causes field losses that follow along the nerve fiber pattern. Thus, Bjerrum's scotomas are the most common nerve fiber layer field loss listed. Hemianopsia, quadrantanopsia, and congruous defects generally occur posterior to the junction of the optic nerve and chiasm. (Retinal detachment is a possible exception.)
171. b) All nerve fibers lead to the disc. Thus, defects in the nerve fiber layer lead to the blind spot (not horizontally and not vertically). There is a definite pattern of progression.
172. d) A left homonymous hemianopsia would occur posterior to the chiasm, not involving the retinal fiber layer as in Answers a) through c).
173. c) Ocular hypertension has no field loss. The definition of ocular hypertension is intraocular pressure that is above normal but where no optic nerve damage or field loss occurs.
174. b) Retinal detachment causes a field loss that is projected to the opposite quadrant. It does not cause enlargement of the blind spot per se, as do the other answers.
175. c) Optic nerve disease other than glaucoma usually causes an enlargement of the blind spot that is more equal in all directions, producing a rounder (concentric) scotoma. In glaucoma, the nerve damage occurs more unequally, usually causing first vertical orientation, and later, horizontal.
176. c) The most common finding in optic nerve damage is a central scotoma. This is because the nerve fibers from the macula move to a central position about 1 cm behind the disc. Thus, any pressure on the disc would affect the macular fibers.
177. a) Optic nerve damage is monocular until the fibers reach the junction between the nerve and the chiasm. Thus, there is an area just anterior to the chiasm that will cause a binocular defect. In addition, the question specifies optic nerve damage. Anatomically, the optic nerve ceases to exist at the chiasm.
178. a) The field loss experienced in optic neuritis can resolve. In fact, about half of all patients with optic neuritis will have normal fields less than 1 year later. Answers b) through d) are true.
179. b) Optic disc drusen can cause a field defect that mimics glaucoma. The important difference is that the drusen nasal step is inferior, while the glaucomatous nasal step is superior.
180. d) The most common field defect seen in optic disc drusen is an inferior nasal step. Defects in Answers a) through c) also can occur but are less common.
181. d) Field loss in patients taking Plaquenil may include paracentral and pericentral scotomas as well as central scotoma. Infrequently, constriction may occur.

182. d) Due to the pattern of glaucoma damage to specific retinal nerve fibers, glaucoma classically causes changes in the nasal field (nasal step), central 20 degrees (Bjerrum's scotoma), and the blind spot (enlargement).

183. c) The pattern of field loss in glaucoma directly corresponds to how the nerve fiber layers are being damaged. This is not related to the pressure, since a person can have elevated intraocular pressure and no damage, or normal intraocular pressure and experience a field loss. The damage is a result of the pressure on the optic disc, not the blood supply in the choroid. In addition, the damage is to the nerve fiber layer itself, not posterior into the visual pathway.

184. b) The nasal step in glaucoma is superior. It generally is not connected to the blind spot, as is a Bjerrum's scotoma.

185. c) Early glaucomatous defects include a paracentral scotoma in Bjerrum's area and a nasal step. Answer b) is correct, but Answer c) is more correct.

186. b) Bjerrum's area is generally in the 15-degree eccentricity.

187. a) Bjerrum's area is between the 10-degree and 18-degree eccentricities, extending from the tip of the physiologic blind spot, arcing over the central vision, and stopping abruptly at the 180-degree meridian.

188. d) In end-stage glaucoma, before total blindness occurs, there remains a temporal crescent of vision. At this point, even the typical glaucoma tunnel vision has been lost.

189. c) The more congruous a defect is, the more posterior it is located (as a general rule). Prechiasmal and optic nerve lesions are monocular, and hence not congruous.

190. d) Macular sparing is a situation where the central vision, which corresponds to the macular area (the central 8 degrees), remains even though much of the right or left hemisphere has been lost. An arcuate (or comet) scotoma is, as the name suggests, an area shaped like a curving comet where there is no vision. A nasal step is where a defect stops abruptly at the 180-degree meridian, and a cecocentral scotoma would be a scotoma that extends from the blind spot toward or into the central vision.

191. a) Sparing of the central (macular) field is most often seen in disorders involving the occipital cortex, the "end of the trail" for the pathway of vision. The cause is often vascular, such as a stroke. Optic nerve head disorders may lead to an enlarged blind spot of the affected eye. A disorder in the optic radiations often cause wedge-shaped defects ("pie"). Disorders at the chiasm (eg, pituitary gland tumor) causes defects in the temporal field of each eye.

192. a) Because of the anatomical location of the retinal nerve fibers, neurological lesions respect (ie, do not cross) the vertical meridian.

193. b) See Answer 192.

194. a) The optic nerve is prechiasmal, hence a defect would be monocular. A homonymous defect is, by definition, binocular.

195. c) Because the only place where the temporal fibers are together is the chiasm, the chiasm is the only place where a bitemporal defect can occur.

196. c) A wedge-shaped field loss is the "pie." A wedge in the upper quadrant ("in the sky") indicates that the fibers to the inferior retinas have been damaged. A wedge in the lower quadrant ("on the floor") indicates that fibers to the superior retinas have been damaged. These kinds of defects occur where the fibers fan out in the optic radiations.

197. d) When there are no specific areas of field loss but a generalized decrease (depression) of the field, a media opacity may be the problem. This includes cataract, posterior capsule opacity, corneal dystrophy, etc. *Note:* In automated field testing, a *pattern deviation analysis* may unmask "hidden" scotomas lurking beneath the overall depressed field.

198. a) A field with the appearance of a "clover leaf" (also called 4-leaf clover) often results when the patient responds well at the beginning of the test but then fatigues or stops paying attention later in the exam. An overall depression can be caused by a media opacity, such as cataract. An enlarged blind spot may be due to swelling of the optic nerve head. A ring scotoma happens when the trial lens is not close enough to the eye.

199. d) Spiral, star-shaped, and tubular fields are all findings in the hysterical patient.
200. c) Hysteria is actually a neurosis, and usually is caused by mental conflict of some sort. A desire to trick the examiner is malingering. Elevated intraocular pressure and pseudotumor do not cause hysteria.
201. d) Nonexpanding (tubular) and spiral fields are more easily detected on the Goldmann or by tangent screen. Also, in these 2 tests, the examiner has the option of moving the patient back from the screen to retest. Increasing the testing distance should geometrically increase the size of the field. If the field does not expand, then the loss is probably functional (ie, without an organic cause; see also Answers 37 and 202).
202. a) A field loss pattern that cannot be reproduced from one testing to another is an indication of nonorganic field loss (ie, not due to any physical problem). Organic patterns (ie, those caused by a physical disorder or injury) generally will resemble each other from one exam to the next.
203. **Matching:**

chiasmal defect	g) Figure 3-13
glaucoma	f) Figure 3-12
nerve fiber layer defect	d) Figure 3-10
nonorganic defect	b) Figure 3-8
optic disc drusen	e) Figure 3-11
post-chiasmal defect	c) Figure 3-9
retinal detachment	a) Figure 3-7

Reference

1. Komagata Y, Nakano T, eda A, et al. Comparison between liquid trial lens and the conventional method for astigmatism correction on the Humphrey Field Analyzer III860. Abstract. *Japanese Orthopic Journal*. Accessed March 12 2023. https://sci-hub.ru/10.4263/jorthoptic.046F203.

Bibliography

Pate CB. Understanding visual field testing. Presented at North Carolina Optometric Society Spring Congress, June 2018. Accessed March 12, 2023. www.nceyes.org/assets/docs/2018SpringCongressHandouts/Pate%20-%20PARA-%20 Understanding%20Visual%20Field%20Testing%20NCEyes%20June%202018.pdf.

Chapter 4

Pupil Assessment

Ledford JK.
*Certified Ophthalmic Technician Exam
Review Manual, Third Edition* (pp 75-85).
© 2023 Taylor & Francis Group.

ABBREVIATIONS USED IN THIS CHAPTER

- CNS   central nervous system
- mm   millimeter
- OD   right eye
- OS   left eye
- OU   both eyes
- RAPD   relative afferent pupillary defect

1. **Your patient's pupils measure 4.0 right eye and 2.5 left eye. This is called:**
   a) anisocoria
   b) anisometropia
   c) aniseikonia
   d) anisoiridius

2. **What is the size range of the average human pupil at rest?**
   a) 1.0 to 2.0 mm
   b) 2.0 to 3.5 mm
   c) 2.5 to 5.0 mm
   d) 6.0 to 9.5 mm

3. **Which patient will generally have the smallest pupils?**
   a) 20-year-old
   b) 73-year-old
   c) patient with myopia
   d) blue irises

4. **You are preparing to perform an automated visual field on a patient. The minimum pupil size required is:**
   a) 1 mm
   b) 3 mm
   c) 5 mm
   d) 7 mm

5. **You will be performing mydriatic fundus photography on your patient. Which of the following is *true* regarding pupil dilation?**
   a) any dilation is acceptable
   b) dilation is not necessary
   c) a minimum pupil size of 4 to 5 mm
   d) a maximum pupil size of 6 mm

6. **Patients with large pupils who are being fit for rigid contact lenses will require:**
   a) a lens with an imprinted iris
   b) larger optical zone and larger lens diameter
   c) smaller optical zone and smaller lens diameter
   d) larger optical zone and smaller lens diameter

7. **If the pupil dilates into the peripheral curves of a rigid contact lens, the patient probably will notice:**
   a) vision is clearer right after a blink, then blurs
   b) vision is blurred right after a blink, then clears
   c) blurred vision due to corneal edema
   d) light streamers (flare)

8. **The pupils of each eye are "linked" so that they normally constrict or expand at the same time. This is known as the:**
   a) light response
   b) accommodative response
   c) direct response
   d) consensual response

9. **Argyll Robertson pupils are often:**
   a) unreactive to direct or consensual light
   b) unreactive to accommodation
   c) reactive to light
   d) sluggishly reactive to accommodation

10. **You might first suspect that the patient has a tonic pupil when:**
    a) the response to direct light is slow
    b) the pupil enlarges in direct light
    c) that eye also has a ptotic lid
    d) the patient is photophobic

11. **A patient with iritis often exhibits:**
    a) a smaller pupil in the unaffected eye
    b) a smaller pupil in the affected eye
    c) no difference in pupil size
    d) no pupillary reaction in the affected eye

12. **A person being chased by a bear will exhibit:**
    a) pupil constriction
    b) pupil dilation
    c) pupil hippus
    d) anisocoria

13. **The pupil evaluation is essentially a test of the nervous system. Which of the following is *true*?**
    a) The afferent system involves a stimulus (light) being transmitted to the brain.
    b) The efferent system involves the brain transmitting to a body part (iris).
    c) The sympathetic and parasympathetic nervous systems are not related to pupil function.
    d) Both a) and b)

14. **The nerve fibers that carry light impulses from the eye to the brain are:**
    a) neurotic
    b) virtual
    c) afferent
    d) efferent

15. **Which of the following statements regarding the iris is *true*?**
    a) The sphincter muscle is innervated by the voluntary nervous system.
    b) The dilator muscle is innervated by the sympathetic system.
    c) The sphincter and dilator muscles are both innervated by the sympathetic system.
    d) The sphincter and dilator muscles are both innervated by the parasympathetic nervous system.

16. **When evaluating the pupils' response to light, the patient is directed to look at a fixation target in the distance to:**
    a) cause maximum miosis
    b) minimize photophobia
    c) avoid stimulating divergence
    d) avoid stimulating accommodation

17. **During pupil exam of a 6-month-old, you notice that the left pupil does not meet at the bottom, creating a "key hole" appearance. This is most likely a:**
    a) sign of prematurity
    b) gestational defect
    c) sign of birth injury
    d) sign of congenital glaucoma

18. **When an iris coloboma is noted, the physician will also specifically evaluate:**
    a) extraocular muscles
    b) visual fields
    c) optic nerve and retina
    d) eyelid position for ptosis

19. **Synechiae are most often seen in cases of:**
    a) chronic allergic reaction
    b) chronic inflammation
    c) open-angle glaucoma
    d) genetic abnormalities

20. **You are evaluating a patient with trauma to the right globe. When you check the pupil, you see that it is drawn up and pointed to the 11 o'clock position. This may be a sign of:**
    a) perforation
    b) posterior synechiae
    c) subconjunctival hemorrhage
    d) endophthalmitis

21. **An abnormal pupil shape may occur after:**
    a) dilation in the eye clinic
    b) cataract surgery if the pupil was stretched mechanically
    c) laser capsulotomy
    d) fluorescein angiography

22. **The pupil in a patient with angle closure may be:**
    a) dilated and oval
    b) miotic and round
    c) peaked
    d) missing a segment of iris

23. **Aniridia is:**
   a) any defect of pupil shape
   b) a growth on the iris
   c) a separation of the iris root from the ciliary body
   d) absence of an iris

24. **Which of the following is used to detect an RAPD?**
   a) cross cover test
   b) interpupillary distance test
   c) swinging flashlight test
   d) direct flashlight test

25. **When performing the swinging flashlight test, it is best to:**
   a) rapidly move from one eye to the other
   b) allow a 2-second recovery between testing one eye and the other
   c) lowering the light when switching
   d) hold the light on each eye for 3 seconds before switching

26. **You might first suspect that the patient has an RAPD when:**
   a) the response to direct light is slow
   b) the pupil enlarges in direct light
   c) that eye also has a ptotic lid
   d) the patient is photophobic

27. **The presence of an RAPD:**
   a) demonstrates a totally blind eye
   b) indicates a problem in the optic nerve
   c) indicates a defect in the facial nerve
   d) indicates a problem in the cerebral cortex

28. **An eye with an RAPD usually has:**
   a) redness and pain
   b) subnormal visual acuity
   c) delayed extraocular muscle responses
   d) irregular astigmatism

29. **Another name for an RAPD is:**
   a) Argyll Robertson pupils
   b) Adie's syndrome
   c) Marcus Gunn pupil
   d) tonic pupil

30. **You are performing a swinging flashlight test. The right pupil does not react at all when you shine the light in it. When you swing over to the left eye, the left pupil constricts rapidly. When you swing back to the right eye, there is again no reaction. This indicates:**
   a) a normal reaction
   b) RAPD OD by reverse
   c) RAPD OS by reverse
   d) a tonic pupil

31.   You are performing a swinging flashlight test. The right pupil seems to constrict normally. When you swing to the left eye, it constricts, but much slower than the right. When you switch back to the right eye again, there is now a very rapid constriction. This may indicate:
       a) a variation of normal
       b) RAPD OD
       c) RAPD OS
       d) poor patient fixation

32.   Your patient has 20/20 vision OD and 20/50 OS. Using the muscle light to check pupils, you are unsure whether OS has an RAPD. To help clarify, you can:
       a) instill a drop of 1% pilocarpine OS to see if the pupil reacts
       b) check the pupils' reaction to accommodation
       c) use the indirect headset at its brightest setting as a light source
       d) have the patient look directly at the muscle light

33.   Which of the following can contribute to the difficulty of detecting RAPD?
       a) the patient fails to understand the test
       b) hippus
       c) performing the test in dim light
       d) having the patient fixate at a distance

34.   Which is the *most* likely to be associated with RAPD?
       a) optic nerve disease
       b) retinal disease
       c) cataracts
       d) blow-out fracture

35.   A patient has a dense cataract, obscuring the view of the retina and optic nerve. Why might the swinging flashlight test be important in such a case?
       a) It could validate the presence of a retinal detachment.
       b) It could validate the presence of glaucoma.
       c) It could indicate the health of the optic nerve.
       d) It has no bearing in a case like this.

36.   A new patient gives a history of using "glaucoma drops" back in the 90s but has not had treatment for years. They have best corrected vision of 20/80 in each eye and an intraocular pressure of 32 in each eye. The left eye has a 2+ RAPD. This most likely indicates:
       a) nothing; the swinging flashlight test is not useful in a case like this
       b) there is a media opacity in the left eye
       c) optic nerve damage is worse in the left eye
       d) the left eye has a retinal detachment

37.   A patient seems to have profound vision loss in one eye following a head injury at work. You perform a very careful pupillary assessment and find *no* RAPD. This probably indicates that the vision loss is:
       a) due to refractive error
       b) due to media opacity
       c) associated with malingering
       d) associated with any of the above

38. **RAPD is usually documented by:**
    a) an objective rating by the patient
    b) a measurement of the pupils' diameter
    c) a subjective rating by the observer
    d) a standardized rating system

39. **An RAPD may actually be quantified by using:**
    a) Bangerter filters
    b) neutral density filters
    c) a pupil gauge
    d) a diffusing filter

40. **To test the pupils' response to accommodation, the evaluator should observe the patient's pupils as the patient:**
    a) tracks a light moved into the positions of gaze
    b) tracks a near object from left to right and back
    c) shifts focus from a distant object to a light and back
    d) shifts focus from a distant to a near object and back

41. **Prior to pupil dilation, one must "check the angles." This is pertinent in a discussion of pupils because dilation can:**
    a) cause a rapid rise in intraocular pressure
    b) precipitate accommodation
    c) cause open-angle glaucoma
    d) cause dilation-induced cataracts

42. **Pupil dilation in the clinic using topical medication is best accomplished when:**
    a) a topical anesthetic is used first
    b) the dilator muscle is stimulated and the sphincter muscle is paralyzed
    c) both sphincter and dilator muscles are paralyzed
    d) accommodation is well controlled

Study Notes

When checking pupils, the basic questions are: (1) Is light getting through the optic nerve (ie, is the afferent system intact)? (2) Is the pupil reacting appropriately to a) light, b) dark, and c) accommodation (ie, is the efferent system of the eye working properly)? (3) Do the pupils react consensually (ie, respond equally to the same stimulus at the same time)?

If the afferent system is damaged, the efferent system is affected. That is, if the optic nerve is damaged and light cannot properly reach the CNS, then the CNS's efferent system will not be able to cause normal pupillary reactions in that eye. Thus we are evaluating the afferent system by observing the efferent response. There are specialized, automated instruments that detect and quantify RAPD, but we will discuss only the swinging flashlight test.

Also important are the questions: (4) Is the pupil round or is the shape abnormal? (5) What size is the pupil, and are the pupils equal in size? (6) Do the pupils react to accommodation?

Suggested reading in *Principles and Practice in Ophthalmic Assisting: A Comprehensive Textbook:*
> Chapter 2: Ocular Anatomy (*Nerve Supply* p 13, *The Anterior Segment* pp 17-20)
> Chapter 3: Ocular Physiology (*Uveal Tract* pp 31-32)
> Chapter 9: Basic Eye Exam (*Pupil Assessment* pp 122-128 through Sidebar 9-11)
> Chapter 22: Pharmacology (*Mydriatics and Cycloplegics* pp 425-426)

Correction Note: If you are using *Principles and Practice in Ophthalmic Assisting* as your study text, Table 9-1, page 124, next to the last entry *CN III palsy (complete)* should be corrected to say <u>Parasympathetic</u> under "Notes."

Explanatory Answers

1. a) Anisocoria is the correct term for pupils of unequal size. The prefix aniso- means unequal. So anisometropia is unequal refractive errors (usually defined as 2 diopter difference between the 2 eyes). Aniseikonia is a difference in image size between the 2 eyes (eg, a corrected myopic eye will see a smaller image than a corrected hyperopic eye). Anisoiridius is a bogus term that I made up just for you.

2. c) When not accommodating and in daylight, the human pupil is usually about 2.5 to 5.0 mm (the number given by different references will vary). Light conditions, drugs, emotions, and age affect pupil size at any given moment. The maximum human pupil range is from < 1.0 to 9.0 mm (2.0 to 8.0 mm would be a more "average" range).

3. b) The size of the pupil decreases with age (called *senile miosis*). Pupils are smaller in infants, hyperopia/emmetropia (as compared to myopia), and dark irises.

4. b) If the pupil is smaller than 3 mm, consider dilating the patient before proceeding with the test.

5. c) Four to 5 mm dilation would be the *minimum* size for decent mydriatic fundus photos.

6. b) A patient with large pupils needs a larger optic zone and a larger diameter lens for best vision.

7. d) If the pupil dilates beyond the optic zone, then light is coming through the peripheral curves into the eye. This causes glare and light flares. Answers a) and b) have to do with the steepness of the lens. A large pupil is not related to corneal edema.

8. d) The term that describes the linked action of the pupils is the consensual (think "both agree") response. The light and accommodative responses are the pupils' reaction to light and near objects, respectively. The direct response is the response of a single pupil to a stimulus.

9. a) The hallmark of Argyll Robertson pupils is their lack of response to direct or consensual light.

10. a) A tonic pupil will have a slow reaction to direct light. A pupil that enlarges in direct light most likely has a Marcus Gunn pupil (ie, RAPD). Horner's syndrome exhibits ptosis on that same side.

11. b) An eye with iritis usually has a smaller pupil. The pupillary margin may also be somewhat irregular, if posterior adhesions to the lens (posterior synechiae) have occurred.

12. b) Fear, as generated when a sane person is being chased by a bear, activates the sympathetic nervous system ("fight or flight") causing a release of adrenaline. Pupil dilation is one of the results. When the parasympathetic system is active ("rest and digest"), the pupils are in a normal state. Hippus is the normal "pulsing" of the pupil as it reacts to light variations in the environment. Anisocoria is when the 2 pupils have a 2 mm or more difference in size.

13. d) Both a) and b) are true. Light traveling through the eye to the brain is part of the afferent system. When the brain sends the iris a response (ie, to constrict or dilate) triggered by the stimulus, this is the efferent system. Regarding Answer c), see Answer 12.

14. c) *Afferent* (sensory) neurons carry information *away* from a sensory organ to the CNS; the optic nerve is generally considered to be purely afferent since its function is to carry a stimulus (light) to the brain. Efferent (motor) nerve fibers carry impulses from the brain to muscle (which is what the iris is), inducing movement (as in pupillary constriction/dilation).

15. b) The dilator muscle is part of the sympathetic nervous system, and the sphincter muscle is part of the parasympathetic. The voluntary nervous system is that which we can control, such as moving our limbs. The involuntary system (which includes both the parasympathetic and sympathetic branches) works automatically, like heartbeat and pupil size.

16. d) If the patient looks at a close object, accommodation may be stimulated. Accommodation is hallmarked by 3 responses: convergence (the eyes move inward, toward each other), accommodation of the crystalline lens (which causes the lens to thicken, increasing "plus" power and thus moving the focal point closer to the macula), and miosis (the pupils get smaller). When evaluating the pupils' reaction to light, we want to prevent the miosis caused by the accommodative response. When looking at a distant object, the eyes are already "diverged" in the sense that they are not converged (as in accommodation). Photophobia is light sensitivity, not affected by looking at distance vs near.

17. b) Coloboma of the iris occurs when the iris tissue does not fuse properly during early gestation. It is a "fusion defect" that develops during the first trimester and thus not associated with prematurity or injury. Nor is it a sign of congenital glaucoma.

18. c) Not only may the iris have failed to fuse, but there may also be a cleft or notch in the retina, optic nerve, and even the lens. Actually, coloboma of the eyelid can occur, creating a notch in the lid margin (usually the upper), but it is not necessarily associated with iris coloboma.

19. b) Synechiae occur when tissue of the iris adheres either to the corneal endothelium (anterior synechiae) or the anterior of the lens (posterior synechiae). They are most commonly seen in chronic inflammation. The adhesions can cause irregularities in the pupil shape, often with tiny jagged edges that are even more visible if the pupil is dilated. The situations in Answers a), c), and d) are not associated with synechiae.

20. a) If the globe is perforated and the uveal tissue prolapses, the pupil may be drawn toward the wound creating a "peak" toward the area of prolapse. In the case of posterior synechiae, parts of the iris's posterior surface are adhered to the anterior surface of the lens. This may create ragged edges but not the dramatic peak that you see in a prolapsed uvea. A subconjunctival hemorrhage is external and would not affect the pupil. Endophthalmitis is a reaction in the fellow/uninjured eye.

21. b) If the pupil is not sufficiently dilated to perform cataract surgery, the surgeon may have to stretch the iris manually. This may cause tears in the iris, affecting pupil shape. Routine dilation for exams, laser, or imaging will not cause abnormal pupil shape.

22. a) The classic appearance of the pupil in angle closure is dilated and oval, although it may be dilated and round. A peaked pupil may appear in cases of globe perforation. Missing a segment of iris might be congenital (coloboma) or surgical (sector iridectomy).

23. d) Aniridia (an- meaning without) refers to the absence (or partial absence) of the iris. This may be congenital or due to injury. The separation of the iris root from its attachment to the ciliary body, usually by blunt trauma is termed *iridodialysis*.

24. c) The swinging flashlight test (or "swinging torch test") is used to test the consensual light response, comparing the light reaction of one pupil to the other. This is how an RAPD is identified. The direct flashlight test is simply shining the light into one pupil to evaluate its reaction. Cross cover testing is used in strabismus evaluation, and interpupillary distance is measured for fitting spectacles.

25. d) Hold the light one eye for 3 seconds, then quickly switch to the other eye, observing its initial response. Hold for 3 seconds then switch back to the other eye. The switch is made directly from one eye to the other, without a break between.

26. b) A pupil that enlarges in direct light most likely has an RAPD defect. A tonic pupil will have a slow reaction to direct light. Horner's syndrome exhibits ptosis on that same side. Photophobia is the patient's aversion to light, not the eye's reaction to it.

27. b) RAPD can be identified by shining the light in one eye, then the other (swinging flashlight test). An eye with an RAPD usually has poorer vision that the normal eye but is not necessarily blind. It generally indicates a problem with the optic nerve.

28. b) RAPD indicates optic nerve damage, so visual acuity is usually compromised to some degree. The other situations do not apply to RAPD.

29. c) Another name you may hear for RAPD is Marcus Gunn pupil (or Marcus Gunn sign); some texts may refer to it as an afferent pupillary defect. Robert Marcus Gunn was a Scottish ophthalmologist in the 19th century.

30. b) Usually an RAPD is identified when the unaffected eye constricts rapidly, and the affected eye dilates or constricts less (as compared to the unaffected eye) when you swing back to it. But one can still identify an RAPD in a fixed pupil by the reaction of the other (reverse), reactive eye, as in this scenario where the right eye is affected.

31. c) We often tend to think that an RAPD eye will not react to light at all, and then we see an obvious "zooming" constriction of the other, normal pupil. RAPD can be much more subtle, however. Your only clue (besides poorer vision in the affected eye, usually) may be the *difference* in a *positive* light reaction in both pupils as in this case, indicating RAPD in the less reactive left eye.

32. c) Try using the light of the indirect ophthalmoscope (at its brightest setting) to check the pupils. Sometimes the muscle light is not strong/bright enough to differentiate between pupils (hence the adage that most cases of RAPD are caused by weak flashlight batteries!). Turning off all room lights may help as well. The pilocarpine drop will cause the pupil to get smaller and is not diagnostic for RAPD. The accommodative response is generally intact. Pupils are checked with the patient looking into the distance so as not to induce accommodative miosis.

33. b) Hippus is a normal pulsating of the pupil. Because this causes the pupil to make tiny enlargement then constricting movements, it can confuse the identification of RAPD. The pupil evaluation is an objective test, not requiring any understanding on the part of the patient. Pupils' light reaction should always be testing in dim lighting with the patient focusing at a distance in order to avoid accommodation. *Note:* Also of interest is *pupillary release* ("the small amount of pupillary dilatation immediately following initial constriction during steady illumination"[1]).

34. a) RAPD is most often seen in optic nerve disorders (eg, optic neuritis, compression of the optic nerve, optic nerve infections, ischemic optic neuropathy, severe glaucoma worse in one eye), or optic nerve trauma (including surgical). Severe retinal disease may exhibit RAPD if one eye is much more affected than the other,[1] but is not the most likely. Cataracts in and of themselves are not associated with RAPD. A blow-out fracture does not cause RAPD unless there is accompanying optic nerve damage.

35. c) In the case of dense media opacity, the finding of an RAPD (via swinging flashlight test) is a strong indication that the optic nerve is not healthy. Even if an RAPD is found, however, you could not specifically validate a retinal detachment or glaucoma without other tests (a B-scan springs to mind).

36. c) In this scenario all other things being equal (vision and intraocular pressure), the presence of an RAPD most likely indicates that the left eye has more optic nerve damage. The swinging flashlight test is extremely useful in a case like this. Media opacity in and of itself does not cause RAPD. While it is possible that there could be a retinal detachment, this is not the most likely of Answers c) and d). Of note: there is probably optic nerve damage in both eyes, so technically both eyes would have an RAPD. But you can only detect this, in this case, because one eye is worse than the other.

37. d) Your first inclination may be to implicate the patient with malingering, where a person "decides" not to see in order to get some type of gain (usually financial). However, refractive error and media opacity could be to blame as well. In these cases, perhaps the patient has had poor vision in one eye for a long time, but only noticed it when comparing one eye to the other post-injury.

38. c) Unfortunately, there is no standardized rating for RAPD. Instead, each observer makes a subjective rating (ie, personal opinion) from 1 to 4, with 4 being the most obvious scenario where the affected pupil dilates and the normal pupil "zoom" constricts during the swinging flashlight test. Thus my +3 RAPD might be your +2. *Note:* Some references grade 1 to 5.

39. b) Neutral density filters are usually mounted in a holder and graduate from least to more opaque. The filter is placed in front of the normal eye, and the swinging flashlight test is performed. The test is repeated with denser and denser filters until the response of the normal eye matches that of the eye with RAPD. The Bangerter filter is used in extraocular muscle testing, a pupil gauge to measure pupil size, and a diffusing filter is used in slit lamp evaluation and photography.

40. d) When focusing on a near object, normal pupils should constrict. When focus shifts to distance, the pupils will dilate somewhat. This occurs because pupil constriction is part of the accommodative response to looking at a close object (see Answer 16). Moving the eyes, as in Answers a) and b), does not affect pupil size per se. The near target should be an accommodative object, not a light.

41. a) When the pupil dilates, the iris draws back and "bunches up." If the angle is not deep enough, the iris might bunch up into it, blocking the exit of aqueous from the eye. In turn, this causes a rise in intraocular pressure, precipitating an angle-closure glaucoma event with subsequent (and perhaps permanent) damage to the eye. The angles are checked (preferably with the slit lamp) prior to dilation to evaluate the possibility of angle closure occurring. If the angles are narrow, dilation would be deferred (at least until the practitioner can take a look).

42. b) For the most effective dilation we (1) paralyze the sphincter muscle (with a parasympatholytic drug such as tropicamide) so it cannot work to make the pupil smaller; and (2) stimulate the dilator muscle (with a sympathomimetic drug such as phenylephrine) so that the pupil will open. Using a topical anesthetic first is more comfortable for the patient because the other drops really sting, but this does not affect dilation. Tropicamide also paralyzes the ciliary muscle so that the eye cannot accommodate, but that is a result of the medication and not a condition of its action.

Reference

1. McGee S. The Pupils. In: *Evidence-Based Physical Diagnosis*. 4th ed. 2018. Accessed March 12, 2023. https://sciencedirect.com/science/article/pii/B9780323392761000214.

Bibliography

Amirhossein V. Relative Afferent Pupillary Defect. EyeWiki, website of The American Academy of Ophthalmology. Accessed March 12, 2023. https://eyewiki.org/Relative_Afferent_Pupillary_Defect

Bell RA, Waggoner PM, Boyd WM, Akers RE, Yee CE. Clinical grading of relative afferent pupillary defects. *Arch Ophthalmol.* 1993;111(7):938-942. Abstract. Accessed March 12, 2023. doi:10.1001/archopt.1993.01090070056019

Broadway DC. How to test for a relative afferent pupillary defect (RAPD). *Community Eye Health.* 2012;25(79-80):58-59. Accessed March 12, 2023. https://pubmed.ncbi.nlm.nih.gov/23520419/

Chapter 5

Tonometry

Ledford JK.
*Certified Ophthalmic Technician Exam
Review Manual, Third Edition* (pp 87-94).
© 2023 Taylor & Francis Group.

Background

1.   **Patients often refer to tonometry as the "glaucoma test." This is a misnomer because:**
     a) it does not contact the eye
     b) it is not accurate on the average cornea
     c) it also tests for optic nerve damage
     d) eye pressure is just one part of diagnosing glaucoma

2.   **At what time of day would you expect a patient's intraocular pressure to be *lowest*?**
     a) during sleep
     b) morning
     c) afternoon
     d) none, it is always the same

3.   **What is the normal fluctuation of intraocular pressure in a 24-hour period?**
     a) 0 to 2 mm Hg
     b) 2 to 6 mm Hg
     c) 4 to 7 mm Hg
     d) 6 to 10 mm Hg

4.   **The characteristic of the toughness of the sclera to affect intraocular pressure readings in some cases is known as:**
     a) scleral rigidity
     b) corneal rigidity
     c) connective rigidity
     d) uveal rigidity

5.   **The characteristic of the cornea's elasticity that affects intraocular pressure readings is:**
     a) corneal hydrops
     b) keratoconus
     c) corneal rigidity
     d) corneal hysteresis

6. The principle that a gas- or fluid-filled sphere will be indented *more* by a given weight if the sphere's internal pressure is low (vs being indented less if the internal pressure is high) is the basis for:
    a) indentation tonometry
    b) applanation tonometry
    c) biotometry
    d) rebound tonometry

7. The principle behind rebound tonometry is that the probe tip:
    a) will expend more energy to measure a harder eye
    b) will bounce back faster from a harder eye
    c) will display a higher curve when measuring a harder eye
    d) is so fast it's not felt

8. If the cornea is extremely thick or scarred:
    a) the intraocular pressure measurements will always be underestimated
    b) the intraocular pressure measurements will always be overestimated
    c) the intraocular pressure measurements can be accepted with reservations
    d) no tonometric measurement will be accurate enough to satisfy clinical needs

Hand-Held*

9. The hand-held tonometer that comes in a case with a set of weights and a test-plate is the:
    a) rebound tonometer
    b) Tono-Pen
    c) Schiøtz tonometer
    d) Perkins tonometer

10. Which of the following might register a *falsely low* reading with the Schiøtz tonometer?
    a) a person with blue eyes
    b) a person with high myopia
    c) a person with nasolacrimal duct obstruction
    d) a person with macular degeneration

11. A disadvantage of the Schiøtz tonometer is that it:
    a) permanently deforms the sclera
    b) is impossible to sterilize
    c) displaces a significant amount of aqueous during use
    d) is complicated to use

12. Which of the following is a type of hand-held applanation tonometer?
    a) Perkins
    b) Goldmann
    c) Icare
    d) Schiøtz tonometer

---

* The criteria says "hand-held applanator." I have elected to cover hand-held tonometers in general.

13.   The tonometer of choice when measuring intraocular pressure in a patient who has had a recent corneal graft is the:
a) Schiøtz
b) Goldmann
c) noncontact
d) Tono-Pen

14.   Which of the following has a sleeve with a central plunger and is not affected by scleral rigidity?
a) Schiøtz
b) Icare
c) Tono-Pen
d) Perkins

15.   Your patient is wearing a soft contact lens for an irregular cornea. Checking intraocular pressure with the Tono-Pen is advantageous in this case because:
a) topical anesthetic is not required
b) no fluorescein is required
c) the mires are more clear
d) the intraocular pressure can be measured through the contact

Applanation Tonometry*

16.   What setting is required on the slit lamp when measuring intraocular pressure using the Goldmann tonometer?
a) cobalt-blue filter
b) diffuser
c) red-free filter
d) no filter

17.   Using the Goldmann tonometer on an edematous or scarred cornea will generally cause measurements that are:
a) higher than the actual intraocular pressure
b) lower than the actual intraocular pressure
c) reliable enough to be accepted
d) unreliable because fluorescein cannot be used

18.   A scarred, irregular cornea is difficult to measure with the Goldmann tonometer because:
a) there is decreased scleral rigidity
b) one cannot instill topical anesthetic because of tissue melt
c) one cannot use fluorescein because it will infiltrate the tissue
d) the mires are irregular, making it difficult to judge the endpoint

19.   One must make an adjustment to the Goldmann or Perkins tonoprism if the patient's corneal astigmatism is:
a) with the rule
b) greater than 1 D
c) greater than 2 D
d) greater than 3 D

* I am interpreting the criteria's "applanation tonometry" as slit lamp–mounted Goldmann tonometry.

Noncontact Tonometry

20. **One disadvantage of an "air-puff" tonometer is that it is:**
    a) more likely to give a false high reading
    b) uncomfortable for the patient
    c) requires the patient to recline
    d) more likely to cause a corneal abrasion

21. **The noncontact "air-puff" tonometer is an example of:**
    a) applanation tonometry
    b) indentation tonometry
    c) fixed force tonometry
    d) pachymetry

Clean and Disinfect Tonometers

22. **Which of the following does *not* use either one-use probes or probe-tip covers?**
    a) Schiøtz tonometer
    b) Tono-Pen
    c) Icare tonometer
    d) None of the above

23. **In the wake of the COVID-19 virus, which of the following tonometry methods might be better avoided?**
    a) Tono-Pen
    b) air-puff tonometry
    c) Icare tonometer
    d) Goldmann

24. **Failure to thoroughly rinse disinfectant from a reusable tonometer tip may result in:**
    a) faded markings
    b) inaccurate readings
    c) corneal burn
    d) transfer of pathogens

25. **Which of the following is *not* recommended when disinfecting a re-usable tonometer tip?**
    a) clean it prior to disinfection
    b) soak in isopropyl alcohol
    c) soak in 1:10 bleach
    d) rinse well after disinfection

Study Notes

Suggested reading in *Principles and Practice in Ophthalmic Assisting: A Comprehensive Textbook:*
    Chapter 9: Basic Eye Exam (*Tonometry* p 127)
    Chapter 13: Tonometry (pp 233-251)

Explanatory Answers

1. d) Although often called "the glaucoma test," tonometry by itself is not adequate to diagnose glaucoma. Applanation, by definition, does touch the ocular surface. The "average" cornea is the ideal for accurate readings; the reading on a thick and/or scarred cornea is much less likely to be accurate.

2. c) Because of the *diurnal curve* (normal fluctuation of intraocular pressure during a 24-hour period), intraocular pressure varies according to when it is checked. It is higher during sleep, and then decreases during the day. The correct answer, of those given, is afternoon.

3. b) The intraocular pressure variation of a normal/average eye in a 24-hour period is 2 to 6 mm Hg. (References do vary a little bit, however.)

4. a) The physical resistance of the sclera to being deformed (as by tonometry) can affect the intraocular pressure readings; this is known as *scleral rigidity*. If the sclera is "tough," then it is has less "give" and a false high intraocular pressure might be read. If the sclera is less rigid, then a false low reading may result.

5. d) Corneal hysteresis is a factor of the cornea's elasticity (ability to return to its original shape after being distorted, as by tonometry) and the viscosity (fluid thickness) of the cornea's base matrix. It is suspected that corneal hysteresis is a more reliable indicator in the progression of glaucoma. Keratoconus is a deformity of the cornea causing high amounts of astigmatism and can be progressive. Corneal hydrops is a corneal disorder seen in keratoconus where aqueous leaks into the stroma. Corneal rigidity is not a term used in this manner.

6. a) Indentation tonometry works on the principle that the soft eye (ie, low or normal pressure) will indent more easily than a hard eye (ie, with elevated intraocular pressure). The Schiøtz is the most common indentation tonometer. And while it might be stretching things just a bit to consider the fingers a tonometer, using the fingers to judge the eye's resistance to pressure does use the principles of indentation. Biotometry is a word I made up.

7. b) A higher pressure makes the eyeball more rigid (harder). If the probe tip of a rebound tonometer (eg, the hand-held Icare) strikes a harder eye, the probe will bounce back more quickly than when it strikes a softer (lower pressure) eye. Think of a ping-pong ball bouncing back after hitting a rock vs a balloon. True, the rebound tonometer is so fast that it's not felt, so no anesthetic drops are needed. But that is not the principle behind the instrument.

8. d) This opinion comes from Brubaker in his excellent article entitled *Tonometry* (see Bibliography). Other sources agree.

9. c) The Schiøtz is a portable, hand-held indentation tonometer that comes with the instrument, a test plate (for verifying calibration), a set of weights (considered unique to that individual instrument), and a conversion chart.

10. b) When using the Schiøtz tonometer, the resistance of the sclera can affect the readings; this is known as *scleral rigidity*. (See also Answer 4.) If the sclera is "tough," then it is has less "give" and a false high introaocular pressure might be read. If the sclera is less rigid, then a false low reading may result. Patients with myopia tend to have a less rigid sclera (as may patients who have had a scleral buckle). Patients with high hyperopia and persons with long-standing glaucoma may have higher scleral rigidity. *Note*: Technically, the term *elasticity* is the wrong word to use when discussing scleral rigidity, because elasticity actually means the ability of a tissue to resume its original shape after physical distortion. Rigidity refers to the tissue's resistance to being physically distorted without mention of its recovery.

11. c) The Schiøtz is a high-displacement tonometer, meaning that when used it displaces an amount of aqueous significant enough to affect the accuracy of the intraocular pressure reading (15 to 20 µl). The applanation tonometer is preferred because it is a low-displacement tonometer, meaning that it does not displace a significant amount of aqueous during the measurement (0.5 µl). Thus, applanation tonometry is considered more accurate.

12. a) The Perkins is basically a hand-held Goldmann tonometer, using the same tonoprism. The Goldmann is mounted on a slit lamp, not hand-held. The Icare is a rebound tonometer, and the Schiøtz is an indentation instrument.

13. d) The Tono-Pen tonometer is the most accurate in this case because corneal elasticity does not figure into the measurement. The Schiøtz was designed for the "normal" eye, and its accuracy must be questioned if the eye is not "average." The Goldmann and NCT are inaccurate if the cornea has edema, scarring, or irregularities (see Answer 17).

14. c) The Tono-Pen is a sort of hybrid indentation/applanation tonometer (ie, it has elements of both types). The sleeve negates any scleral rigidity issues, and the central plunger measures the force required to flatten (not indent) a tiny area of the cornea. The Schiøtz is notoriously affected by scleral rigidity. The Icare and Perkins do not involve a central plunger.

15. d) Because the Tono-Pen measures electrically (rather than optically, as with the noncontact or Goldmann/Perkins) and is not affected by corneal elasticity, the intraocular pressure can be taken through a soft contact lens. Anesthetic is used and fluorescein is not, but these factors make no difference in this case.

16. a) Because fluorescein dye is used during Goldmann tonometry, the cobalt-blue filter is required to excite the dye and make it visible.

17. b) The cornea with edema or scarring generally tends to be more elastic than normal. Thus, it takes less pressure (from the tonoprism) to applanate the required 3.06 mm. Therefore, the measurement would be lower than actuality. On a "regular" cornea, it is possible (although more difficult) to get accurate readings without fluorescein.

18. d) If the cornea is irregular, the mires will also be irregular. This makes it tough to tell when the inner edges are meeting. Besides scarring, corneal distortion can be seen in pterygium and keratoconus.

19. d) The "magic number" is 3 D when it comes to resetting the tonoprism. Failure to do so may result in an erroneous measurement. Axis position is not a factor.

20. a) The air-puff tonometer is more likely to give a false high reading. The puff may startle some patients, but it is not uncomfortable. The test is administered with the patient sitting up. Since no part of the instrument makes physical contact, the chance of a corneal abrasion is pretty much nil.

21. a) The noncontact tonometer is a form of applanation tonometry. This may not be apparent at first, since there is no physical contact between the tonometer and cornea. However, the noncontact tonometer does measure the amount of force (generated by the puff) required to flatten a given area of the cornea (detected by the instrument's optics).

22. d) I was surprised to find, during research, that there are actually one-use tip covers for the Schiøtz. The Tono-Pen, of course, uses latex-free tip covers, and the Icare probes are one-use and disposable. There are also one-use tips for the Goldmann tonometer (which did not appear in this question).

23. b) It has long been known that the puff of air from the noncontact tonometer causes a tiny burst of air-borne particles known as a *microaerosol*. With COVID-19 on the scene, there is concern that the virus could be suspended in the air following intraocular pressure measurement with the noncontact tonometer.[1] The Perkins (not listed) may be of concern as well, as it requires the examiner to come very close to the patient, as does the hand-held noncontact tonometer.

24. c) If the tonometer tip is not well-rinsed after disinfection, residual disinfectant may cause a painful chemical burn to the patient's cornea.

25. b) Isopropyl alcohol is a good disinfectant but tends to damage the tips. Clean the tip first, to remove any surface debris. Then soak in 1:10 bleach or 0.3% hydrogen peroxide for 10 minutes. Rinse in clean drinking water for 10 to 15 minutes, then dry and store.

Reference

1.   The College of Optometrists Website. Coronavirus (COVID-19) pandemic: guidance for optometrists. Updated May 19, 2020. Accessed May 24, 2020. www.college-optometrists.org/the-college/media-hub/news-listing/coronavirus-covid-19-guidance-for-optometrists.html.

Bibliography

Aref AA, Piltz-Seymour J, Albis-Donado OD, Salim S. IOP and tonometry. Eyewiki Website of American Academy of Ophthalmology. Updated June 22, 2022. Accessed March 12, 2023. https://eyewiki.aao.org/IOP_and_Tonometry

Brubaker RF. Tonometry. In: Tasman W, Jaeger EA, eds. Duane's Ophthalmology on CD-ROM 2006 edition. Accessed March 12, 2023. www.oculist.net/downaton502/prof/ebook/duanes/pages/v3/v3c047.html

Gautam S, Patel P. Tonometry. SlideShare Website. Published March 13, 2016. Accessed March 12, 2023. www.slideshare.net/siddarthgautam16/different-types-of-tonometry

Chapter 6

Keratometry*

* Originally the term *keratometer* was a trade name but this has fallen into
common use. The generic name of the instrument is ophthalmometer. At the time
of publication, *keratometry* on the COA® exam lists only *automated* keratometry.
Thus, questions formerly in *Certified Ophthalmic Assistant Exam Review Manual,
Third Edition* have been move to this edition of *Certified Ophthalmic Technician
Exam Review Manual.*

Ledford JK.
*Certified Ophthalmic Technician Exam
Review Manual, Third Edition* (pp 95-102).
© 2023 Taylor & Francis Group.

ABBREVIATIONS USED IN THIS CHAPTER

- K   keratometry reading
- mm   millimeter

---

1. **Unequal corneal curvature where the flattest and steepest curves are 90 degrees apart is known as:**
    a) myopia
    b) presbyopia
    c) astigmatism
    d) hyperopia

2. **Corneal curvature can be recorded as:**
    a) millimeters/diopters
    b) milliliters/diopters
    c) millimeters/cylinder
    d) centimeters/decibels

3. **The curvature of the average human cornea is:**
    a) 38.0 mm
    b) 40.0 mm
    c) 44.0 mm
    d) 48.0 mm

4. **When performing any type of keratometry, it is important to:**
    a) read all peripheral curves
    b) maintain centration
    c) make sure the eye is as dry as possible
    d) instill topical anesthetic

5. **The keratometer:**
    a) helps us to monitor changes in corneal curvature at the apex and in the periphery
    b) is the only way to accurately measure the cornea of a patient with keratoconus
    c) enables the user to view microscopic defects on a rigid lens
    d) can be used to identify corneal warpage and rigid lens edema

6. **A keratometry reading of 42.0 mm in the vertical and 44.0 mm in the horizontal indicates:**
    a) the presence of lenticular astigmatism
    b) the presence of residual astigmatism
    c) the presence of corneal astigmatism
    d) a spherical cornea

7. **Manual keratometry would *not* be the most appropriate method for reliable measurements in which of the following cases?**
    a) fitting contact lenses
    b) monitoring keratoconus
    c) calculating intraocular lens power
    d) evaluating after cataract surgery

8.   **Keratometry would be useful in evaluating all of the following *except*:**
   a) keratoconus
   b) preoperative cataract surgery
   c) contact lens fitting
   d) corneal ulcer

9.   **Label the parts of the keratometer (Figure 6-1):**
   __ barrel
   __ chin rest
   __ chin rest adjustment
   __ eye piece
   __ focus adjustment
   __ forehead adjustment
   __ horizontal mires adjustment
   __ lock
   __ occluder
   __ vertical barrel adjustment
   __ vertical mires adjustment

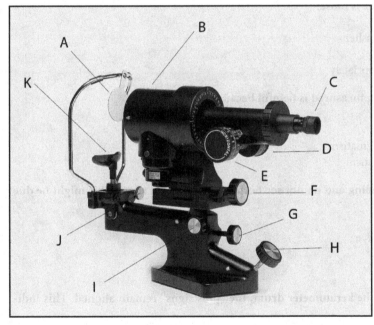

Figure 6-1. Keratometer.

10.   **Number the following steps of using a keratometer in chronological order:**
   __ occlude the eye not being tested
   __ turn the drum so that the horizontal plus signs are aligned exactly tip to tip
   __ turn the dials to superimpose the horizontal plus and vertical minus signs
   __ position the patient
   __ focus the mires and center the crosshairs in the lower right-hand circle
   __ focus the eye piece

11. **You are adjusting the keratometer eye piece by looking at the occluder through the ocular. The mires are distorted. You should:**
   a) calibrate with metal balls
   b) spray cleaner into the instrument
   c) clean the instrument with compressed air
   d) return to the manufacturer for cleaning

12. **When calibrating the keratometer with the metal balls, all of the following are done *except*:**
   a) using chrome balls of known radius
   b) placing holder on the headrest
   c) setting the eye piece for your refractive error
   d) placing the chrome ball in the holder with your fingers

13. **If calibration of the keratometer reveals a discrepancy:**
   a) adjust the drums
   b) tighten the headrest
   c) loosen the top screw
   d) have the manufacturer repair it

14. **If the keratometer's occluder is loose:**
   a) simply remove it
   b) re-bend or replace the washer
   c) tape it up out of the way
   d) adjust the headrest appropriately

15. **Occluding the eye not being measured is helpful because it:**
   a) reduces reflections
   b) aids in fixation
   c) eliminates lenticular astigmatism
   d) reduces irregular astigmatism

16. **You are attempting a K reading and do not see both horizontal plus signs. This might be due to:**
   a) a drooped upper lid
   b) the patient closing their eye
   c) the occluder is in the way
   d) improper focusing

17. **No matter how you rotate the keratometer drum, the "plus signs" remain aligned. This indicates that there is:**
   a) irregular astigmatism
   b) poor tear film
   c) poorly focused eye piece
   d) no astigmatism

18. **Which of the following types of astigmatism is *not* obvious when measuring with the keratometer?**
   a) astigmatism at 180 degrees
   b) irregular astigmatism
   c) lenticular astigmatism
   d) oblique astigmatism

19. The patient's keratometry mires are very oval-shaped. This means that there is:
    a) no astigmatism
    b) high emmetropia
    c) significant astigmatism
    d) inaccurate alignment

20. The patient's keratometry mires are squiggly looking and change when the patient blinks. You should try:
    a) instilling topical anesthetic
    b) instilling artificial tears
    c) re-explaining the procedure
    d) realigning the patient

21. Matching, one answer:

Probable Condition	Keratometer Mires Appear
__ astigmatism	a) small
__ corneal warpage	b) round
__ dry eye	c) elliptical
__ flat cornea	d) very large
__ keratoconus	e) clear, then quickly blur
__ spherical cornea	f) wavy, blurred, discontinuousr
__ steep cornea	g) distorted, small, cannot superimpose

22. In order to determine the base curve for a patient's contact lenses, one must perform:
    a) keratometry
    b) lensometry
    c) refraction
    d) slit lamp exam

23. If the crosshairs of the keratometer are *not* centered during the initial reading for contact lens fitting:
    a) you may select a lens that is too strong
    b) the resulting fit may be too tight
    c) the resulting fit may be too loose
    d) you may select a lens that is too small

24. You have removed the patient's contacts and are evaluating the corneas with the keratometer. You note that the K readings are steeper than at the last visit, several months ago. This could indicate:
    a) corneal neovascularization
    b) mechanical molding of the cornea
    c) corneal edema
    d) corneal ulcer

25. K readings in a contact lens-wearing patient may be used to evaluate all of the following *except*:
    a) progressive corneal steepening
    b) lens fit
    c) lens coverage
    d) corneal warpage

26. **Keratometry readings should be taken over a period of time in a contact lens wearer in order to:**
    a) indicate the need for refractive surgery
    b) be prepared for future cataract surgery
    c) detect over-wear syndrome
    d) monitor for progressive corneal flattening or steepening

27. **Which of the following would be *most* useful in fitting a keratoconus patient with contact lenses?**
    a) corneal pachymetry
    b) corneal topography
    c) keratometry
    d) Placido's disk

Study Notes

Suggested reading in *Principles and Practice in Ophthalmic Assisting: A Comprehensive Textbook:*
      Chapter 5: Ophthalmic Equipment (*Keratometer* p 60)
      Chapter 21: Contact Lenses (*Keratometer* pp 389-391)

Explanatory Answers

1.   c) Astigmatism occurs when the cornea is more curved in one direction and less in the other. (Think of the back of a spoon or the surface of an egg.) These curves are almost always 90 degrees from each other, a situation called *regular astigmatism*, which is easily corrected using cylindrical lenses. If the curves are not 90 degrees from each other, the situation is *irregular astigmatism*, which cannot be entirely corrected with cylinder lenses.

2.   a) Corneal curvature can be designated in both millimeters and diopters. (Did you notice that Answer b was in milli *liters*?)

3.   c) The average human cornea is around 44.0 mm. Anything less than 40.0 mm is considered very flat, and anything over 48.0 mm is very steep.

4.   b) Keratometry measures only 3 mm, so it is vital to make sure that the patient's eye is centered, and that fixation is maintained. The keratometer is not used to read peripheral curves. The eye surface should be hydrated as normal; have the patient blink frequently to distribute the tear film. An artificial tear may be used if the eye is dry, gently blotting the excess. Topical anesthetic is not required.

5.   d) In addition to measuring the curvature of the central cornea, the keratometer can be used to identify warped and edematous corneas (the mires appear wavy, blurred, or discontinuous). A keratometer does not measure the corneal periphery (its main drawback), nor can one directly view a contact lens through it. Keratoconus is better evaluated via corneal topography.

6.   c) The keratometer measures corneal astigmatism. Lenticular astigmatism is caused by irregular curvature of the crystalline lens. Residual astigmatism is a factor in contact lens fitting, where the contact lens does not fully correct the patient's astigmatism. A spherical cornea has no astigmatism, and the vertical and horizontal numbers are the same.

7.   b) This was a tough one; did you catch the phrase "most appropriate"? Because the keratometer evaluates only a tiny section of the cornea (3 mm), it would be more accurate to follow keratoconus using corneal topography. This is not to say that one cannot use manual keratometry in this case, but the question asked for "most appropriate."

8.   d) The keratometer is definitely useful in measuring the curvature of the central cornea for contact lens fitting and intraocular lens calculations. Keratoconus is better followed by corneal topography, although one can use the keratometer. The best Answer is d), corneal ulcer, which would cause irregular keratometry mires and is best evaluated at the slit lamp.

9.   **Labeling:**
   <u>B</u> barrel
   <u>K</u> chin rest
   <u>G</u> chin rest adjustment
   <u>C</u> eye piece
   <u>F</u> focus adjustment
   <u>J</u> forehead adjustment
   <u>E</u> horizontal mires adjustment
   <u>I</u> lock
   <u>A</u> occluder
   <u>H</u> vertical barrel adjustment
   <u>D</u> vertical mires adjustment

10.   **Order:**
   <u>3</u> occlude the eye not being tested
   <u>5</u> turn the drum so that the horizontal plus signs are aligned exactly tip to tip
   <u>6</u> turn the dials to superimpose the horizontal plus and vertical minus signs
   <u>2</u> position the patient
   <u>4</u> focus the mires and center the crosshairs in the lower right-hand circle
   <u>1</u> focus the eye piece
   Note: Steps 5 and 6 may be reversed, but most examiners prefer to set the axis before completing alignment. In addition, some keratometers have plus sign mires at both horizontal AND vertical, rather than plus at horizontal and minus at vertical.

11.   d) Distorted mires are caused by problems with the internal filters and lenses. Only the manufacturer can handle that.

12.   d) Do not handle the chrome balls with your fingers. Use a tissue or magnet. Oils from the fingers can cause the chrome to corrode, changing the readings.

13.   d) If you test the keratometer and the readings are not true, the manufacturer will have to repair it.

14.   b) A loose occluder can be re-bent, or you can replace the washer. It is important to use the occluder, however, because it helps keeps the eye centered for the reading.

15.   b) The occluder forces the patient to fixate with the eye being measured. This helps hold that eye steady for an accurate reading.

16.   c) The plus sign is projected on the side, and the main thing that might obstruct the mires from the side is the occluder on the keratometer. A common vertical obstruction (which would obstruct the minus signs) is the patient's upper lid.

17.   d) If the corneal surface is spherical (ie, no astigmatism), the "plus signs" will stay aligned no matter where the barrel is positioned, because the curve is the same in every meridian.

18.   c) Situations a) and d) are evident by the axis readings on the keratometer. Irregular astigmatism can be detected by the fact that the sections of the mires do not focus together, and there seems to be several "axes," although an accurate measurement is not possible. Lenticular astigmatism is caused by the crystalline lens, which is not detected with the keratometer, but rather by noting a difference in the amount of astigmatism found on keratometry and that found on refraction.

19.   c) Oval mires indicate the presence of significant astigmatism. Actually, this makes the reading easier, as even a tiny turn of barrel or dial makes an obvious difference. An eye with no astigmatism would have very round mires. Emmetropia is lack of refractive error, so it cannot be classified as high, low, or in between. Inaccurate alignment is evident when the crosshair is not centered in the lower right circle.

20. b) "Squiggly" mires that change when the patient blinks indicate a problem with the tear film. Instill some artificial tears, have the patient blink a lot, and blot gently with a tissue. Then, try the readings again. There is no need to use an anesthetic.

21. **Matching:**

astigmatism	c) elliptical
corneal warpage	f) wavy, blurred, discontinuous
dry eye	e) clear, then quickly blur
flat cornea	d) very large
keratoconus	g) distorted, small, cannot superimpose
spherical cornea	b) round
steep cornea	a) small

22. a) The keratometer measures the curvature of the cornea. The base curve of the contact lens is then selected to complement this measurement.

23. c) If the crosshairs are not centered, you are not reading the corneal apex. Because the corneal periphery is flatter, the resulting fit will be too loose when placed on the steeper apex.

24. c) Corneal edema causes steepening of the corneal curvature. Corneal molding, or warpage, generally causes flattening. Neovascularization has no direct effect on K readings. A corneal ulcer might cause distortion of the mires.

25. c) The keratometer can be used to evaluate corneal steepening by taking a series of readings over time. Corneal warpage is evident by distorted mires. By using the keratometer to look at contacts on the patient, the fit can be evaluated by the appearance of the mires and whether they clear/blur before or after a blink. (Of course, a slit-lamp exam is still required to complete the evaluation.) Lens coverage of the cornea is evaluated at the slit lamp, not with the keratometer.

26. d) Any progressive change in the K readings of a contact lens wearer may need to be dealt with by changing lens material or design.

27. b) Corneal topography shows the curvature of the entire cornea. The keratometer only measures the corneal apex, which is only moderately useful. Placido's disk gives a picture of the curves, but no measurements. Pachymetry measures corneal thickness.

Chapter 7

Ocular Motility Testing

Ledford JK.
Certified Ophthalmic Technician Exam
Review Manual, Third Edition (pp 103-134).
© 2023 Taylor & Francis Group.

ABBREVIATIONS USED IN THIS CHAPTER

- BD   base down
- BI   base in
- BO   base out
- BU   base up
- C   central
- CN   cranial nerve
- E   eso
- ET   exotropia
- HT   hypertropia
- IO   inferior oblique
- IR   inferior rectus
- L   left
- LR   lateral rectus
- M   maintained
- MR   medial rectus
- NPA   near point of accommodation
- NPC   near point of convergence
- OD   right eye
- OS   left eye
- P&C   prism and cover
- R   right
- S   steady
- SO   superior oblique
- SR   superior rectus
- T   tropia
- UC   uncentral
- UM   unmaintained
- US   unsteady
- W4D   Worth 4-dot
- X   exo
- XT   exotropia

Part I*

Versions and Ductions

1. **Ductions refer to:**
    a) muscles that work against each other during eye movements
    b) movements of one eye
    c) movements of both eyes in the same direction
    d) movements of both eyes in the opposite direction

2. **Testing ductions is useful in differentiating cases of:**
    a) restrictive strabismus
    b) accommodative strabismus
    c) congenital esotropia
    d) pseudostrabismus

3. **All of the following are involved in ductions *except*:**
    a) agonist
    b) antagonist
    c) synergist
    d) yoke

4. **In what direction do you have the patient look if testing the function of the right inferior oblique muscle?**
    a) up and medial
    b) up and lateral
    c) down and lateral
    d) straight up

5. **Versional movements are those that:**
    a) result in fusion
    b) move one eye
    c) move both eyes in the same direction
    d) move both eyes in a different direction

6. **Basic version testing evaluates:**
    a) how well a pair of yoke muscles work together
    b) over and under action of antagonists
    c) how well synergists and agonists work together
    d) under and over action of an agonist

7. **Matching, one answer:**

    dextroversion   looking right
    infra-/deorsumversion   looking left
    laevoversion   looking up
    supro-/sursumversion   looking down

* Sections have been inserted into this lengthy chapter for ease of study, to allow for a logical "break" point.

8. **If the eyes have normal version movements, all of the following will exist *except*:**
    a) each eye will move with equal speed
    b) each eye will move smoothly
    c) the eyes will diverge equally
    d) each eye will be at the same position with respect to the other

9. **Which of the following is *not* considered a cardinal position of gaze?**
    a) down and left, or up and left
    b) up and right, or down and right
    c) straight ahead, or straight up or down
    d) directly left, or directly right

10. **When testing a patient's versions, it is important to:**
    a) test in dim lighting
    b) keep the patient's head still
    c) use an opaque occluder to break fusion
    d) keep the patient's eyes in primary position

11. **You are testing versions, and the patient cannot move the left eye laterally. Which nerve is involved?**
    a) left CN II
    b) left CN III
    c) left CN IV
    d) left CN VI

12. **Vergence testing examines the ability of the eyes:**
    a) to move in opposite directions in order to maintain stereopsis as an object moves closer or farther away
    b) to move in opposite directions to maintain fixation as an object moves closer or farther away
    c) to move together in the same direction to maintain fixation as an object moves closer or farther away
    d) to judge spatial relationships as an object moves closer or farther away

13. **Your patient has an esodeviation that is worse at near than at a distance. This is classified as:**
    a) convergence insufficiency
    b) convergence excess
    c) divergence excess
    d) divergence insufficiency

Functions

14. **The main "goal" in extraocular muscle function is:**
    a) diplopia
    b) depth perception
    c) 20/20 vision
    d) binocular single vision

15. The ability to hold the eye(s) steady so that an image falls on the macula is known as:
a) objectivity
b) fixation
c) vergence
d) maintenance

16. How many extraocular muscles are innervated by CN III?
a) 1
b) 2
c) 4
d) 6

17. Which of the following extraocular muscles is innervated by CN VI?
a) LR
b) MR
c) SO
d) IR

18. Which of the following extraocular muscles is innervated by the trochlear nerve?
a) IO
b) IR
c) SR
d) SO

19. The only extraocular muscles that do not have either a secondary or tertiary action are:
a) IO and SO
b) LR and MR
c) IR and SR
d) IR and IO

20. Which of the following extraocular muscles have the primary action of torsion?
a) SO and IO
b) LR and MR
c) IR and SR
d) SO and SR

21. Which of the following extraocular muscles have the secondary action of torsion?
a) LR and MR
b) SO and IO
c) SR and IR
d) SO and SR

22. In abduction of the right eye, the RLR has what function?
a) yoke
b) agonist
c) synergist
d) antagonist

23. In abduction of the right eye, the RMR has what function?
a) agonist
b) antagonist
c) yoke
d) synergist

24. **In right gaze, which muscle is yoked to the RLR?**
    a) LMR
    b) RMR
    c) LLR
    d) LIO

25. **The law that states that an equal amount of innervation goes to the yoke muscles of each eye is:**
    a) Herring's law
    b) Sarah's law
    c) Panum's law
    d) Snell's law

26. **You are evaluating ductions of the right eye and direct the patient to look to the left. To do this, the MR must contract and the LR must relax. The law that applies to this occurrence is:**
    a) Herring's law
    b) Sherrington's law
    c) Prentice's law
    d) Snell's law

27. **You are conducting a binocular range of motion test and direct the patient to look up and right. Which law says that the RSR and LIO are receiving the same amount of stimulation?**
    a) Herring's law
    b) Sherrington's law
    c) Panum's law
    d) Snell's law

Anomalies

28. **You are shopping and run into an old friend and her 2-year-old. Looking at the child you can see that his left eye is obviously turning out while the right eye is straight. This anomaly is a:**
    a) tropia
    b) phoria
    c) pseudostrabismus
    d) Bell's palsy

29. **The difference between a phoria and an intermittent tropia is:**
    a) the patient experiences diplopia with the phoria but not with the intermittent tropia
    b) the phoria rarely is controlled and the intermittent tropia always is controlled
    c) the phoria usually is controlled and the intermittent tropia always is uncontrolled
    d) the phoria usually is controlled and the intermittent tropia sometimes is controlled

30. **An adult patient with a tropia has either:**
    a) amblyopia or anisometropia
    b) prism or slab-off lenses
    c) diplopia or suppression
    d) fusion or stereopsis

31. **Vertical deviations are conventionally described by indicating:**
    a) the higher eye
    b) the lower eye
    c) the preferred eye
    d) the eye with best vision

32. **The most common patient complaint in a new nerve palsy is:**
    a) decreased vision
    b) diplopia
    c) an ache in the affected muscle(s)
    d) an inability to read at near

33. **Nerve palsies cause the affected muscle(s) to become:**
    a) overactive
    b) underactive
    c) spasmodic
    d) responsive

34. **Brown syndrome affects which extraocular muscle?**
    a) inferior oblique
    b) inferior rectus
    c) superior oblique
    d) superior rectus

35. **The most common finding of the affected eye in Brown syndrome is:**
    a) limitation in looking up and in
    b) limitation looking down and out
    c) limitation in left gaze
    d) limitation in right gaze

36. **Most commonly, Duane syndrome affects which extraocular muscle?**
    a) MR
    b) LR
    c) SR
    d) SO

37. **Duane syndrome is caused by:**
    a) uncorrected amblyopia
    b) abnormal insertion of an extraocular muscle
    c) abnormal development of muscle tissue
    d) mis-wiring of cranial nerves

38. **In the most common form of Duane syndrome, in primary position the patient will display:**
    a) hypertropia
    b) exophoria
    c) esotropia
    d) hypotropia

39. **In thyroid eye disease the most common type of deviation is in downgaze. The affected extraocular muscle is the:**
    a) IR
    b) SR
    c) SO
    d) IO

40.   **The main cause of extraocular muscle deviation in thyroid eye disease is:**
      a) CN nerve damage
      b) thickening and fibrosis of the extraocular muscle(s)
      c) expansion of orbital fat
      d) birth trauma

Near Point of Convergence

41.   **The NPC is reached when a test object:**
      a) gets so close that one eye deviates inward
      b) gets so close that one eye deviates outward
      c) gets so close that it blurs
      d) is so far away that one eye deviates inward

42.   **Judging the NPC by having the patient report diplopia may not always be accurate because the patient might be:**
      a) amblyopic
      b) accommodating
      c) suppressing
      d) monocular

43.   **Which of the following is required in order to perform the NPC test?**
      a) at least 20/40 vision
      b) depth perception
      c) normal color vision
      d) normal fusion

44.   **Which of the following regarding NPC is *not* true?**
      a) It tends to become more remote with age.
      b) It is more remote with children vs adults.
      c) It is more remote in convergence insufficiency.
      d) It can be tested objectively and subjectively.

Near Point of Accommodation

45.   **The NPA measures the:**
      a) amount of bifocal add the patient requires
      b) distance at which fusion breaks
      c) distance at which an object doubles
      d) diopters available for accommodation

46.   **To test the NPA:**
      a) small print is brought closer until it blurs
      b) small print is brought closer until it doubles
      c) plus lenses are added until the print clears
      d) a pen light is brought closer until its image blurs

47. **The most accurate way to measure NPA is to:**
     a) use distant vision correction only in patients with hyperopia
     b) have the patient wear full distance correction
     c) have the patient wear full near correction
     d) correct every patient with a +2.50 lens

48. **NPA should be measured:**
     a) with both eyes together
     b) separately for each eye
     c) only if the patient has fusion
     d) only if the patient has depth perception

Measure and Record Fusional Amplitudes*

49. **A patient's ability to overcome induced prism in their glasses is a product of their:**
     a) strabismus
     b) stereopsis
     c) fusional amplitudes
     d) convergence insufficiency

50. **Which of the following fusional amplitudes are strongest in the normal patient?**
     a) convergence at distance
     b) convergence at near
     c) divergence at distance
     d) divergence at near

51. **When testing fusional amplitudes, the prism that *first* causes diplopia is recorded as the:**
     a) break point
     b) recovery point
     c) doubling point
     d) maximum prism

Part II

Cover Tests

52. **The purpose of covering one eye with an occluder for strabismus testing is to:**
     a) determine if the patient is suppressing
     b) perform monocular testing
     c) disrupt fusion
     d) determine if the patient is malingering

* Fusional convergence amplitude is listed as a COMT® level item in the Ocular Motility Testing area. However, it appears at the COT® level under Supplemental Testing as "Measure and record fusional amplitudes." I have chosen to include it here.

53.   Cover testing can be performed even on an infant because:
a) it is nonthreatening
b) it is painless
c) it is objective
d) it is brief

54.   Cover testing can be useful in all of the following patients *except*:
a) the patient with bilateral aphakia
b) the patient with bilateral pseudophakia
c) the patient with suppression
d) the monocular patient

55.   The cover/uncover test is used to determine the presence of:
a) phoria vs a tropia
b) amblyopia
c) suppression
d) stereopsis

56.   The cover/uncover test can also reveal the presence of:
a) E vs X
b) vergence insufficiency
c) depth perception
d) visual acuity

57.   You have covered the patient's right eye. When you uncover it, the right eye moves inward. Now you cover the left eye. When you uncover it, the left eye moves inward. You can deduce that the patient has an:
a) exophoria
b) exotropia
c) exodeviation
d) esodeviation

58.   The patient's vision is 20/20 OD and OS. You cover the patient's right eye and note that when you do so, the left eye moves outward. When you uncover the right eye, neither eye moves. When you cover the left eye, the right eye moves outward. When you uncover the left eye, neither eye moves. This indicates:
a) alternating exotropia
b) esophoria
c) intermittent esotropia
d) alternating esotropia

59.   During the cover/uncover test, if a patient has a phoria, the response of the eye that is *not* covered is to:
a) take up fixation
b) move in the same direction as the covered eye
c) remain straight
d) deviate in or out

60.   The alternate (cross) cover test does *not* reveal:
a) exodeviations
b) esodeviations
c) hyper deviations
d) a phoria vs a tropia

61.   **When performing the alternate (cross) cover test, it is important to:**
a) momentarily remove the cover from one eye before covering the other
b) move the cover rapidly from one eye to the other
c) allow the patient to look at the target with both eyes before covering again
d) move the cover from one eye to the next every half-second

62.   **If there is no movement of either eye during any part of the alternate (cross) cover test, one has determined that:**
a) the patient is amblyopic in one eye
b) the eyes are orthophoric
c) the patient has stereo vision
d) the patient has equal vision in either eye

63.   **You have performed the alternate (cross) cover test and notice that each eye moves inward when uncovered. What is your next step?**
a) record exodeviation in the chart
b) record exotropia in the chart
c) record esodeviation in the chart
d) perform a cover/uncover test

Strabismus With Prisms

64.   **The alternate (cross) cover test can be used to measure the size of a deviation *if*:**
a) the patient can fuse
b) the corneal reflex can be seen
c) it is combined with prisms
d) polarized glasses are used

65.   **Which of the following will give the *most* accurate measurement of strabismus in a patient with good fixation?**
a) Hirschberg test
b) prism and cross-cover
c) Krimsky measurement
d) swinging flashlight test

66.   **All of the following are true regarding the prism and cover test *except*:**
a) the prism may be split between the 2 eyes
b) the prism must be placed in front of the deviated eye
c) prisms may be stacked base-to-base and added together
d) alternate (cross) covering is used, not cover/uncover

67.   **To properly place the prism to measure deviations:**
a) the prism apex should point in the same direction as the deviation
b) the prism apex should point in the opposite direction as the deviation
c) always split the amount of prism between the 2 eyes
d) always place the prism over the deviating eye

68. **On cross-cover testing, the left eye moves up when the cover is shifted to the right eye. In order to measure this deviation, how would you orient the prism?**
    a) base up over the right eye
    b) base down over the left eye
    c) base up over the left eye
    d) base in over the right eye

69. **The endpoint of the prism and cover test is reached when:**
    a) the amount of movement is equal in both eyes
    b) no movement is seen on alternate covering
    c) the patient reports that the target is single
    d) the patient reports that the target is double

70. **When measuring a patient with an RHT, the correcting prism could be placed:**
    a) BO, OD
    b) BU, OD
    c) BD, OS
    d) BD, OD

71. **Which of the following is *true* when using P&C to measure a deviation?**
    a) Measuring can be done using the phoropter.
    b) Fresnel prisms can be used.
    c) Best correction should be used.
    d) Vertical deviations should be measured first.

72. **When performing P&C measurements at distance, the target should be:**
    a) easily seen
    b) the smallest the patient can recognize
    c) the 20/40 optotype
    d) a Snellen letter optotype

73. **When performing initial P&C, the patient should be positioned:**
    a) 6 ft from the target
    b) with their head in primary position
    c) allowing them to turn or tilt the head naturally
    d) allowing them to assume a chin-up position

74. **An advantage of using the prism bar is:**
    a) it is more accurate
    b) it is easier for the patient to tolerate
    c) prisms are additive
    d) it is easier to change

75. **Each of the following regarding P&C testing is true *except*:**
    a) position bar in front of one eye, with apex pointing in direction of the deviation
    b) cover one eye then the other, allowing fixation in between
    c) if movement in the original direction is seen, shift the bar to the next strongest prism
    d) a prism correction that is too strong will cause the direction of the deviation to reverse

76. **The deviation of a patient with a tropia is neutralized with a 10-diopter prism, base out, in front of the right eye and a 5-diopter prism, base out, in front of the left eye. This patient has a:**
    a) 5-diopter ET
    b) 5-diopter XT
    c) 15-diopter XT
    d) 15-diopter ET

Worth 4-Dot Test*

77. **The W4D test is used to determine:**
    a) suppression and fusion
    b) fusional amplitudes
    c) tropia vs phoria
    d) E- vs X- deviation

78. **In order for a patient to be able to perform the W4D test, they must:**
    a) have normal color vision
    b) be able to interpret their responses
    c) be able to count objects
    d) be able to read

79. **The test screen or flashlight used in the W4D test has:**
    a) 4 white lights
    b) 2 green, 1 red, and 1 white light
    c) 1 green, 1 red, and 2 white lights
    d) 1 green, 2 red, and 1 white light

80. **The W4D flashlight should normally be held with:**
    a) the white light on bottom
    b) the red light on bottom
    c) the green light on bottom
    d) a red light to left and right

81. **With the red lens over the right eye, a patient with fusion will report seeing:**
    a) 3 lights
    b) 4 lights
    c) 5 lights
    d) 6 lights

82. **A patient with fusion might report all of the following on W4D testing *except*:**
    a) the bottom light switches back and forth from red to green
    b) only the top light is red, the rest are green
    c) only the bottom light is red, the rest are green
    d) the top and bottom lights are red, and the left and right lights are green

* For all questions on W4D, the red lens is over the right eye.

83. **With the red lens over the right eye during W4D testing, the patient reports seeing only 2 red lights. This represents:**
    a) crossed diplopia
    b) uncrossed diplopia
    c) a vertical deviation
    d) suppression OS

Maddox Rod*

84. **The Maddox rod is composed of:**
    a) glasses with green lenses
    b) polarized lenses
    c) cylinders made of red plastic
    d) rotary prisms

85. **The Maddox rod is used to measure:**
    a) tropias
    b) phorias
    c) tropias and phorias
    d) horizontal deviations only

86. **The Maddox rod test will be accurate in which of the following situations?**
    a) the malingering patient
    b) the patient with suppression
    c) the binocular patient
    d) the monocular patient

87. **The Maddox rod test can be done:**
    a) only with the eyes in primary gaze
    b) in all fields of gaze
    c) only at a distance, to avoid accommodation
    d) as an objective measurement

88. **If the Maddox rod is held so that the ridges run up and down, the light coming through it will appear as a:**
    a) red dot
    b) white dot
    c) red horizontal line
    d) red vertical line

89. **You are measuring a patient with a vertical deviation. The Maddox rod should be placed so that the light forms a:**
    a) horizontal line
    b) vertical line
    c) diagonal line
    d) dot

*At printing, Maddox rod is listed as a COMT® item, but also under Supplemental Testing at the COT® level. For COT®, I have elected to include it here under extraocular muscle evaluation.

90. **When measuring a patient with the Maddox rod:**
    a) the correcting prism goes over the uncovered eye
    b) the fixing eye is underneath the Maddox rod
    c) be sure to use an opaque occluder
    d) only a rotary prism can be used

91. **The endpoint of the Maddox rod test occurs when:**
    a) the red dot is superimposed on the light source
    b) the red line goes through the light
    c) the red line is just above or to the right of the light
    d) the red line disappears

Krimsky

92. **Which of the following regarding the Hirschberg test is *false*?**
    a) It is an objective test.
    b) Interpreting results is somewhat subjective.
    c) It grossly evaluates strabismus.
    d) It requires using prisms.

93. **The Krimsky measurement combines the Hirschberg method with:**
    a) a prism and cover test
    b) correcting prisms
    c) a prescription for reading
    d) a Maddox rod

94. **The idea behind the Krimsky measurement is to move the deviated corneal reflex so that:**
    a) there is no movement when you alternate the cover
    b) both eyes are fixating at the same time
    c) the Hirschberg estimate matches the Krimsky measurement
    d) it falls on the same relative spot as the reflex on the fixating eye

Stereoacuity

95. **Stereopsis is recorded in:**
    a) Snellen fractions
    b) degrees of arc
    c) seconds of arc
    d) degrees of field

96. **Bifoveal stereopsis is defined as:**
    a) 20/20
    b) better than 67 seconds of arc
    c) better than 450 degrees of arc
    d) better than 1000 degrees of arc

97. **Which of the following indicates the better stereo vision?**
    a) 50 degrees of arc
    b) 25 degrees of arc
    c) 50 seconds of arc
    d) 25 seconds of arc

98. **Stereopsis can be measured in which of the following patients?**
    a) 60-diopter ET
    b) 45-diopter XT
    c) 8-diopter intermittent XT
    d) monocular

99. **Stereopsis differs from depth perception in that:**
    a) depth perception is monocular or binocular
    b) stereo vision involves judging spatial relationships
    c) depth perception involves seeing in 3 dimensions
    d) stereopsis is a learned experience

100. **While it does not give a measurement, a simple stereo test that can be done at bedside is the:**
    a) Hirschberg test
    b) confrontation stereo test
    c) pencil point to pencil point test
    d) Amsler grid stereo test

101. **The Titmus test, Wirt test, random dot E, Randot test, and AO distance vectograph slide all utilize:**
    a) polarized glasses
    b) glasses with one red and one green lens
    c) dissociating prisms
    d) a red filter

102. **You ask a cooperative 3-year-old to touch the wings of the Titmus fly. They recoil and refuse. You can assume that most likely they:**
    a) are tired and cranky
    b) do not fuse
    c) do fuse
    d) have an intermittent deviation

103. **You are testing an intelligent 12-year-old with the Titmus dots and suspect that they are either a good guesser or a cheater. You should:**
    a) turn the test 90 degrees
    b) turn the test 180 degrees
    c) switch the glasses around
    d) record the patient's responses regardless

Part III

Nystagmus

104. **The root cause of nystagmus is thought to be:**
    a) fixation confusion due to eccentric fixation
    b) extraocular muscle imbalances due to neurological defect(s)
    c) "searching" movements by eyes with poor vision
    d) a neurological feedback problem that results in poor control of the fixation mechanism

105. **Adult-onset nystagmus will frequently cause the patient to complain of:**
    a) diplopia
    b) oscillopsia
    c) photophobia
    d) extraocular muscle pain

106. **Which of the following is *not* true regarding congenital nystagmus?**
    a) It is often associated with maternal infections.
    b) The child may adopt a specific head position.
    c) The child will frequently outgrow the condition.
    d) It is often associated with visual impairment and/or lesions in the optic system.

107. **A head position in which nystagmus is quietest (least) is known as the:**
    a) null point
    b) near point
    c) angle of deviation
    d) cyclic amplitude

108. **Nystagmus movements where the movements are equal in speed, equal in amplitude, and have equal duration in each direction are referred to as:**
    a) jerk
    b) spasmus nutans
    c) pendular
    d) congenital

109. **The patient with nystagmus should be refracted using:**
    a) no special adaptations
    b) the astigmatic dial
    c) +6.00 lens instead of an occluder
    d) −3.00 lens instead of an occluder

110. **To further study a patient's nystagmus, the practitioner may request a(n):**
    a) electro-oculogram
    b) B-scan ultrasound
    c) potential acuity test
    d) optical coherence tomography

Amblyopia Therapy

111. **Amblyopia may be manifested as:**
    a) an eye that learns to see with a retinal point other than the fovea
    b) poor vision in one eye that can be improved with lenses
    c) poor vision in both eyes that can be improved with lenses
    d) poor vision in a healthy eye that cannot be improved with lenses

112. **Clinically, amblyopia is diagnosed when the:**
    a) best corrected vision of each eye differs by 2 or more acuity lines
    b) best corrected vision of each eye differs by 4 or more acuity lines
    c) uncorrected vision of each eye differs by 4 or more acuity lines
    d) patient cannot appreciate binocular/stereoscopic vision

113. **The evaluation of fixation and vision in an infant or very young child is appraised by each of the following *except*:**
    a) central
    b) maintained
    c) steady
    d) strabismic

114. **Which of the following is *most* likely to develop amblyopia in the right eye?**
    a) a 3-year-old with a refractive error of –3.00 sphere OD and +0.50 sphere OS
    b) a 3-year-old with a refractive error of +4.00 sphere OD and +1.25 sphere OS
    c) a 12-year-old with convergence insufficiency type exodeviation
    d) a 1-year-old with 1 mm of ptosis on the right

115. **A child with uncorrected/undetected high myopia in both eyes may develop:**
    a) reverse amblyopia
    b) reflex amblyopia
    c) refractive amblyopia
    d) anisometropic amblyopia

116. **A child with one myopic eye and one hyperopic eye:**
    a) is guaranteed to develop anisometropic amblyopia
    b) does not have normal fusion while uncorrected
    c) generally develops nonalternating strabismus
    d) does not require refractive correction

117. **You are evaluating an 18-month-old child. Of the following scenarios, which might be evaluated as CSM in each eye alone and UCSM when both eyes are viewed simultaneously?**
    a) esotropia with amblyopia in one eye
    b) pseudostrabismus
    c) esophoria
    d) alternating exotropia

118. **In a child with congenital ptosis that obscures the pupil, even after the lid is repaired it is likely that the child will need to be treated for:**
    a) alternating amblyopia
    b) nocturnal amblyopia
    c) crossed amblyopia
    d) amblyopia ex anopsia

119. **Which of the following is both a cause of amblyopia as well as a sign that amblyopia exists in a particular child patient?**
    a) freely alternating strabismus
    b) nonalternating strabismus
    c) intermittent strabismus
    d) phoria

120. **In the child with strabismic amblyopia, optimizing the vision in the amblyopic eye is generally attempted:**
    a) prior to any alignment surgery
    b) following any alignment surgery
    c) instead of alignment surgery
    d) by using glasses only

121. **When using a conventional stick-on patch to treat amblyopia, all of the following are true *except*:**
    a) it may be applied to either the glasses or directly to the face with equal results
    b) wearing the patch during sleep does not count as treatment time
    c) the younger the child, the more frequent the follow-up
    d) there are psychological factors to consider

122. **In patching therapy, once the vision in the eyes is equal or stable:**
    a) patching can be discontinued
    b) the patch is switched to the other eye
    c) patching is gradually decreased
    d) patching continues in the same manner

123. **A child being patched to treat amblyopia has been faithfully wearing the patch as directed but has missed the last 2 appointments. This creates concern that:**
    a) treatment will take longer than necessary
    b) reverse amblyopia will occur
    c) glasses may become necessary
    d) pharmacologic penalization may become necessary

124. **Which type of topical medication is used in amblyopia treatment?**
    a) miotic
    b) spasmotic
    c) anesthetic
    d) cycloplegic

125. **The most common agent used in pharmacologic penalization for amblyopia treatment is:**
    a) atropine
    b) phenylephrine
    c) tropicamide
    d) pilocarpine

126. **Examples of optical penalization include use of:**
    a) full refractive correction for both eyes
    b) full prism correction for both eyes
    c) blurring the lens of the stronger eye
    d) tarsorrhaphy on the stronger eye

127. A 4-year-old patient has been successfully treated for amblyopia and now has equal vision in both eyes. The parents may be told that:
    a) their problems and worries are over
    b) it is not guaranteed that optimal vision will be maintained
    c) there will be a definite need for future treatment
    d) the child may require further treatment around puberty

128. If amblyopia in a child does not respond to treatment, the amblyopia is referred to as:
    a) suppressive
    b) organic
    c) functional
    d) dense

129. Which group of children would require the *most frequent* follow-up during amblyopia treatment?
    a) ages 5 to 9 years patching < 6 hours a day
    b) ages 5 to 9 years using penalization
    c) ages 0 to 2 years patching > 6 hours a day
    d) ages 3 to 5 years patching < 6 hours a day

130. Once maximum vision is obtained and patching/penalization discontinued, which group of children would require the most frequent maintenance follow-up?
    a) ages 0 to 4 years
    b) ages 5 to 9 years
    c) those treated by patching
    d) those treated with penalization

131. You are doing an exam on a 14-year-old patient who has never been seen in your practice before. The physician has diagnosed amblyopia OD. Which of the following is *true*?
    a) Amblyopia treatment won't work because the patient is beyond visual maturity.
    b) With proper treatment, the patient will be able to achieve 20/20 in the amblyopic eye.
    c) If the patient was treated for amblyopia at age 4, there is a great chance that repeating therapy will work again.
    d) If therapy improves vision in the amblyopic eye, the recurrence rate is lower than that of a 6-year-old.

Convergence Training

132. Patient complaints associated with convergence insufficiency include:
    a) headaches after prolonged periods of looking into the distance
    b) letters on street signs jumping/swimming
    c) closing one eye to watch a movie at the theater
    d) falling asleep after several minutes of reading

133. Initial therapy of convergence insufficiency may consist of:
    a) bilateral LR resections
    b) a reading add
    c) vision exercises
    d) base in prisms

134. **A patient with which of the following might be taught how to do "pencil push-up" eye exercises?**
    a) amblyopia
    b) convergence insufficiency
    c) divergence insufficiency
    d) exotropia

135. **The purpose of pencil push-ups is to:**
    a) strengthen the NPC
    b) increase the near point of divergence
    c) relax accommodation
    d) treat pseudostrabismus

136. **For pencil push-up exercises:**
    a) any object can be used
    b) only a pencil or pen can be used
    c) any small accommodative target can be used
    d) only a red pencil can be used

137. **For pencil push-ups, the patient is instructed to begin with the target:**
    a) at arm's length
    b) 1 meter away
    c) 6 inches from eyes
    d) to the extreme right

138. **For pencil push-ups, the patient is instructed to move the target:**
    a) rapidly from right to left
    b) slowly away
    c) rapidly closer
    d) slowly closer

139. **For pencil push-ups, the patient is instructed to:**
    a) stop the exercise when the target doubles
    b) try to fuse when the target doubles
    c) continue to move the target closer after it doubles
    d) restart the exercise when the target doubles

140. **In pencil push-ups, what is actually happening when the target doubles is that:**
    a) accommodation has reached its limit
    b) exophoria is at its maximum
    c) fusion has broken
    d) any remaining V pattern is manifest

141. **Stereogram cards are used to treat:**
    a) abnormal retinal correspondence
    b) convergence insufficiency
    c) monocular vision
    d) parallax diplopia

Study Notes

Suggested reading in *Principles and Practice in Ophthalmic Assisting: A Comprehensive Textbook:*
    Chapter 9: Basic Eye Exam (*Stereopsis Assessment* p 128)
    Chapter 10: Ocular Motility, Strabismus, and Amblyopia (pp 137-177)
    Correction Notes: In Table 10-1 the primary actions of the medial rectus and lateral rectus are reversed. The correct notation is medial rectus- adduction, lateral rectus- abduction.
    On page 150, right column, first full paragraph, second sentence should read* "A blowout fracture is a break in one or more of the bones in the orbit, usually the <u>floor or medial wall</u> because these bones are very thin."

Explanatory Answers

Part I

1.   b) Ductions refer to movements of one eye. Muscles that work against each other in the same eye are antagonists. Movements of both eyes in the same direction are versions. Movements of both eyes in opposite directions are vergences.
2.   a) Testing ductions is useful when one eye is at fault for a deviation, as in restrictive strabismus. In Answers b) through d) it would be more helpful to test versions.
3.   d) Yoked muscles are muscles in both eyes that act to move the eyes in the same direction (ie, versions rather than ductions). For example, the RMR is yoked to the LLR for left gaze. The other answers are in the same eye (see Answer 1). The agonist is the muscle in one eye that is the primary mover for a given gaze.
4.   a) To test the function of the RIO, direct the patient to look up and medially (ie, toward the nose). See Figure 7-1.

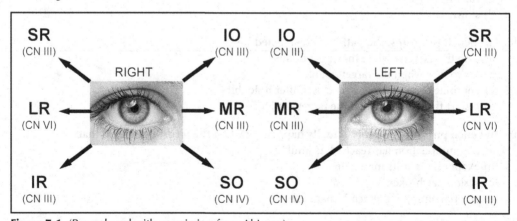

Figure 7-1. (Reproduced with permission from Al Lens.)

5.   c) Versions move both eyes in the same direction. Fusion does not necessarily occur; for example, the muscles in a blind eye are still innervated and linked to those of the other (seeing) eye.
6.   a) Versions evaluate the function of yoked muscles. The other items are monocular.

* Correction underlined.

7. **Matching**:

dextroversion	looking right
infra-/deorsumversion	looking down
laevoversion	looking left
supro-/sursumversion	looking up

8. c) Divergence is when the eyes move in opposite directions, away from each other. In versions, the eyes are moving together in the same direction.

9. c) Straight ahead (primary gaze), straight up, and straight down are not cardinal positions of gaze. In any of these positions, the action of one muscle can be masked by the action of another, so these positions are not considered diagnostic.

10. b) When testing versions (range of motion), it is important that the patient keep their head still. If the patient moves the head to follow the target, you are not able to test the full motion of the eyes, but rather the range of motion of the neck. The test is done in room light so you can see the eyes as they move. An occluder is not used when testing versions. If the eyes remained in primary position, they would not move at all.

11. d) Moving the left eye laterally is abduction. The muscle that abducts is the left lateral rectus, which is innervated by the left sixth cranial nerve (CN VI). CN II is the optic nerve, CN III is the oculomotor nerve, and CN IV is the trochlear nerve.

12. b) Vergence is the ability of the eyes to fuse on the same object, whether it is close or far away, by moving the eyes inward or outward (that is, in the opposite direction). There may or may not be stereopsis. Versions move the eyes in the same direction; depth perception is judging spatial relationships.

13. b) A convergence excess means that the eyes over-converge for near viewing. Thus, an esotropia would be worse at near in this situation.

14. d) The end result of balanced extraocular muscle function is binocular single vision. This means that both eyes are situated and functioning so that a slightly different image falls on each macula, is merged by the brain, and results in a single image that appears in stereopsis. Remember, even a monocular person can have a level of depth perception; that's not the same as stereopsis.

15. b) Fixation results when the image of regard falls on the macula. It can be monocular or binocular. Binocular fixation is required in order to have binocular single vision (see Answer 14).

16. c) A branch of the facial nerve, CN III, supplies 4 of the extraocular muscles: MR, SR, IR, and IO. Remember the mnemonic LR6SO4. All the rest are CN III.

17. a) The LR is innervated by CN VI, also called the abducens nerve. (ABducens ABducts)

18. d) The SO is the only extraocular muscle that is supplied by the trochlear nerve, or CN IV. (Remember, the SO goes through the *trochlea* before it inserts into the eye.)

19. b) The LR and MR have only a primary action: that of abducting and adducting, respectively. Each of the other extraocular muscles have primary, secondary, and tertiary actions.

20. a) The primary action of the SO and IO are intorsion and extorsion respectively. The SR and IR intort and extort (respectively) as well, but only as secondary actions. Remembering that the SO and IO attach to the eye at an angle may help you visualize them and remember that they are torsionists.

21. c) While the primary action of the SR and IR are elevation (upgaze) and depression (downgaze) respectively, their secondary actions are intorsion and extorsion respectively.

22. b) The agonist is the muscle that is contracting: the "prime mover."

23. b) The antagonist is the muscle(s) that must relax in order for the agonist to move the eye.

24. a) A yoke muscle is the muscle(s) in the fellow eye that move(s) the eyes together in the same direction. In the situation given, the "reference" eye is the right. The agonist for right gaze (ABduction) in the right eye is the RLR. When OD ABducts, OS ADducts. The muscle (agonist) that ADducts the left eye is the LML. Thus in right gaze, the LMR is yoked to the RLR.

25. a) Herring's law says that equal innervation is applied to the yoke muscles of each eye. It applies to versions (ie, both eyes moving together in the same direction).

26.   b) Sherrington's law applies to ductions. It states that the amount of innervation supplied to the agonist muscle is balanced by an equal amount of relaxation to the antagonist muscle.

27.   a) Herring's law applies to binocular eye movements (versions). See Answer 25.

28.   a) A strabismic deviation that can be seen without any type of testing is a tropia. Phorias are usually discovered only by cover testing or when fusion is broken. With pseudostrabismus, the shape of the child's face is causing an optical illusion that the eyes are crossed. Bell's palsy in a 2-year-old would be highly unlikely and causes a lid/facial droop on one side.

29.   d) A phoria usually is controlled unless fusion is disrupted. When the disruption is removed, the eyes will fuse again. An intermittent tropia comes and goes; sometimes the patient is fusing and sometimes they're not. When they're not fusing, the deviation appears.

30.   c) An adult with a crossed eye either has learned to suppress the image from the eye that is not fixating or has double vision (if they have not learned to or are unable to suppress). It is not a given that amblyopia or anisometropia exist, although they might. Fusion and stereopsis can occur only when both eyes are working together, looking at the same object.

31.   a) Conventionally, vertical deviations are described as a hypertropia of the higher eye. Thus, if the patient was fixating with the right eye and the left eye was deviated downward, the right eye is higher. So this situation would be designated as an RHT.

32.   b) An adult or child with a *new* nerve palsy notices double vision. (A child with a congenital nerve palsy learns to suppress one image and does not see double.)

33.   b) If the muscle is not getting a full nerve supply, it will not be able to react properly (if at all). It thus will be underactive. This might manifest itself as an over-action of the muscle's antagonist.

34.   c) In Brown syndrome (you will sometimes see it referred to as *Brown's*), the superior oblique muscle is affected. It is a mechanical restriction, where the SO cannot move smoothly through the trochlea. Normally this is congenital, but it can be acquired due to injury (including surgical) or inflammation.

35.   a) The secondary action of the SO is depression (eye looking down) and the tertiary action is abduction (looking out/away from the midline). So the deviation is most noticeable when the patient is trying to look up and in with the affected eye. (Remember: in versions testing this occurs when the patient is attempting to look up and out with the unaffected eye.) The patient may adopt a chin up and/or head turn to avoid diplopia.

36.   b) Duane syndrome (you will sometimes see it referred to as *Duane's*) occurs when CN VI (the abducens nerve) is not "connected" properly to the lateral rectus muscle.

37.   d) See Question 36. In rare cases a branch of CN III may also be mis-wired, causing a problem with the medial rectus as well.

38.   c) There are 3 types of Duane syndrome. The most common (75% to 80%)[1] involves only the lateral rectus, so the affected eye will have difficulty abducting. This will present as an esotropia. The patient may also have a head turn in the direction of the affected eye.

39.   a) The most commonly affected extraocular muscle in thyroid eye disease (also called Graves's disease) is the IR. After the IR, the next most common are (in order) MR, SR, and LR. The obliques aren't usually involved.[2]

40.   b) Thyroid disease is an autoimmune condition. Strabismus occurs as the extraocular muscles become thick and more fibrous (less stretchy) and can no longer move the eye properly. There is also expansion of orbital fat in the disorder, but this causes exophthalmos, not strabismus. It is not caused by nerve damage or birth trauma.

41.   b) NPC is the point at which the eyes cannot maintain fusion on an object at near. The closer an object is to the eyes the more convergence is required to fuse. Eventually fusion is no longer possible and breaks down, one eye drifting out.

42.   c) NPC is measured objectively by bringing a small test object closer, usually alongside a ruler, and observing when fusion breaks and one eye drifts outward. Bringing an object closer and asking the patient to report diplopia is a subjective test for NPC. However, if a patient is suppressing, they will

not notice the extra image when fusion breaks. Because of this, the examiner must watch for one eye to drift out in these cases (making this an objective test). An amblyopic or monocular patient cannot do the subjective NPC because they do not have fusion. Accommodation does not contaminate the NPC measurement.

43. d) Of the items listed, only fusion is required. (A monocular patient, who has no fusion, will still have depth perception.)

44. b) NPC is more remote in adults. Children may measure from 5 to 10 cm, but adults may be more remote than 10 cm, and it tends to move further back with age. Patients with convergence insufficiency may have an NPC even greater than 25 cm. The test can be done objectively or subjectively (see Question 42).

45. d) NPA measures the amount of accommodation, in diopters, that a patient has available for near viewing. It is not a measurement of the bifocal add. Answer b) relates to NPC.

46. a) To test NPA, bring small print (J3, for example) closer to the patient until the patient reports that the letters have blurred.

47. b) Normally the patient (whether hyperopic or myopic) should wear full distance correction for the test. If the patient is too presbyopic to be able to see the test object from arm's length, you may test with their bifocals and subtract the add from the test result. Another option is to fully correct at distance and use a +2.50 lens over this, then subtract 2.50 from the test result. Every patient does not need a +2.50 lens, however, only those who are too presbyopic to test otherwise.

48. b) NPA should be checked in each eye. Fusion and depth perception are not required.

49. c) Fusional amplitude refers to the amount of prism that the patient can overcome to maintain single vision (ie, avoid diplopia).

50. b) Normal convergence amplitudes at near are 20 prism diopters (break point) and 18 prism diopters (recovery point). This is about double the distance convergence amplitudes and the near divergence amplitudes. It is over 3 times the distance divergence amplitude.

51. a) When enough prism has been added to finally cause fusion to break down (resulting in diplopia), this is recorded as the break point. Once the break point has been reached, the recovery point is that prism where the patient can first re-fuse.

Part II

52. c) The occluder is used in strabismus cover tests to disrupt fusion (ie, to prevent the eyes from being locked onto the same target). Fusion will hold a phoria and often an intermittent deviation in check, so fusion must be disrupted in order to determine if these deviations exist.

53. c) The cover tests are objective; they are based on the observations of the examiner rather than on the responses of the subject. Thus, they can be performed on an infant or any other patient who cannot or will not give a verbal response.

54. d) There is no point in doing cover tests on a monocular patient because there is no vision in the second eye with which to fuse. The patient must always fixate with the single, seeing eye.

55. a) The cover/uncover test differentiates between a phoria and a tropia.

56. a) The cover/uncover test also indicates the direction of any deviation (ie, E, X, or vertical).

57. c) The eyes must have drifted *out* under the cover if they make *inward* movements when uncovered, so an exodeviation is present. You were not given enough information to differentiate between a phoria and tropia. For that, you need to know what the uncovered eye is doing, as well.

58. d) An *outward* motion upon uncovering indicates that the eye has drifted *in*, denoting an esodeviation. In this case, regardless of which eye is covered, the covered eye drifts in. When the eye is uncovered, it does not move to take up fixation (indicating a tropia). This further indicates that the patient is willing to use either eye to fix, revealing an alternating esotropia.

59.   c) In a phoria, the eye under the cover drifts. The eye that is not covered is fixating. When you remove the cover, the resulting diplopia causes the deviated eye to move in order to pick up fixation. The eye that was not covered is fixating already, so it does not need to move. Be sure to read the questions carefully; the answer would have been different if this had been a cross-cover test.

60.   d) The alternate (or cross) cover test will reveal horizontal and vertical deviations but does not differentiate between a phoria and a tropia.

61.   b) When performing the alternate (cross) cover test, move the cover rapidly from one eye to the other, but every half-second is too fast. The important thing is to prevent the patient from seeing with both eyes at once, thus regaining fusion.

62.   b) If no motion is seen during the alternate (cross) cover test, it is logical to assume that the patient is orthophoric. You cannot, however, assume that amblyopia does or does not exist, that the patient has stereopsis, or that vision is equal in both eyes.

63.   d) The only thing you know at this point is that there is some type of exodeviation. (For the eye to move inward when it is uncovered, it must have drifted outward under the cover.) Once you have found movement on the alternate (cross) cover test, use the cover/uncover test to determine if it is a tropia or a phoria.

64.   c) The alternate (cross) cover test combined with prisms to measure the size of a deviation (phoria or tropia) becomes the "prism and cover test" (P&C). The deviation can be measured in a patient with fusion because the test itself disrupts fusion. The corneal reflex and polarized glasses are not used in the prism and cover test.

65.   b) Of the tests listed, the prism and cross-cover will give the most accurate measurement of a tropia. The Hirschberg test is a "guesstimate." The Krimsky, while it does provide a measurement in prism diopters, is not as exact as the prism and cross-cover. The swinging flashlight test is for evaluating pupils for afferent pupillary defects.

66.   b) If vision is equal in both eyes, it doesn't matter over which eye the prism is held. (If vision is not equal, hold prism in front of eye with BEST vision.) Statements a), c), and d) are true.

67.   a) The prism's apex should point in the same direction as the deviation. You've probably been taught that the base goes in the opposite direction as the deviation. That's just a different way to say the same thing. (Think of the prism as an arrow in order to help you remember which way to use the prism.) For measuring, it is not necessary (or practical) to split the prism amount between the 2 eyes. The prism may be placed over either eye. *Note:* If you hold the prism in the wrong direction, when you do the cross-cover, the deviation will appear even larger and in the original direction.

68.   c) If the left eye shifts up when the cover is moved to the right eye, that means that the left eye was down under the cover. This is a (vertical) hypo-deviation, neutralized with a base up prism (ie, with the apex "arrow" pointing down) over the left eye. Base down over the left or base up over the right will make the deviation look worse on cross-cover. Base in or out is used to measure horizontal deviations.

69.   b) The endpoint is reached when you have added prism sufficient enough so that neither eye moves when you cross-cover. (Except for paralytic strabismus, the eyes move an equal amount anyway.) Answers c) and d) are wrong because the prism and cover test is objective, not subjective. *Note:* Sometimes when you neutralize a deviation in one direction (horizontal is most common), you will suddenly see a deviation in another direction (ie, vertical). This is measured in the same way, holding the prism(s) or bar with the apex pointed in the direction of the new deviation. HINT: If using loose prisms, you can hold up the prism that neutralized the original deviation and add a prism (with THIS base positioned appropriately) to it. That way the original deviation doesn't get you confused.

70.   d) The patient has an RHT; the right eye is deviated up, so the prism apex ("arrow") should point up. This puts the base *down*. You could put the prism in front of the left eye, too, but the left is the lower eye so the apex would point down (ie, base up). This was not offered as an answer.

71.   c) Ideally, use best corrected vision. (If using patient's glasses, make sure you know whether or not there's already prism in the glasses.) When testing near deviation, presbyopic patients will need an appropriate add. For prism and cover testing, the phoropter would obscure the examiner's vision. Fresnel press-on prisms are not used for measuring deviations. There is no "rule" that dictates whether one should measure horizontal or vertical deviations first; horizontal deviations are much more common, so most of us neutralize the horizontal first. There may be no need to measure vertical.

72.   a) For distance P&C, use a target you know the patient can see easily (maybe 1 or 2 lines above best vision). The 20/40 may be too small for some patients. Any optotype (number, letter, etc) can be used as long as the patient can see it easily and maintains fixation on it.

73.   b) Have the patient look at the fixation point, *head in primary position* (ie, straight on). Do not allow head turn, tilt, or tip. There are situations where the P&C would done with the patient's head positioned in various positions (this is COMT® level stuff), but the initial testing is done in primary position. Any other positions (if needed) will be compared to this. For distance testing, the standard 20 ft is used.

74.   d) Unlike loose prisms, where one must put down one prism to select another, the prism bar is easy to use because one need only move the entire bar up or down while measuring. The prism bar is not more accurate, and patients seem equally tolerant of either method, although the bar would be faster and thus perhaps preferred for children. Prisms *are* additive, but that is not an advantage for the prism bar but rather loose prisms (where one can stack prisms together in case of a large deviation).

75.   b) The cross-covering should *not* allow for fixation between; you need each eye to take up fixation on its own. Start with a weaker prism and cross-cover, watching each eye for movement. If there is still movement, shift the bar to the next strongest prism and repeat the cross-cover. Continue, moving to stronger prisms until there is no movement: this is the dioptric measurement of the deviation. If you go too far (ie, position a prism that is too strong), the deviation will reverse direction.

76.   d) The patient has a 15 diopter ET. The prisms are base out, with the apexes "pointing" to the nasal. This indicates that you are dealing with an esodeviation. The power of the prisms is additive, hence 15 diopters.

77.   a) Properly performed, the W4D can identify suppression and fusion. Fusional amplitudes are the patient's vergence ability.

78.   c) If the patient can distinguish between the 2 colors, the W4D can be performed. Additionally, they must be able to count objects ("How many dots do you see?"). However, being able to count is not enough; the patient must be able to *reliably* count objects. Believe it or not, normal color vision is not required because even the red/green color deficient patient can distinguish between the colors. It is the examiner's job to interpret the patient's responses. Even knowing left from right isn't needed if you tap the patient's right hand and say, "Are the red lights on this side," then tap the left hand and say, "or on this side?" Literacy is not required, either.

79.   b) The standard test screen or flashlight has 2 green, 1 red, and 1 white light.

80.   a) By convention, the flashlight is held with the white light at the bottom. This puts the red light on the top, and a green light on either side ("Red Rising" to remember that the red light is at the top).

81.   b) Again, by convention, the glasses are placed on the patient with the red lens over the right eye (I remember this by the Rs: Right, Red). The patient with fusion will report seeing 4 lights.

82.   c) A patient who fuses may report any of the listed combinations *except* for seeing one red light on the bottom and 3 green lights (on top, left, and right). Additionally, sometimes the bottom light might be seen as yellowish, a sort of blended red and green.

83.   d) The eye looking through the red lens (OD) will see the red light as red, and the white light as red. The 2 green lights are not seen with that eye. The eye looking through the green lens (OS) will see the 2 green lights as green, and the white light as green. The single red light is not visible with the left eye. Thus, the patient in the example is suppressing with the left eye.

84.   c) The Maddox rod is a red plastic disk made up of cylinders that appear as ridges. When a pen light is observed through the Maddox rod, the light appears as a red line that runs perpendicular to the direction of the ridges.

85.   b) The Maddox rod test is used to measure phorias (because it disrupts fusion). It is used to evaluate horizontal and vertical deviations.

86.   c) The Maddox rod test requires a cooperative, honest patient who does not suppress. A patient who suppresses would not see the red line, nor would a monocular patient when the rod was placed over the suppressed or blind eye.

87.   b) The Maddox rod test can be performed in all positions of gaze at distance and at near. It is a subjective measurement, not objective, because it depends on the response of the subject.

88.   c) The red line appears perpendicular to the direction of the rods. If the rods are vertical, the line is horizontal.

89.   a) A horizontal line is used to measure a vertical deviation, because the line can then be moved up and down. A vertical line is used to measure a horizontal deviation, because the line can then be moved left and right.

90.   a) The Maddox rod is placed over the nonfixating eye and the prism is placed over the other eye. An occluder is not used. A rotating prism is easiest to use during testing, but loose prisms or a prism bar can also be utilized.

91.   b) The eye behind the Maddox rod sees a red line (not a dot!), while the other eye sees the light source. Orthophoria is reached when the red line goes through the light.

92.   d) The Hirschberg test does not use prisms. It is an objective test in that it does not require a response from the patient. Interpreting it, however, can be somewhat subjective (ie, left to the opinion of the examiner vs a more exact measurement). It is used to grossly evaluate strabismus, useful for determining if there is a deviation and if so, what direction.

93.   b) The Krimsky measurement involves moving the Hirschberg reflexes by means of prisms. No occluder, special glasses, or Maddox rod are needed. It is also an objective test.

94.   d) In the Krimsky test, prisms are used to move the displaced reflex to a position that is relative to the reflex on the fixating eye. No cover testing is used, nor is fixation of both eyes required. The Krimsky will likely give a more accurate measurement than the Hirschberg estimation, so the numbers may not match exactly.

95.   c) Stereopsis is measured in seconds of arc. The smaller the number, the finer the stereopsis.

96.   b) Bifoveal stereopsis is indicated when the patient can distinguish test items of less than 67 seconds of arc.

97.   d) Twenty-five seconds of arc indicates finer stereo discrimination than 50 seconds of arc. Stereo vision is not measured in degrees of arc as given in Answers a) and b).

98.   c) A patient with a constant ET or XT *over* 10 degrees will not have stereo vision. Nor will a monocular patient. A binocular patient with an intermittent deviation, phoria, or deviation of 10 degrees or less should have a stereo acuity test performed.

99.   a) Stereopsis is present only in binocular individuals. Depth perception exists in binocular and monocular patients. Answers b) and c) are backward: stereo vision involves seeing in 3 dimensions, and depth perception involves judging spatial relationships. Stereopsis is not learned; depth perception is.

100.   c) Having the patient touch one pencil point to another is an indicator of gross stereopsis. (Try it on yourself: once with both eyes opened and once with one eye closed.) The Hirschberg estimates the size of a deviation, not stereopsis. Answers b) and d) are contrived.

101.   a) Each of the tests listed utilized polarized glasses.

102. c) The fly was chosen as a test object because it is repulsive. An otherwise cooperative child may refuse to touch the fly because it is ugly and appears to be real. When the child sees it in 3-D, the huge fly seems to be standing on the page. Refusal is considered a positive indication that gross stereopsis exists.

103. b) Turning the test around 180 degrees will change the location of the stereo dots and make them appear sunken instead of elevated. If you turn the test 90 degrees it will not be stereopic. Polarized glasses are usually designed to be worn only one way. It is in the patient's best interest to get the most accurate measurement possible.

Part III

104. d) Cassin, McDavid, and Shamis note that "the underlying defect appears to be disturbed feedback to the gaze centers in the brain stem that interferes with control of the fixation mechanism."[3]

105. b) Oscillopsia is where objects of regard seem to move, jerk, or wiggle when the patient concentrates on them. This phenomenon occurs only in acquired nystagmus; patients with congenital nystagmus do not have this symptom.

106. c) In some cases (notably spasmus nutans), the nystagmus will resolve as the child grows; however, that is not the case with most types of nystagmus. The other statements are true. The head position is adopted in order to move the eyes into a position where the jerking is quieter or stopped, giving the patient clearer vision. The patient "finds" this position (which varies from patient to patient) at an early age, generally when beginning to sit up or stand.

107. a) The null point is when the head is in a position where the jerking is "most nullified" or lessened (ie, quieter).

108. c) In evaluating nystagmus, the speed of each movement, its amplitude, and its duration in each direction are considered. Pendular nystagmus could be compared to the pendulum of a clock: each movement extends equally to either side, takes as long, and lasts as long. In jerk nystagmus, the movement in one direction is slow, but the movement in the opposite direction is rapid. In spasmus nutans, the movements of the 2 eyes do not occur together but are dissociated. See Table 7-1 for classifications of nystagmus.

109. c) Occluding one eye may make the nystagmus worse. Fog the untested eye with +6.00 of plus; using minus would probably stimulate accommodation. (*Note:* References differ in the strength of fogging lens to be used. I've seen everywhere from +3 to +10.) Just do not forget to switch when you go to measure the other eye and to remove the +6.00 when doing that final vision check and documenting your results. Fogging should also be used instead of an occluder when checking visual acuity.

110. a) When used to evaluate eye movement, the electro-oculogram procedure is known as electronystagmography. Electrodes are attached to the skin at the nasal and temporal canthi. The electrodes detect electrical changes in the eye(s) caused by movement. The practitioner is thus given a visual representation of the patient's nystagmus patterns.

111. d) Amblyopia occurs in an eye that never learns how to see. Even after any organic problem is resolved, corrective lenses still will not improve vision. Answer a) is the definition of abnormal retinal correspondence.

112. a) If the eyes are best corrected and there is a difference of 2 or more acuity lines in the vision of the eyes, the diagnosis is amblyopia. An amblyopic patient will have difficulty with the stereo test, but so will other patients with other eye problems.

TABLE 7-1

CLASSIFICATIONS OF NYSTAGMUS

I. Normal Physiologic
    a. End-Point
    b. Induced
        1. Drugs
        2. Optokinetic
        3. Caloric
        4. Rotational
II. Congenital
    a. Motor
    b. Sensory
    c. Latent
III. Acquired
    a. Convergence Retraction
    b. Cerebellar

Adapted from Cassin B, ed. *Fundamentals for Ophthalmic Technical Personnel*. WB Saunders; 1995.

113. d) When evaluating fixation in an infant or small child, you want to answer these questions: Is the vision central (is the corneal reflex central or slightly nasal)? Does the eye hold steady (are there "searching" movements or jerking)? Does the eye continue to look at the light or small toy (does it maintain fixation)? If the answer to any of the questions is *no*, then a "U" (for un-) is added before the negative element (eg, *US* would mean *unsteady*). We use these same questions to make assumptions about vision. If both eyes together seem to be CSM, then we assume that vision is roughly equal in each eye.

114. b) In situation b, the brain will only accommodate enough to focus the least hyperopic eye, leaving the +4.00 eye in a constant blur and in danger of becoming amblyopic. The 3-year-old in Answer a) is likely to use the –3.00 eye for near (as it requires no accommodation) and the +0.50 eye for distant visual activities. Although amblyopia *could* occur in such a scenario, it is much more likely in hyperopic anisometropia. Amblyopia develops by age 12 years, not after. A single mm of ptosis is not enough to drop the lid over the pupil. (If the lid covers the pupil, then deprivation amblyopia could develop.)

115. c) Refractive amblyopia is generally bilateral and due to high, uncorrected refractive errors. Reverse amblyopia occurs when the "stronger" eye, which has been covered or penalized during treatment, becomes amblyopic due to disuse. Reflex amblyopia is caused by an injury or other insult to the eye. Anisometropic amblyopia develops when there is a refractive difference between the eyes.

116. b) The child in this scenario has "natural" monovision. In such a case, even if the child is anisometropic, amblyopia might not develop. The child often uses the myopic eye for near and the hyperopic eye for distance. However, because the eyes do not see a clear image at the same time, the patient does not have perfect fusion (maybe in the neighborhood of 400 seconds). Because of the desirability of promoting fusion in childhood, the refractive correction will generally be given in some form.

117. d) Let's break down the results. Each eye on its own is CSM, so you know that you have central fixation in each eye. But when you look at both eyes together, the corneal reflexes are uncentered (UC) at the same time. If this were a phoria, the binocular observation would also be CSM as long as fusion was not interrupted. A pseudostrabismus would also be CSM for each eye as well as both eyes together. The fact that fixation is UC but *maintained* for binocular testing rules out amblyopia, because in that case fixation would be *unmaintained* by the amblyopic eye. The remaining answer, alternating exotropia, is the correct answer.

118. d) Amblyopia ex anopsia is another name for amblyopia of disuse. It is also called stimulus deprivation. This is the type of amblyopia that remains once the organic cause of the poor visual development has been removed (such as congenital ptosis, congenital cataract, or anything that obscures the visual axis for a sufficient period of time). The other answers are actually types of amblyopia; see SLACK Incorporated's *Quick Reference Dictionary of Eyecare Terminology* latest edition or some other reference for the definitions.

119. b) In nonalternating strabismus, only one eye is being used. The other eye does not have a chance to develop visually, thereby causing amblyopia. However, when you test a child and find nonalternating strabismus, this is also a *sign* that you can expect the nonpreferred eye to be amblyopic.

120. a) By optimizing the vision in the amblyopic eye prior to alignment surgery, the physician increases the chances that the eyes will be able to fuse and "lock" together, holding the eyes straight. However, if the amblyopia is caused by deprivation (cataracts, for example), where the causative problem is surgically repairable, surgery is done prior to amblyopia treatment.

121. a) The patch is best applied to the face, because the child will usually look around the glasses. Regarding the age of the child, the younger the child the more frequent the follow-up.[4] Also to be considered are psychological factors (the stigma of "the patch," the responses of other children and family members, etc).

122. c) Patching is gradually decreased, not abruptly discontinued. Abruptly stopping the patch is associated with a higher rate of recurrence. This is especially true during the first 13 weeks after treatment is stopped.[5] If the same patching regimen is continued once the vision is equal (or as good as it's going to get), there is a chance that the occluded, previously stronger eye, will develop amblyopia itself.

123. b) If the "good" eye is patched too long, its visual development may become impaired. This results in reverse amblyopia in the formerly "good" eye. Another term for this is occlusion amblyopia.

124. d) A cycloplegic is used to dilate the "stronger" eye because it will blur the vision, forcing the "weak" eye to work harder. A miotic would make the pupil smaller, nor would it blur the vision. An anesthetic would numb the eye, never recommended for home use for any purpose. Spasmotic is a bogus term.

125. a) Topical atropine is the most commonly used drug for amblyopia treatment via pharmacologic penalization. Phenylephrine and tropicamide wear off too quickly. Pilocarpine is a miotic.

126. c) Optical penalization refers to blurring the stronger eye by optical means. A tarsorrhaphy is a surgery where the eyelids are sewn together to close the eye.

127. b) Continued monitoring is needed to watch for possible reversal of any visual improvement following treatment (at least with patching or atropine). One study found that there was a 24% chance of losing 2 or more lines of acuity following successful treatment.[6] There is a good chance to catch this if the patient is being followed.

128. b) If the eye looks normal yet has decreased vision despite treatment at an early age, the amblyopia is classified as organic. The term functional amblyopia implies that the poor vision is treatable.

129. c) In general, the younger the patient the more frequent the follow-ups. The longer the patching session (> 6 hours daily vs < 6 hours daily), the more frequent the follow-up. Penalization also requires less frequent follow-up than the patching > 6 hours a day group.[4]

130. a) The younger the patient the more frequent the maintenance exams, regardless of treatment type.[4]

131. d) Surprised? The Amblyopia Treatment Studies (ATS) run by the Pediatric Eye Disease Investigator Group found that even teens could have a vision improvement after optical correction and patching/atropine therapy. Apparently, a teen's brain still has some *neuroplasticity*; in other words, there is still enough flexibility (virtually speaking) for some chance that amblyopia therapy will help. The outcome was better if the teen had not been treated for amblyopia before. The study also found that of the teens who improved, regression (defined as a loss of 2 lines or more) was seen in only 5% vs 24% in children.[6]

132. d) Answers a), b), and c) are just the *opposite* of what you would expect. The real symptoms are headaches after near work, letters on the page swimming or jumping, losing their place when reading, closing one eye when reading, double vision at near, and/or falling asleep soon after starting to read. All activities at near require convergence, which is insufficient in this patient's case. Also worth noting: Some of these patients start out with an exodeviation of some kind. Symptoms may occur at any age. Exercises work well as therapy.

133. c) Vision exercises ("pencil push-ups," stereogram cards, etc) are the initial line of therapy. Base-in prism is somewhat controversial; it may relieve the symptoms but is generally advised only when exercises fail. Surgery is rarely considered.

134. b) "Pencil push-ups" (convergence training) involves training the eyes to increase and hold convergence.

135. a) In pencil push-ups, the goal is to strengthen the patient's ability to converge the eyes.

136. c) While the name of the exercise is pencil push-ups, any small accommodative target/object will do. A pencil is usually readily available.

137. a) The correct starting point for pencil push-ups is arm's length.

138. d) The correct manner to move the accommodative target in pencil push-ups is slowly from arm's length, closer to the eyes.

139. b) When the pencil push-ups target doubles, the patient is to hold the target at that point and attempt to force the eyes to converge (fuse), making the target single again. If fusion is achieved, the target is brought even closer until diplopia again occurs, at which point fusion is again attempted.

140. c) When the target gets so close that it doubles, it is at this point that fusion breaks (which is actually the near point of convergence). In this case one eye maintains fixation on the target but the other eye drifts out, creating the diplopia.

141. b) Stereogram cards are used to treat convergence insufficiency.

References

1. Barry BJ, Whitman MC, Hunter DG, Engle EC. Duane Syndrome. GeneReviews website. Published May 25, 2007. Updated August 29, 2019. Accessed March 12, 2023. www.ncbi.nlm.nih.gov/books/NBK1190/

2. Schreiber C. Ocular motility, strabismus, and amblyopia. In: Ledford JK, Lens A. *Principles and Practice in Ophthalmic Assisting*. SLACK Incorporated; 2018:173-174.

3. Cassin B, McDavid D, Shamis D. Eye Disorders. In: Cassin B. *Fundamentals for Ophthalmic Technical Personnel*. WB Saunders Company; 1995.

4. International Council of Ophthalmology (ICOPH). Amblyopia (Initial and follow-up evaluation). Accessed April 5, 2019. www.icoph.org/dynamic/attachments/resources/icoamblyopia_2.pdf

5. Coats DK, Paysse EA. Amblyopia in children: Management and outcome. UpToDate website. Accessed March 12, 2023.www.uptodate.com/contents/amblyopia-in-children-management-and-outcome

6. Petroysan T. Amblyopia: The pathophysiology behind it and its treatment. The American Optometric Association website. Published 2016. Accessed January 16, 2020. www.aoa.org/Documents/optometric-staff/Articles/Amblyopia%20-The%20Pathophysiology%20Behind%20It%20and%20Its%20Treatment%20FINAL%20-%20Google%20Docs.pdf

Chapter 8

Lensometry

Ledford JK.
Certified Ophthalmic Technician Exam Review Manual, Third Edition (pp 135-142).
© 2023 Taylor & Francis Group.

Neutralize Spectacles

1. **An automated lensometer may be disadvantageous in identifying:**
    a) optical centers
    b) add powers
    c) prisms
    d) warped lenses

2. **The best method for reading the add on a no-line progressive lens using a manual lensometer is to:**
    a) mark the lens first using the template from that manufacturer
    b) use the least plus reading for the distance and the most plus reading for the add
    c) take the distant lensometry reading at a point between the laser marks on the lens
    d) center the target in the lensometer

3. **To check a manual lensometer for accuracy:**
    a) adjust the eye piece then read a trial lens
    b) set the target lines for your refractive error, then see if they are clear
    c) set the eye piece at zero, then read a trial lens
    d) set the eye piece at zero, and see if the target lines clear at plano

4. **Which of the following regarding the green filter on the lensometer is *not* true?**
    a) It is more accurate.
    b) It is more comfortable for viewing.
    c) It is rarely used.
    d) It is not used for dark lenses.

5. **You are reading a pair of glasses. The single line focuses at +1.25. The triple lines clear at –1.25. Axis reads 035. The power of this lens is:**
    a) +1.25 – 2.50 x 035
    b) +1.25 – 1.25 x 035
    c) +1.25 + 1.25 x 125
    d) Plano – 1.25 x 035

6. **A lens reads –2.25 – 1.00 x 180. This indicates the presence of:**
    a) simple myopic astigmatism
    b) mixed astigmatism
    c) compound myopic astigmatism
    d) simple hyperopic astigmatism

Fresnel Prism

7.   **Fresnel prisms are often used:**
     a) following a blepharoplasty
     b) in congenital strabismus
     c) the first 6 months of a new paralytic strabismus
     d) to improve visual acuity

8.   **All are *true* regarding Fresnel prisms *except*:**
     a) they can be placed vertically or horizontally
     b) they are affixed to the lens with acrylic glue
     c) power can be read on lensometer
     d) they can be cut to fit the spectacle lens

9.   **Advantages of Fresnel prisms include:**
     a) they are useful in testing extraocular muscles
     b) they are easy to remove
     c) they can be incorporated onto gas-permeable contact lenses
     d) the refractive power is adjustable

10. **The best way to read the Rx of a lens with press-on prism is to:**
     a) center the mires and read as usual
     b) remove the prism from the lens first
     c) make sure there are no air bubbles in the prism
     d) use the prism compensation device

11. **You had removed a press-on prism to read the glasses then put it back on. Now the patient complains that "something's not right" with the glasses. What could have happened?**
     a) When you removed and reapplied the prism, the optics were stretched.
     b) The lensometer foot scratched the lens.
     c) The optical center of the lens was somehow changed.
     d) You misapplied the press-on prism.

Ground-In Prism

12. **You are neutralizing a pair of glasses with the manual lensometer, and the mires won't center no matter where you move the lens. This indicates:**
     a) the presence of a no-line multifocal
     b) the lenses are polarized
     c) the presence of ground-in prism
     d) the lenses are coated

13. **In order to determine the amount of ground-in prism present in a pair of glasses, one must:**
     a) use Prentice's rule to calculate it
     b) use a rotating chart to calculate it
     c) use a template to mark the lenses
     d) use the circles in the reticle

14. **How does one determine the orientation of the base of a ground-in prism, using the lensom-eter?**
    a) by the position of the center of the mires
    b) by evaluating image jump
    c) by the ring in the reticle where the mires center
    d) this cannot be evaluated with a lensometer

15. **You have determined that a lens has 3.5 prism diopters of ground-in lens. The mires are dis-placed to the left. This indicates that:**
    a) the prism is base-in
    b) the prism is base-out
    c) the prism is vertical
    d) not enough information to determine

16. **You are reading a pair of glasses, and you can't get any mires to move onto the instrument where you can see them. Your next action should be:**
    a) use the prism compensation device
    b) let the practitioner know that these lenses cannot be read
    c) tape a +1.50-sphere trial lens to the instrument's eye piece
    d) send the instrument for repair

17. **In order to use the prism compensation device, one must:**
    a) rotate the device until the mires appear on the screen
    b) observe the mires as you rotate the entire instrument by 180 degrees
    c) use the knob of the device to move the mires to the center of the reticle
    d) count the number of rings that the mires are displaced from center

18. **In order to measure the amount of prism using the prism compensation device, one must:**
    a) count the number of rings by which the image is displaced
    b) read the amount off the device itself
    c) calculate the difference between the sphere and cylinder of the lens
    d) convert the lens to spherical equivalent and then use a calculator

Slab-Off

19. **You are about to neutralize a pair of bifocal glasses. You notice that one lens has a fine line across the entire lens that extends horizontally beyond the bifocal segment. This indicates that the lens:**
    a) has been damaged
    b) is a slab-off lens
    c) is crown glass
    d) is a trifocal

20. **Slab-off (bicentric) lenses are most useful in:**
    a) high myopia
    b) presbyopia
    c) anisometropia
    d) ametropia

21.   **A presbyopic patient with anisometropia might experience which of the following at near?**
      a) vertical diplopia
      b) horizontal diplopia
      c) pseudostrabismus
      d) torsional diplopia

22.   **Which of the following is *false*?**
      a) A slab-off lens induces vertical prism.
      b) A slab-off is placed in the most minus of the 2 lenses.
      c) A reverse slab-off induces horizontal prism.
      d) A reverse slab-off is placed in the most plus of the 2 lenses.

23.   **In order to evaluate slab-off prism in a lens using the lensometer:**
      a) you must use the prism compensation device
      b) center the mires in the usual way
      c) place the lens on the stage straddling the slab-off line
      d) slab-off can only be evaluated with an automated lensometer

24.   **When a slab-off lens is placed properly in the lensometer:**
      a) you will see 2 sets of mires
      b) the mires will not be visible
      c) the mires will look distorted
      d) only half of the mires will be visible

25.   **When a slab-off lens is properly aligned in the lensometer, the prism power is determined by:**
      a) centering the mires
      b) reading directly off the power drum
      c) counting the number of prism rings separating the 2 sets of mires
      d) finding the difference between the sphere and cylinder

Miscellaneous

26.   **Which instrument is used to measure the base curve of a glasses lens?**
      a) radiuscope
      b) keratometer
      c) lensometer
      d) Geneva lens clock

27.   **You are reading a rigid contact lens with the lensometer. In what case might an error be induced if you hold the lens on the stage by hand?**
      a) bandage lens
      b) lens with a brown tint
      c) monovision contact
      d) +12.00 sph power lens

Study Notes

Suggested reading in *Principles and Practice in Ophthalmic Assisting: A Comprehensive Textbook*:
    Chapter 5: Ophthalmic Equipment (*Lensometer* pp 65-66)
    Chapter 19: Optical Procedures (various topics pp 347-356, *Geneva Lens Clock* pp 360-361)
    Chapter 20: Eyewear: Spectacles and Lenses (*Lens Forms* pp 369-374)

Explanatory Answers

1.   d) The automated lensometer is not very useful in identifying a warped lens. Characteristics of the lens itself (aside from the numerical measurements) are better identified with a manual lensometer.

2.   a) Each manufacturer of a progressive add lens (PAL) has a template for their lens. Once you identify and notate the lens markings nasal and temporal, you can match these marks up with the template and draw on the central cross and reading circle using a wax pencil. The reading circle is positioned on the lensometer (automated or manual) and the lens is read as usual.

3.   a) An accurate lensometer should read a trial lens exactly. Be sure to adjust the eye piece first, however.

4.   c) The green filter should be left in place all the time unless reading sunglasses/dark lenses. The green color is more comfortable for the viewer, with less glare. The measurement is more accurate if the green filter is used.[1]

5.   a) The single line focuses at +1.25. To get to –1.25, you must turn the drum away from you, indicating minus cylinder. There are 2.50 "steps" from +1.25 to –1.25, so the cylinder power is –2.50. The axis is read right off the dial. Result: +1.25 – 2.50 x 035. *Note*: Transposed, this would be –1.25 + 2.50 x 125. Read answers carefully.

6.   c) In the example given, both focal points are in front of the retina, indicated compound myopic astigmatism. In simple myopic or simple hyperopic astigmatism, one focal point is on the retina and the other in front of or behind it, respectively. In compound astigmatism (myopic or hyperopic) both focal points are in front of or behind the retina (respectively). Finally, in mixed astigmatism, one focal point is in front of and the other is behind the retina.

7.   c) Fresnel prisms are generally considered temporary, making them ideal for new-onset paralytic strabismus (most often seen in adults). Blepharoplasty is a "lid lift," and Fresnels do not improve visual acuity. It is also unlikely that they would be used in congenital strabismus.

8.   b) The Fresnel prism is quite adaptable. It is cut to fit the patient's lens and can be positioned for vertical or horizontal effect. They can be read on a lensometer because they displace the optical center the same way as ground-in prism. However, they are not glued on. To apply, some advocate putting glasses and prism under warm water, laying the prism onto the lens, and gently pressing out any bubbles.

9.   b) Fresnel prisms are easy to apply and remove, see Answer 8. They are not used in extraocular muscle testing, cannot be placed onto contact lenses, and do not have refractive power (ie, they have "prism power").

10.   b) To read the lens Rx, it is easiest to remove the press-on prism then read the lens as usual. Otherwise, the mires may be blurry and difficult to interpret. (It may also be a good idea to check visual acuity, contrast sensitivity, etc, while the prism is off, too.)

11.   d) If you remove a press-on prism for any reason, make a note of what surface it came off of (outer or inner), the direction of the base, and whether it was on the left or right lens. Otherwise, the patient will possibly see double and/or experience asthenopia (uncomfortable vision).

12.   c) Ground-in prism will not center in the lensometer no matter where you move the lens. If there is prism in the lenses by decentration, you should still be able to center the mires, even though the lens may have to be moved around quite a bit to do so. A no-line progressive lens (without any prism, which was not indicated in the answer/choice) will center. Polarization cannot be identified with a lensometer, and a coating will not displace the optical centers.

13.   d) The concentric circles in the reticle of the lensometer ocular indicates the power of the prism present, up to (usually) 5 diopters. Each ring stands for one prism diopter. Thus if the center of the mires falls on the third ring, there are 3 diopters of prism in the lens. Prentice's rule is used to calculate induced prism when the lenses are decentered.

14.   a) The orientation (ie, up, down, left, right) of the mires indicates the direction of the base of ground-in prism as seen in the lensometer.

15.   d) In order to determine base in or out, one must know if it is the right or left lens being read. In the case given, if this is the right lens then it is base out. If you are evaluating the left lens, then it is base in.

16.   a) Actually, the FIRST thing I would do is check and be sure that the last person who used the instrument didn't leave the prism compensation device in place. Once you've got that settled, use the prism compensation device to search for the mires. If the device's knob is on the left or right, then you'll be searching for horizontal prism. If you then rotate the device by 90 degrees (so the knob is up at the top of the eye piece), you'll be looking for vertical prism. Be sweet: when you're done, set the compensation device back to zero.

17.   c) The knob of the prism compensation device is turned until the mires are moved to the center of the field. The rings are always visible in the lensometer reticle; they can be rotated if desired by turning the knurled sleeve below the eyepiece.

18.   b) The prism compensation device has marks and numbers on it that indicate the amount of prism. Once you have the mires centered, you can read the prism power directly off the device, where a little arrow or mark indicates the reading.

19.   b) Slab-off lenses are a type of prism for near/close-up use only. In multifocals with a segment, you can see a fine line extending all the way across the lens from the top of the reading segment. (Thus, in a segmented trifocal, the slab-off line will be between the 2 segments, which is still at the top of the reading [vs the intermediate] segment.) A progressive lens with slab-off will also have a faint line across it.

20.   c) Anisometropia (a difference of over 1.00 diopter between eyes) can induce prism and unwanted diplopia for near vision. Slab-off prism may be needed when the difference between the power of the 2 lenses is 1.50 D or more (some references may say 1.25). The purpose is to prevent double vision at near. *Note:* The difference does *not* have to be plus in one eye and minus in the other (a situation known as *antimetropia*).

21.   a) The difference in power between the lenses in an anisometropic patient can cause vertical diplopia. Pseudostrabismus does not cause double vision.

22.   c) A reverse slab-off still induces vertical prism. The regular slab-off lens is place in the most minus (or least plus) of the right and left lenses. A reverse slab-off is placed in the most plus (or least minus) of the right and left lenses. BOTH induce vertical prism; the slab-off is base up and the reverse slab-off is base down. The reverse slab-off is most commonly used because the lens blanks are molded in the factory. A regular slab-off must be hand-ground by someone very skilled in the technique.

23.   c) Place the lens on the lensometer stage so that the slab-off line "splits" the opening.

24.   a) If you have put the lens into the lensometer so that the slab-off line bisects the opening, you will see 2 sets of mires, one above the other.

25.   c) Because you are bisecting the slab-off line, neither set of mires will be centered. But you can still count the number of prism rings between the 2; this is the amount of prism created by the slab-off. If you want, you can use the prism compensation device, knob rotated up for vertical prism, to center one set of mires. Then you can easily visualize the number of prism rings between the 2 sets. If you use this method, however, do NOT read the prism amount on the compensation device! You are not using it to measure with, just moving a set of mires to center for convenience!

26.   d) The Geneva lens clock is used to read the base curve of spectacle lenses. It is actually possible to figure out the lens Rx with it as well. A radiuscope is used to read the base curve of a contact lens; the keratometer reads corneal curvature. The lensometer is used to read the glasses Rx, but not the base curve.

27.   d) A high-powered lens (whether a contact lens or glasses lens) that is not flush on the stage may cause an erroneous reading. The stronger the lens, the more this comes into play. A bandage lens is a soft lens. Lens tint would make no difference, nor would the lens' being part of a monofit system.

Reference

1.   Marco LM-100 & LM-201 Standard Lensmeters Instruction Manual. Accessed March 12, 2023. https://opticianworks.com/wp-content/uploads/2015/10/LM-101-1021.pdf

Bibliography

Bruce A. Slab-off, Reverse Slab-off and Bi-centric Grinding. 20/20. Published February 2015. Accessed March 12, 2023. www.2020mag.com/article/slaboff-reverse-slaboff-and-bicentric-grinding

Chapter 9

Refraction*, Retinoscopy, and Refinement**

* The term "refractometry" has now gone out of vogue. The word "refraction" is basically an easier, catch-all term used to refer to measuring the patient's refractive error. ·

** In order to more closely follow the order that one would use in the clinic, I have changed the order of the criteria items in this chapter. All the material is here, however.

Ledford JK.
Certified Ophthalmic Technician Exam Review Manual, Third Edition (pp 143-166).
© 2023 Taylor & Francis Group.

```
┌─────────────────────────────────────────────────────────┐
│          ABBREVIATIONS USED IN THIS CHAPTER               │
│   • AR          automated refractor                       │
│   • cm          centimeter                                │
│   • mm          millimeter                                │
│   • PD          pupillary distance                        │
│   • RAM/GAP     red add minus/green add plus              │
└─────────────────────────────────────────────────────────┘
```

Part I*

Automated Refractor

1. **Using an AR to analyze a patient's refractive error would be which type of analysis?**
    a) signatory
    b) symptomatic
    c) objective
    d) subjective

2. **Which type of light does an AR use to analyze the patient's refractive error?**
    a) infrared
    b) ultraviolet
    c) blue ray
    d) low-level laser

3. **The patient asks if the doctor will prescribe the reading from the AR. Which is the best response?**
    a) Yes, this is a very accurate method of getting a prescription.
    b) We'll use this as a starting point in determining your prescription.
    c) No, only fools do that.
    d) No, it's not accurate enough.

Accommodation

4. **If the patient is accommodating during retinoscopy or refraction, this may result in:**
    a) a prescription that has over-plus
    b) a prescription that has over-minus
    c) a prescription without necessary cylinder correction
    d) a prescription that will cause the eyes to relax too much

---

* Sections have been inserted into this lengthy chapter for ease of study, to allow for a logical "break" point.

5.   **All of the following may be used to reduce or eliminate accommodation *except*:**
     a) duochrome test
     b) bringing the distant eye chart closer
     c) fogging
     d) topical cycloplegics

6.   **A patient whose prescription is inaccurate due to accommodation will have to:**
     a) relax accommodation in order to see clearly when wearing the correction
     b) have prism in the lenses to reduce diplopia
     c) accommodate in order to see clearly when wearing the correction
     d) have a bifocal for near vision

7.   **If a patient is known to be myopic:**
     a) one need not worry about accommodation
     b) one must still reduce or eliminate accommodation
     c) the eye has no ability to accommodate
     d) avoiding too much minus is not critical

Retinoscopy

8.   **In order to avoid contaminating the measurements, retinoscopy and refraction should be performed prior to:**
     a) contact tonometry
     b) dilation
     c) pupil exam
     d) muscle balance testing

9.   **A slit lamp exam is useful before retinoscopy and refraction in order to:**
     a) determine if astigmatism is present
     b) measure the intraocular pressure
     c) check the clarity of the media
     d) determine if refraction is needed

10. **The retinoscope provides information on the patient's refractive status by:**
     a) reflecting light off the patient's cornea
     b) reflecting light off the patient's retina
     c) reflecting light off the patient's lens
     d) projecting light from the examiner's retina

11. **The streak retinoscope permits:**
     a) no comparison of principal meridians
     b) neutralization of individual ocular meridians
     c) subjective measurement of nonverbal patients
     d) correction of plus cylinder only

12. **All of the following are components of the streak retinoscope *except*:**
     a) light and power sources
     b) condensing lens and mirror
     c) rotating lens system
     d) focusing sleeve

13. **If a streak retinoscope is habitually placed flat on the table:**
    a) this is an acceptable practice
    b) the lenses may get scratched, causing a distorted reflex
    c) the mirror will be jarred out of alignment
    d) the filament may bend, causing a distorted streak

14. **Raising or lowering the focusing sleeve of a streak retinoscope:**
    a) rotates the streak to evaluate all meridians
    b) changes the vergence of the light leaving the instrument
    c) permits measurement of hyperopia or myopia
    d) adjusts for the examiner's own refractive error

15. **The plane mirror effect is used in streak retinoscopy because:**
    a) it is easier to use the instrument with the sleeve up
    b) it is easier to use the instrument with the sleeve down
    c) this projects parallel light rays into the eye
    d) this projects converging light rays into the eye

16. **A working lens is required in retinoscopy in order to:**
    a) simulate working at infinity
    b) simulate working at 10 m
    c) simulate working at 66 cm
    d) simulate working at 14 inches

17. **Standard retinoscopy working distance is:**
    a) 50 cm
    b) 66 cm
    c) 75 cm
    d) 88 cm

18. **If you use a retinoscopy working distance that is closer than the standard, your working lens will need to be:**
    a) the same at any working distance
    b) more plus power than standard
    c) more minus power than standard
    d) one should work at the standard distance only

19. **In streak retinoscopy, the *intercept* is:**
    a) that part of the streak that is reflected from the pupil
    b) when the streak is swept at 90 degrees
    c) when the streak is swept at 180 degrees
    d) the part of the streak that falls on the patient's iris

20. **Moving the streak back and forth across the pupil and evaluating the reflex is called:**
    a) sweeping
    b) aligning
    c) refracting
    d) neutralizing

21. **In streak retinoscopy, if the streak is vertical, you should:**
     a) sweep the streak up and down
     b) sweep the streak left to right
     c) sweep the streak in a circle
     d) turn the streak to the horizontal

22. **Which of the following can be determined with the most accuracy using a streak retinoscope?**
     a) sphere power
     b) sphere axis
     c) cylinder power
     d) cylinder axis

23. **The magnitude of a refractive error can often be evaluated by noting all of these streak qualities *except*:**
     a) brightness
     b) width
     c) speed
     d) height

24. **If you sweep the retinoscope streak across the patient's pupil and the reflex travels in the same direction as the intercept, this is known as:**
     a) neutrality
     b) "with" motion
     c) "against" motion
     d) luminosity

25. **Most retinoscopists prefer to neutralize "with" motion because:**
     a) they work in plus sphere
     b) they work in minus sphere
     c) "against" motion can be difficult to evaluate
     d) "with" motion can be difficult to evaluate

26. **One can convert any refractive situation to "with" motion by adding:**
     a) plus cylinder
     b) minus cylinder
     c) enough plus sphere
     d) enough minus sphere

27. **One matches the retinoscope streak to the axis of the refractive error by:**
     a) rotating the sleeve until there is an unbroken line
     b) raising the sleeve until there is an unbroken line
     c) lowering the sleeve until there is an unbroken line
     d) turning the instrument until there is an unbroken line

28. **As the measurement approaches neutrality, the reflex will become:**
     a) dimmer, slower, and longer
     b) brighter, wider, and faster
     c) brighter, narrower, and faster
     d) brighter, wider, and slower

29. **At the point of neutrality, the reflex will:**
    a) be clearer to the patient
    b) appear as a fine line
    c) seem to blink on and off
    d) disappear entirely

30. **Which of the following might cause "scissors" reflex?**
    a) dry eye
    b) keratoconus
    c) corneal ulcer
    d) cataract

31. **All of the following regarding use of the streak retinoscope are true *except*:**
    a) keep the room lights low
    b) keep both of your eyes open
    c) observe the patient's right eye with your right eye
    d) when using your right eye, hold the retinoscope in your left hand

32. **To help stabilize the retinoscope and maintain alignment:**
    a) rest it against your brow or spectacle frame
    b) rest the handle against your cheek
    c) rest your elbow on the exam chair arm rest
    d) rest it against the phoropter

33. **If your patient is *not* dilated for retinoscopy, instruct them to look at:**
    a) your nose
    b) the retinoscope light
    c) a target on the near card
    d) a target on the distance chart

34. **If your patient is fully dilated for retinoscopy, you should:**
    a) evaluate the full reflex
    b) concentrate on the peripheral portion of the reflex
    c) concentrate on the central portion of the reflex
    d) instill dilation reversal drops until the pupil is 3 mm

35. **Which of the following patients would probably be the easiest to retinoscope?**
    a) a patient who has had a corneal graft
    b) a patient with a posterior subcapsular cataract
    c) a patient with an intraocular lens implant
    d) a patient who has had refractive surgery

36. **In your initial retinoscopy evaluation (using the proper working lens), you note that the patient has "against" motion in every meridian. This indicates:**
    a) myopia
    b) hyperopia
    c) mixed astigmatism
    d) compound hyperopic astigmatism

37. **In your initial retinoscopy evaluation (using the proper working lens), you note that the patient has "with" motion in one meridian and "against" motion in the other. This indicates:**
    a) simple hyperopic astigmatism
    b) mixed astigmatism
    c) compound hyperopic astigmatism
    d) compound myopic astigmatism

38. **In your initial retinoscopy evaluation (using the proper working lens), you note that the patient seems to be neutralized already. You should:**
    a) record your measurement as Plano sphere
    b) double check for a high refractive error
    c) retinoscope through the cross cylinder
    d) remove the working lens and check again

39. **You are working in plus cylinder using a working lens. You see "with" motion at 090 degrees and neutralize this with +1.50 sphere. You now see "with" motion at 180 degrees. Next you should:**
    a) set the cylinder axis at 180 and add cylinder until the reflex is neutralized
    b) set the cylinder axis at 090 and add cylinder until the reflex is neutralized
    c) neutralize the horizontal meridian with sphere, then the vertical meridian with cylinder
    d) convert the "with" motion at 180 degrees to "against," and neutralize with sphere

40. **You are working in minus cylinder using a working lens. You have neutralized "with" motion at 045 degrees. You turn to 135 degrees and now see "with" motion. You should:**
    a) give cylinder at 135 degrees until the reflex is neutral
    b) give cylinder at 045 degrees until the reflex is neutral
    c) neutralize at 135 degrees by giving more plus sphere, then neutralize at 045 degrees with cylinder
    d) neutralize at 135 degrees by removing sphere, then neutralize at 045 degrees with cylinder

41. **If not using the built-in retinoscopy lens on the refractor, when the measurement is complete you must:**
    a) record the refractor setting in the patient's chart
    b) add 1.50 sphere for the working distance
    c) subtract 1.50 sphere for the working distance
    d) fog the patient and re-evaluate the reflex

Part II

Measuring Refractive Error

42. **Before beginning the refraction, it is important to:**
    a) explain the procedure
    b) have an auto-refractor reading
    c) make sure the patient can read 20/20
    d) instill artificial tears to clear the tear film

43.   **Which of the following will give the refractionist the most useful information regarding the patient's refractive status?**
    a) The history
    b) The muscle balance check
    c) The slit lamp exam
    d) The fundus exam

Gross Spheres

44.   **All of the following are appropriate adjustments to the refractor (phoropter) before starting the distance measurement *except*:**
    a) set to the patient's PD
    b) set to an appropriate vertex distance
    c) converge the apertures
    d) make sure the instrument is level

45.   **In general, the first step in the refraction is to:**
    a) correct as much of the refractive error as possible with cylinder
    b) correct as much of the refractive error as possible with sphere
    c) find the cylinder power using the cross cylinder
    d) find the cylinder axis using the cross cylinder

46.   **When offering the patient changes in the spheres, a good general rule is to:**
    a) refine the axis before the power
    b) offer more plus first
    c) offer more minus first
    d) always use minus cylinder

47.   **The "gross spheres" step of refracting involves all of the following *except*:**
    a) causing the optotypes to appear smaller
    b) offering plus first
    c) using 0.50 diopter steps
    d) adding plus until the optotypes blur

48.   **You have no prior record on your young patient, and they have never worn glasses. Their vision is 20/80 uncorrected, 20/20 with pinhole. A correction of –1.50 sphere brings their vision up to 20/30. –2.00 and –2.50 sphere gives no improvement in vision. Your next step should be:**
    a) record the final measurement as –1.50 sphere
    b) see if –1.75 or –2.25 sphere will help
    c) use the duochrome test
    d) check for astigmatism

49.   **The astigmatic dial is useful for:**
    a) finding the exact cylinder power
    b) refining astigmatic correction
    c) finding the exact cylinder direction
    d) estimating the cylinder axis

50. **The astigmatic dial looks like:**
    a) a rotary telephone dial
    b) a clock face
    c) a circular grid
    d) a circle with horizontal lines

51. **When using plus cylinder, if the patient says that all the lines on the astigmatic dial seem to be equally clear:**
    a) proceed directly to cross cylinder refinement
    b) turn the cylinder axis knob 45 degrees and ask again if any lines are darker
    c) add +0.50 sphere and ask again if any lines are darker
    d) open the aperture and try the test with both eyes together

52. **In plus cylinder, if the patient says that the lines on the astigmatic dial running from 12:00 to 6:00 are clearer, you will set your axis cylinder at:**
    a) 090 degrees
    b) 180 degrees
    c) 0 degrees
    d) 045 degrees

53. **In minus cylinder, if the patient says that the lines on the astigmatic dial running from 12:00 to 6:00 are clearer, you will set your axis cylinder at:**
    a) 045 degrees
    b) 090 degrees
    c) 135 degrees
    d) 180 degrees

54. **When using the astigmatic dial, once you have set your axis, you should:**
    a) add cylinder until all lines are equally clear
    b) add sphere until all lines are equally clear
    c) use the cross cylinder until all lines are equally clear
    d) remove the dial and refine with the cross cylinder

Cylinder Refinement

55. **The cross cylinder is used:**
    a) to refine cylinder axis and power
    b) to refine sphere axis and power
    c) to refine sphere and cylinder power
    d) to refine sphere and cylinder axis

56. **Before cross cylinder testing, it is important to:**
    a) be close to the sphere power endpoint
    b) refine sphere power to the endpoint
    c) measure for bifocal add
    d) balance the 2 eyes

57. **On cross cylinder testing:**
   a) the power of the sphere should always be measured first, then its axis
   b) the axis of the sphere should be measured first, then its power
   c) the power of the cylinder should be measured first, then its axis
   d) the axis of the cylinder should always be measured first, then its power

58. **When refining the axis using minus cylinder, you should follow which dot on the cross cylinder?**
   a) red
   b) white
   c) blue
   d) there are no dots on the cross cylinder

59. **You are using plus cylinder and are refining cylinder power. The present cylinder power is +0.50. The patient says that the letters are more clear when the white dot is showing on the cross cylinder. What should you do now?**
   a) rotate the axis toward the white dot
   b) change the cylinder power to zero
   c) change the cylinder power to +1.00
   d) stop because you are at the endpoint

60. **You are using minus cylinder and are refining cylinder power. The present cylinder power is −1.00. The patient says that the letters are more clear when the white dot is showing on the cross cylinder. What should you do now?**
   a) switch to plus cylinder
   b) change the cylinder power to −1.50
   c) change the cylinder power to −0.50
   d) change the sphere power by +0.50

61. **The generally accepted endpoint for the cross cylinder test (for either axis or power refinement) is:**
   a) when the first choice is better than the second choice
   b) when the second choice is better than the first choice
   c) when the 2 choices appear equal
   d) when the patient states their vision is most comfortable

62. **If your patient has more than 6.00 diopters of astigmatism:**
   a) you cannot use the refractor
   b) the cross cylinder will not work
   c) the fogging technique must be used
   d) an auxiliary cylinder lens must be used

Fine Spheres

63. **In the "fine spheres" step of refraction, one should:**
   a) change the sphere by 0.25 diopter steps
   b) change the sphere by giving minus
   c) change the sphere by reducing plus
   d) fog with +3.00

64. If during refinement of cylinder axis and power you increased the cylinder power by 0.50 diopters, you should keep in mind that this will probably require:
a) a 0.25-diopter change in sphere power
b) a 0.50-diopter change in sphere power
c) a 5-degree change in axis
d) a stronger add

65. Your patient reads 20/20 with the following setting: –2.00 + 1.25 x 065. To refine the sphere, you first change the sphere setting to –1.75. The patient says the 20/20 line is now a bit blurred. You show them –2.00 again, and they say it is clearer. Now you change the sphere to –2.25. The patient says the letters are smaller but clearer. What is your next step?
a) see if –2.50 helps
b) record the final measurement as –2.25 + 1.25 x 065
c) record the final measurement as –2.00 + 1.25 x 065
d) record the final measurement as –1.75 + 1.25 x 065

Fogging

66. Fogging during refraction is intended to:
a) evaluate cylinder power and axis
b) measure the reading add
c) prevent giving too much plus
d) control/relax accommodation

67. Fogging is accomplished by:
a) placing a polarized lens in front of the eye to blur the vision
b) placing the Bagolini lens in front of the eye to blur the vision
c) placing enough plus power in front of the eye to blur the vision
d) placing a Maddox rod in front of the eye to blur the vision

68. Fogging makes the patient artificially:
a) more myopic
b) more hyperopic
c) dilated
d) binocular

Duochrome

69. Before beginning the duochrome test, you should:
a) occlude one eye
b) get an accurate distance correction
c) fog with +0.50 sphere
d) all of the above

70. The duochrome test is based on the fact that:
a) the colors red and green are easily recognized
b) shorter wavelengths are refracted more by the eye
c) polarized light is refracted more than nonpolarized light
d) accommodation does not affect the refraction

71. **If the patient says that the letters in the red panel are sharper, you should:**
    a) record this as your endpoint
    b) add more cylinder
    c) add more plus power to the sphere
    d) add more minus power to the sphere

72. **The endpoint for the duochrome test generally is accepted to be when the letters:**
    a) in the red panel are clearer
    b) in the green panel are clearer
    c) are equally clear in both panels
    d) in both panels no longer are visible

73. **If a patient is red-green color blind:**
    a) the duochrome test cannot be used
    b) place a Maddox rod in front of the right eye
    c) place a Bagolini lens in front of the right eye
    d) refer to left and right sides instead of red and green

Binocular Balance

74. **The purpose of balancing is:**
    a) to ensure that the vision is the same in each eye
    b) to make sure that the eyes are accommodating equally
    c) to ensure that the measurement in each eye is as nearly the same as possible
    d) to make sure that the eyes are not crossing

75. **Which of the following regarding binocular balancing is *not* true?**
    a) It is performed once the distance refraction has been determined.
    b) It is valid if the acuity of the eyes is similar.
    c) It is performed at 14 inches.
    d) Fogging is used during the test.

76. **When using the alternate occlusion method of binocular balancing, it is important to:**
    a) fog the dominant eye
    b) fog the nondominant eye
    c) fog the right eye
    d) fog both eyes

77. **When using the alternate occlusion method of binocular balancing, suppose your patient says that the vision in the right eye is sharpest. What is your next step?**
    a) blur the left eye with +0.25 sphere
    b) blur the right eye with +0.25 sphere
    c) blur the left eye with -0.25 sphere
    d) blur both eyes with +0.25 sphere

78. **You are using the alternate occlusion method of binocular balancing and have reached the endpoint. Your next step is to:**
    a) reduce the sphere by −0.25 steps in both eyes until best acuity is obtained
    b) record the measurement as the final refraction
    c) remove the +1.50 working lens from the phoropter
    d) use the binocular balancing formula to make the final calculation

79. **When performing binocular balance, it may be helpful to know:**
     a) which eye is dominant
     b) if stereo vision is present
     c) the near point of accommodation
     d) the near point of convergence

Determine Near Add

80. **To test for the reading add, the standard near card is placed:**
     a) at the distance preferred by the patient
     b) at 10 inches
     c) at 14 inches
     d) at 20 inches

81. **The general rule for determining the reading add is to:**
     a) give the least amount of plus possible
     b) give the maximum amount of plus
     c) go by the standard age chart
     d) never give more than +3.00

82. **When evaluating the patient for a near add, it is important to:**
     a) explain to the patient they'll have to hold reading at 14 inches
     b) make a note of the patient's working distance(s)
     c) use a fogging lens
     d) measure at 6-inch intervals

83. **Your 65-year-old patient plays percussion and needs to be able to see a music stand from 24 inches away. The practitioner will prescribe:**
     a) a stronger add than the one found at 14 inches
     b) a weaker add than the one found at 14 inches
     c) the same add as the one found at 14 inches
     d) distance glasses only, without an add

Part III

Miscellaneous

84. **All of the following patients could have alterations to their refractive status related to their condition *except*:**
     a) a patient with diabetes
     b) a patient who is pregnant
     c) a patient with cataracts
     d) a patient taking allergy shots

85. **Each of the following procedures can affect the refraction *except*:**
    a) pterygium removal
    b) blepharoplasty
    c) nasolacrimal probing
    d) chalazion removal

86. **A patient with a cataract probably will show evidence of what type of refractive shift?**
    a) increased myopia
    b) decreased myopia
    c) increased presbyopia
    d) increased hyperopia

87. **All of the following can cause a hyperopic shift in the refraction *except*:**
    a) orbital mass
    b) macular swelling
    c) elevated blood sugar
    d) corneal edema

88. **The disease/condition that is most likely to cause refractive shifts from one exam to the next is:**
    a) diabetes
    b) hypertension
    c) hyperthyroid
    d) gout

89. **The ocular disease/condition that is most likely to cause refractive shifts from one year to the next is:**
    a) astigmatism
    b) keratoconus
    c) soft contact lens over-wear
    d) glaucoma

Vertex Distance

90. **If a patient with aphakia is corrected with glasses, they might require +12.00. If they wear a contact lens, they might need +14.00. This increase in power with a decrease in distance to the cornea is a product of:**
    a) axial length
    b) vertex distance
    c) pupillary distance
    d) spherical equivalence

91. **Vertex distance is defined as:**
    a) the distance between the back of the glasses lens and the front of the eye
    b) the distance between optical centers
    c) the distance between the front and back of the spectacle lens
    d) the distance between the visual axis of the right and left eye

92. **Vertex distance becomes increasingly important:**
    a) the more compulsive the patient is
    b) the worse the patient's vision is
    c) the stronger the correction is
    d) the weaker the correction is

93. **Vertex distance should be included with the refraction if:**
    a) the patient's vision is 20/20
    b) the patient's vision is 20/40 or worse
    c) the correction is 4.00 diopters or more
    d) the correction is 4.00 diopters or less

94. **Which of the following statements about vertex distance is *correct*?**
    a) Patients with myopia may require more minus power in a soft lens than in spectacles.
    b) Patients with hyperopia may require less plus power in a soft lens than in spectacles.
    c) Patients with aphakia may require less plus power in a soft lens than in spectacles.
    d) Patients with hyperopia may require more plus power in a soft lens than in spectacles.

95. **Your patient wears +8.75 in glasses, for each eye. Vision was 20/20 last exam with these glasses, 10 weeks ago. Today their vision is 20/40. They say, "But look! If I move my glasses out here like this … " (moving them away from their face) " … I can see lots better! E-V-O-T-Z!" This occurs because of:**
    a) a change in vertex distance changes the effective power of the lens
    b) a change in vertex distance changes the power of the lens
    c) induced prismatic effect
    d) induced astigmatism

96. **In addition to the prescription itself, it is vital to include which of the following measurements for aphakic eyewear?**
    a) front and back surface powers
    b) base curve and refractive index
    c) lens material and size limitations
    d) vertex distance and pupillary distance

97. **The device used to measure vertex distance is most properly called a:**
    a) lensmeter
    b) vertex conversion chart
    c) distometer
    d) vertometer

98. **Prior to using the distometer, one must:**
    a) check calibration
    b) determine the lens material
    c) check the patient's corneal sensitivity
    d) sanitize the fixed caliper arm

99. **When positioning the distometer, one should:**
    a) place the plunger on the patient's closed lid
    b) place the moveable caliper arm on the patient's cornea
    c) place the fixed caliper arm on the patient's closed lid
    d) place the fixed caliper arm on the back of the lens

100. **While measuring vertex distance, the patient is told to:**
    a) keep the eye gently closed and the eye is positioned straight ahead
    b) maintain fixation on the muscle light
    c) close the eye gently and roll the eyes up
    d) keep both eyes open at all times

101. **Once the foot plate of the distometer is in place, the plunger is pushed until it:**
    a) beeps twice
    b) aligns with the lens bottom
    c) begins to pulsate
    d) contacts the back of the lens

102. **In order to take a reading from the distometer, one must:**
    a) read the scale on the device
    b) connect the device to a computer
    c) make sure you use the correct weights
    d) calibrate the conversion chart

103. **The reading on the distometer is given in:**
    a) inches
    b) diopters
    c) Ångstroms
    d) millimeters

104. **Which of the following might affect the vertex distance measurement?**
    a) brow ptosis
    b) lid ptosis
    c) blepharitis
    d) dermatochalasis

Conversion

105. **When using the distometer conversion scale, one must:**
    a) use the appropriate scale for plastic or glass
    b) use the appropriate scale for plus or minus lenses
    c) convert the distometer reading to fractions of an inch
    d) use the appropriate scale for toric or nontoric lenses

106. **In order to convert the change of lens power required as one goes from the vertex distance of a trial frame to the vertex distance of the patient's spectacles, one must:**
    a) use a conversion scale
    b) read the numbers on the caliper
    c) use the spherical equivalent
    d) transpose to minus cylinder

107. **If the optician adjusts the lens to account for vertex distance:**
    a) the lens power may not match the original prescription
    b) the patient will complain of diplopia
    c) the vision will not be as good as in the patient's record
    d) there will be induced prism

Transposition

108. Transpose +1.75 – 3.25 x 037
     a) –1.75 + 1.50 x 127
     b) –1.50 + 3.25 x 127
     c) –1.50 + 3.25 x 097
     d) –3.25 – 1.75 x 037

109. Transpose -2.50 + 6.25 x 082
     a) +2.50 – 4.25 x 172
     b) –4.25 – 6.25 x 172
     c) +4.25 – 2.50 x 122
     d) +4.25 – 6.25 x 172

110. Transpose +3.25 + 3.25 x 163
     a) Plano – 3.25 x 073
     b) +6.50 – 3.25 x 073
     c) –3.25 – 3.25 x 073
     d) Plano – 6.50 x 163

Spherical Equivalent

111. If, for some reason, you need to reduce an astigmatic correction to sphere only, the procedure to use is:
     a) transposition
     b) induced prism
     c) bicentric grinding
     d) spherical equivalent

112. Determine the spherical equivalent of –5.75 + 2.50 x 178.
     a) –4.50
     b) –8.20
     c) –4.50 – 1.25 x 178
     d) –2.75 – 2.50 x 088

113. You are about to perform a visual field test on a 20-year-old patient with the following prescription: –0.50 – 2.50 x 090. You open the trial lens box and all the cylinders are missing. Which spherical lens would be best to use?
     a) –3.00 sph
     b) –2.00 sph
     c) –1.75 sph
     d) +0.75 sph

114. You are selecting a contact lens for a patient with the following prescription: +3.25 – 1.00 x 072. What power lens would you choose?
     a) +3.75
     b) +2.75
     c) +4.25
     d) +4.25 – 1.00 x 072

Study Notes

Suggested reading in *Principles and Practice in Ophthalmic Assisting: A Comprehensive Textbook:*
  Chapter 4: Optics (*Transposition* pp 51-52, *Spherical Equivalent* p 52)
  Chapter 11: Retinoscopy and Refractometry (pp 179-211)
  Chapter 19: Optical Procedures (*Transposition* p 348, *Measuring Vertex Distance* pp 359-360)
  Chapter 20: Eyewear: Spectacles and Lenses (*Vertex Distance* pp 374-375)
  Appendix B: In-Office Training (*Vertex Distance* p 757)

Explanatory Answers

Part I

1.   c) The AR is an objective method of testing: it requires no response from the patient. Retinoscopy is another example. Subjective methods involve asking the patient to respond and using the response to determine the measurement. (I remember this by thinking that objective methods treat the patient like an object.)

2.   a) Just like your TV remote, the AR uses harmless infrared light to evaluate the refractive status of the patient's eye. (*Note:* "Blue ray" is not an actual term. The name "Blu-ray" is a trademark.)

3.   b) The best response is to say that the reading will be used as a starting point. This is assuming that the reading will be entered into a phoropter or trial frame and refined subjectively. I have heard that some practices do prescribe the AR. But the norm, and the best Answer, is b). I hope Answer c) made you laugh!

4.   b) If the patient accommodates, they have added plus power to the eye. This is neutralized with minus sphere (or the removal of plus sphere) during the measurement. If prescribed by the practitioner, this spectacle lens won't have enough plus, and the eye will have to strain when wearing it (and even *more* accommodation will be required for near vision).

5.   b) Methods to control or reduce accommodation include the duochrome test, fogging, and topical cycloplegics. Bringing the distant chart closer will stimulate accommodation.

6.   c) See Answer 5.

7.   b) It is a common misconception that if the patient is known to be myopic, you need not worry about accommodation. This isn't true. You might easily refract a young person with myopia who only needs −2.00 sphere as a −4.00 or more.

8.   a) Refractometry should be done prior to contact tonometry or any other procedure that applanates the cornea (A-scan, B-scan, pachymetry, cell count, etc). With any of these tests there is the possibility of some corneal abrasion and/or edema, which can affect the patient's vision and thus the measurement. The pupil test might dazzle the patient for a minute, but you can proceed once they recover. Dilation should be done after distance and near testing but will not "contaminate" the distance measurement.

9.   c) The slit lamp exam will indicate the clarity of the tear film, cornea, aqueous, lens, and vitreous (collectively called the *optical media*), giving you an idea of the prognosis of the measurement. Unless the patient has marked keratoconus, astigmatism will not be seen with the slit lamp. Applanation tonometry was ruled out in Answer 8. The necessity for a refraction is normally determined by factors other than the slit-lamp exam.

10.   b) The light from the retinoscope is refracted by the cornea and lens but reflected by the retina (specifically the pigment epithelium and choroid).

11.   b) Rotating the streak of the streak retinoscope allows neutralization of individual meridians. You also can compare the meridians or use minus cylinder if you want. Retinoscopy is an objective, not subjective, technique.

12. c) The streak retinoscope consists of a light source, power source, condensing lens, mirror, and focusing sleeve. There are no rotating lenses.
13. d) If a streak retinoscope is laid on its side while the bulb is hot, the filament can warp. This causes a C-shaped bend in the reflex.
14. b) Moving the sleeve up and down changes the vergence of the light. One position has a plane mirror effect; the other has a concave effect. The position of the sleeve and its vergence varies from one brand of retinoscope to another.
15. c) When using the plane mirror effect, the light leaving the retinoscope is parallel. A concave mirror will focus the light in front of the instrument.
16. a) Use of a working lens simulates infinity. This allows the technician to work at arm's length from the patient instead of 20 ft away.
17. b) Standard retinoscopy working distance is 66 cm (about 26 in) from the patient.
18. b) If your working distance is closer than 66 cm, you will need a stronger plus-power working lens.
19. d) The intercept is the part of the streak that falls on the patient's iris, or on the phoropter. It always travels in the direction in which you "sweep" (refers to moving the instrument back and forth) the scope. The light that shines from the pupil is called the *reflex*.
20. a) Sweeping is moving the streak across the pupil while evaluating the reflex for with and against motion. This may be done in any meridian, where the sweep should be parallel to the direction of the streak. Neutralizing begins when you start using lenses to manipulate the reflex.
21. b) The streak should be moved ("swept") perpendicular to the intercept's direction. If the intercept is vertical, you move horizontally, and vice versa.
22. d) The streak retinoscope allows for very accurate estimation of the cylinder axis.
23. d) The height of the streak is constant. Brightness, width, and speed of the moving reflex vary according to the patient's refractive error. A higher error will have a dull, narrow, and slow reflex.
24. b) If the intercept and the reflex travel in the same direction, they are moving with each other. This is "with" motion. In "against" motion, the reflex moves in the opposite direction from the intercept. Neutrality just blinks on and off, while luminosity simply refers to the glow.
25. c) "With" motion is easier to see and interpret, regardless of what type of cylinder you use. Answers a) and b) refer to sphere sign, not cylinder.
26. d) Any situation can be converted to "with" motion. If you reduce the sphere enough (remove plus or add minus), "against" motion will convert to friendly "with."
27. a) In order to align the axis of the intercept with the angle of the reflex, turn the sleeve until there is an unbroken line (ie, the intercept and the reflex are aligned). Raising and lowering the sleeve changes the vergence of the scope's light.
28. b) A reflex that is approaching neutral will get brighter, wider, and faster.
29. c) At neutrality, the reflex will be its brightest, widest, and fastest. It will fill the whole pupil and appear to blink on and off as you sweep.
30. b) "Scissors" reflex is basically caused by irregular astigmatism, and it may be the first indication that a patient has keratoconus. The reflex seems to have both with and against motion, and may seem V shaped, or to open and close like a pair of scissors.
31. d) Hold the scope with the right hand when using the right eye, and with the left hand when using the left eye. This makes it easier to turn the dials on the refractor. Statements a) through c) are true, although it takes some discipline to learn to work with both eyes open.
32. a) Rest the head of the retinoscope on your brow or against your glasses frame. This will help stabilize the instrument, keeping the peephole from wobbling around. It would be hard to manipulate the handle (raise, lower, or turn) if it were against your cheek. If you lean on the patient's chair, you are going to be too close. Resting it on the phoropter makes it impossible to work.
33. d) The undilated patient should look at a distant object in order to relax accommodation as much as possible. Options a) through c) are too close to the patient and will stimulate accommodation. Looking at the retinoscopy light also will cause the pupil to constrict, making it harder to see the reflex.

34.   c) A fully dilated patient can have some confusing reflexes. Concentrate on the central reflex, ignoring the periphery. There is no need to reduce the pupil size.

35.   c) None of these situations is ideal, but the patient with the intraocular lens probably will be the easiest of the 4 to scope.

36.   a) "Against" motion in all meridians (with the working lens in place) indicates myopia (it also could indicate compound myopic astigmatism, which wasn't given as an option).

37.   b) Mixed astigmatism has one focus in front of the retina (yielding "against" motion) and one behind the retina (giving "with" motion). Simple hyperopic astigmatism would have one neutral and one "with" meridian. Compound hyperopic astigmatism would have 2 "with" meridians. Compound myopic astigmatism would have 2 "against" meridians.

38.   b) A high refractive error can masquerade as pseudo neutrality. Put in +5.00, +10.00, –5.00, and –10.00 spherical lenses and re-evaluate the reflex. The retinoscope is not used with the cross cylinder. Removing the working lens will only make a difference of 1.50 (or whatever the proper power is for your working distance), not enough to change the reflex much if evaluating a high refractive error.

39.   a) One meridian is neutralized with plus, and the other meridian still has "with." Since you are using plus cylinder, and plus is used to neutralize "with," set your cylinder axis at 180 degrees and give plus cylinder until this meridian also is neutral.

40.   c) The first "with" meridian is neutralized, and the other meridian still has "with" motion. Since you are using minus cylinder, you cannot neutralize "with" motion by using cylinder. If you neutralize the 135 meridian with sphere, this will convert the 045 meridian to "against." So neutralize 135 by adding more plus (or reducing minus). Then set your cylinder axis and retinoscope streak to 045. You will see "against." Give enough minus cylinder to convert this to "with," then reduce the amount of minus cylinder slowly until the meridian is neutralized.

41.   c) If you are not using the built-in retinoscopy lens on the refractor, you must remember to subtract 1.50 sphere (or the appropriate amount for your personal working distance) from the measurement indicated on the refractor (ie, rotate the sphere wheel UP 6 "clicks" if your distance is 1.50).

Part II

42.   a) Patient education is one of the keys to successful measurements and should be given if the patient is able to understand. An auto-refractor reading might be nice but is not necessary. Obviously not everyone can read 20/20 (or they wouldn't need us). If the tear film is cloudy, teardrops may be needed, but they are not needed on every patient.

43.   a) The history will tell you much that can affect the measurement: the presence of any systemic or ocular disease that may affect vision, any medications that can affect vision, past vision history, past problems with glasses, visual symptoms, etc. The option of doing a slit lamp exam prior to refraction is preferable, but not as necessary as knowing the patient's history.

44.   c) Always set the PD, vertex distance, and level before measuring. The apertures are converged to test the reading (near) vision, not distance.

45.   b) The measurement starts by working with spheres. You want to correct as much of the refractive error with spheres (instead of sometimes poorly tolerated cylinder) as possible.

46.   b) Always offer more plus first, whether you are going from +2.00 to +2.50, or from –6.25 to –5.75. This is true in both "gross spheres" (0.50-diopter steps) and "fine spheres" (0.25-diopter steps). More minus always will look better to an eye that is accommodating. Sphere has no axis.

47.   a) In the gross spheres step, you should offer plus first and move in +0.50-diopter steps ("2 clicks"), until the print blurs. Adding minus (reducing plus) may make the optotypes seem smaller/minified. This is a sign that you have gone too far in the minus direction.

48. d) If sphere alone does not correct a patient to 20/20, it is not time to stop. Start looking for astigmatism. If –2.00 and –2.50 sphere did not improve the vision, it is a waste of time to try –1.75 and –2.25. The duochrome test is performed once best visual acuity has been obtained using spheres and, if necessary, cylinder.

49. d) The astigmatic dial, or *clock*, is useful in estimating the cylinder axis. You still should refine with the cross cylinder.

50. b) The astigmatic dial looks like a clock face, with lines radiating from a central point. At their endpoints, each line is separated by 10 or 30 degrees.

51. c) If the lines on the dial appear equally black, add a little sphere (or move in a more plus direction) and ask again. Either way, you are moving the image off the retina enough to see if there is another meridian of focus.

52. a) For plus cylinder, set the cylinder axis parallel to (in line with) the darkest lines as the patient sees them.

53. d) In minus cylinder, first select the lowest/least clock hour. In our example, that is 6. Then multiply that by 30 and use this as your axis. 6 x 30 = 180. Set your axis at 180.

54. a) After setting your axis, slowly give the patient cylinder power until the lines appear to be equally clear.

55. a) Use the cross cylinder (also known as the Jackson cross cylinder) to refine cylinder axis and power.

56. a) If the spherical component of your measurement is too far off, your cylinder won't be correct. You'll be trying to correct things with cylinder that would be corrected better with sphere. (Spheres don't have an axis.)

57. d) Always measure the cylinder axis first. (This is one of the few exceptions to my warning about the word *always*.) If the axis isn't refined first, you can't get the accurate power. Doing this in the wrong order used to be grounds for failing the refraction section of the practical.

58. a) If you are using minus cylinder and are refining axis, follow the red dot. (There are no blue dots.)

59. c) When refining power, the red dot means subtract (same as "giving minus") and the white dot means add (same as "giving plus"), regardless of whether you are working in plus or minus cylinder. If you are at cylinder power +0.50 and the patient likes the white dot choice better, you are going to move to +1.00-cylinder power. (In reality, you could alternately choose to go to +0.75, adding just +0.25, but that was not offered as an answer in this question.)

60. c) See Answer 59. The white dot means give plus, so you should move from –1.00 to –0.50.

61. c) The cross cylinder actually straddles a setting, so on one choice the patient sees the setting with a little "plus," and on the other choice with a little "minus." When straddling the correct reading, each choice is equidistant from that setting and the choices will look about the same.

62. d) Cylinder power in most refractors goes up to 6.00 diopters, but there is an auxiliary cylinder lens that you can snap into the aperture to add more. The cross cylinder is not dependent on a certain amount of astigmatism.

63. a) At the beginning of the gross spheres step we used 0.50-diopter steps. Now we are done with astigmatic correction and ready for the final step. Offer 0.25-diopter steps, starting with plus first.

64. a) For every 0.50-diopter change in cylinder power, there will probably be the need to change the sphere power by 0.25. If you are working in plus cylinder and increase the cylinder power, you will change the sphere 0.25 diopters in the minus direction. If you use minus cylinder, then each 0.50 diopters of minus cylinder given will be offset by 0.25 diopters sphere in the plus direction. The axis or add should not be changed.

65. c) Remember that a minus lens minifies. (You also could say that, compared to a +6.00, a +2.00 minifies.) The patient's impression that the letters have gotten smaller is an indication of too much minus. Therefore, you return to the previous setting of –2.00 + 1.25 x 065 as your endpoint.

66. d) Fogging is used to reduce accommodation during the refraction, which helps prevent giving too much minus (not plus!). It also can be used instead of occlusion.

67. c) To fog, add enough plus sphere to blur the vision. (There is no set amount, but I prefer +3.00.)

68. a) This might sound backward, but think about it. If you neutralize myopia with minus power, that means that the eye has "too much plus." When fogging, you "add" more plus, creating myopia (or decreasing hyperopia).

69. d) Fogging the eye with +0.50 should make the letters in the red darker, so you can move toward the green by –0.25 steps. When used as a final check after distance refraction, the duochrome is a monocular test, so one eye is occluded. The duochrome test is sometimes called the *bichrome* test. Be aware that the term "red-green test" is usually applied to color vision testing.

70. b) Technically, the test is based on chromatic aberration. The shorter the wavelength, the more the eye's optics will refract the light rays. Thus, green is refracted more than red. Fogging moves both green and red in front of the retina; red will be closest. That means the letters in red will move onto the retina first (because they are not refracted as much, they are brought to the macula first). Each 0.25 click in the minus direction moves the red off the macula retro-orbitally and moves the green out of the vitreous and closer to the macula.

71. d) If the letters in the red are sharper and more distinct, remove 0.25 diopters of sphere (ie, reduce plus or increase minus). Go in 0.25 steps so you don't miss the endpoint and over minus. Remember the mnemonic RAM/GAP: red add minus, green add plus. But it's best if the starting point is sharper in the red (ie, fogged with enough plus/less minus so that the red is on or just in front of the macula).

72. c) The endpoint is generally accepted to be when the letters in red and green appear equally dark/clear. (Some prefer to leave the patient "one click" in the green, but this is not "textbook.")

73. d) Even a red-green color-blind patient who cannot distinguish between vivid hues can be tested using the duochrome if you refer to the left and right halves of the screen instead of the colors. No special lenses or tricks need to be used.

74. b) The goal of balancing the prescription is to make sure that each eye is accommodating the same amount. This keeps vision much more comfortable because if one eye is trying to accommodate, so is the other, whether it needs to or not. This results in blurry, fluctuating, uncomfortable vision.

75. c) Binocular balancing is performed after the distance refraction has been determined, and where the vision between the 2 eyes is close to the same. There are several methods; the main 2 (Risley prism and alternate occlusion) involve fogging before the testing starts. It is performed at distance.

76. d) Both eyes are fogged during binocular balancing. (Even if you didn't know what it is, the term binocular would clue you in that it's a binocular [ie, 2-eyed] procedure.)

77. b) Blur the clearest eye with +0.25 sphere. Remember, "adding" minus sphere would make the vision more clear because you fogged the patient to begin with.

78. a) Once balanced (ie, vision is blurred equally in each eye) you must remove the fogging 0.25 diopters at a time, in a MINUS direction. Be careful not to over-minus! No working lens is used for fogging, and there is no formula involved.

79. a) If you are attempting to balance and cannot find a point where the eyes are the same, leave the dominant eye as the clearest one.

80. c) The refractionist should measure the add at the standard 14 inches.

81. a) In general, be cautious with giving plus and also leave half of the patient's accommodation in reserve. If you give the maximum plus that the patient will tolerate, you totally eliminate natural accommodation at near. The age chart may be a guide, but each patient should be measured. Some patients will need more than +3.00. (The word "never" should have indicated that d) was not correct.)

82. b) While refracting for the add is done at the standard 14 inches, it is vital to make a note for the practitioner concerning the patient's actual working distances. The practitioner can then make a determination for the proper add for that patient and for specific tasks. We don't dictate the patient's reading distance, fogging is not needed for near measurements, and we don't measure at intervals.

83. b) If the distance for close-up work is closer than 14 inches, then more plus is required. If the close-up distance is farther away than 14 inches (as in this case), then less plus (a "weaker" add) is needed. At 65, if emmetropic or fully corrected for distance, the patient will need some sort of correction to focus at 24 inches. If the patient is given the add from 14 inches or stronger, they'll have to lean forward into the music stand; that won't make them very happy!

Part III

84. d) As a general rule, taking allergy shots does not affect the measurement. Items a), b), and c) can change the measurement.

85. c) Of the listed procedures, a nasolacrimal probing is least likely to produce a change in refraction. Pterygium removal may alter the cornea. Heavy lids may press on the globe, as may a chalazion.

86. a) A patient with a progressive cataract usually begins to take more minus (or less plus).

87. c) Elevated blood sugar causes a *myopic* shift. Fluid leaves the lens as the body attempts to neutralize the sugar in the blood. This dehydration causes an increase in the lens's curve, resulting in a myopic shift. The items in a), b), and d) can cause a hyperopic shift.

88. a) See Answer 87.

89. b) Keratoconus causes shifts in astigmatism as it progresses. Astigmatism itself, in the absence of keratoconus or physical alteration of the cornea, generally remains stable. Contact lens over-wear causes more pain than refractive change. Glaucoma does not generally cause a change in the refraction.

90. b) The closer one gets to the cornea (or retina, for that matter), the higher the lens power must be. This occurs because the focal length has been shortened. See Answers 94 and 95.

91. a) Vertex distance is the distance from the back of the corrective lens to the front of the cornea.

92. c) Vertex distance is more crucial in high-powered lenses. The weaker the lens, the more "play" there is in the allowable vertex distance.

93. c) If the patient's refractive error is 4.00 diopters (plus or minus) or more, you should measure vertex distance and record this in the chart for the prescriber. *Note:* some references say 3.00 diopters or more.

94. d) The closer you get to the retina, the more plus power it takes to converge and focus the image. So a patient with hyperopia may need more power in the contact than in the glasses. Patients with aphakia also have hyperopia. A patient with myopia might need more plus, too (translating to *less* minus).

95. a) When the vertex distance of a lens is changed, the effective (not actual) power of the lens is also changed. This is especially noticed in stronger lenses. By increasing the vertex distance of a plus lens, the effective power of the lens moves in a minus direction. For an extreme example, a +8.75 lens, if moved from 12 mm to 23 mm now has the refracting effect of a +8.00 lens. This indicates a myopic shift.

96. d) The higher the power of the lens, the more critical it is to provide an accurate PD and vertex distance. Without the PD, you may have induced prism. Without the correct vertex distance, the lens power may not be adequate.

97. c) Distometer is the best term for the device used to measure vertex distance. The instrument includes a conversion chart, which is used to calculate lens power changes associated with various vertex distances. The lensmeter is more commonly known by trade names Lensometer (which has fallen into common, generic use) and Vertometer (a trade name by Bausch & Lomb). One will see the term *vertexometer* applied to *both* the lensmeter and the distometer.

98. d) Because the foot plate of the fixed caliper arm contacts the patient, it must be sanitized between each use; an alcohol swab is sufficient. The device does not require calibration.

99. c) The foot plate on the fixed caliper arm is placed gently on the patient's closed lid. The moveable arm will touch the back of the lens, and the plunger is under your thumb.

100. a) The patient should be cautioned to keep the eyes closed without squeezing. In addition, the eye should be pointed straight ahead, not up or down. You want the measurement approximately over the apex of the cornea.

101. d) Once the foot plate is in place against the lid, the plunger is pushed until the tip of the moveable arm contacts the back of the lens, preferably at the optical center.

102. a) The reading is taken directly from the device. No computer or weights involved.

103. d) The distometer scale uses the metric system and is a linear measurement. The scale is calibrated in millimeters.

104. d) In dermatochalasis, there is redundant skin over the lid itself. Gently use a thumb to pull the lid taut (while still keeping the eye closed) so that you are only measuring through one layer of skin.

105. b) The conversion scale is calibrated in millimeters (on the rotating dial) and diopters (on the stationary part of the dial). The millimeter scales are in red for minus lenses and black for plus lenses.

106. a) If you want to convert a lens power for a given vertex distance (or vice versa), you must use a conversion scale. Some are tables and others are rotary-type charts.

107. a) The lens may not read as being exactly what the doctor ordered if the optician had to adjust for vertex distance. Diplopia and induced prism are a function of optical center alignment. Vision should be just as good regardless.

108. b) The formula for transposition is (1) algebraically add the sphere and cylinder powers, (2) change the sign of the cylinder [without changing the power], (3) rotate the axis by 090 degrees. Algebraically add +1.75 – 3.25 = –1.50, sphere power. Change cylinder power sign +3.25. Rotate axis 90 degrees 037 + 090 = 127.

109. d) Algebraically add –2.50 + 6.25 = +4.25. Change cylinder power sign –6.25. Rotate axis 90 degrees 082 + 090 = 172.

110. b) Algebraically add +3.25 + 3.25 = +6.50. Change cylinder power sign – 3.25. Rotate axis 90 degrees 163 – 090 = 073.

111. d) Spherical equivalent is used when converting an astigmatic correction (ie, with sphere and cylinder) to spheres only. It is determined by adding half of the cylinder power to the power of the sphere. Transposition is used to convert minus to plus cylinder and vice versa. The formula for induced prism is used when determining the prismatic power of a decentered lens. Bicentric grinding is another term for slab-off lens.

112. a) Divide the cylinder power in half: +1.25. Add this to the sphere power: –5.75 + 1.25 = –4.50. Answer d) was the transposition of the original Rx. Read questions carefully!

113. c) While less than desirable, if you just had to get the field done right then, the lens to use would be –1.75 sphere, the spherical equivalent of the given Rx: Half of the cylinder power –2.50 ÷ 2 = –1.25, added to the spherical power –0.50 + (–1.25) = –1.75.

114. b) In most cases where astigmatism is 1 diopter, the contact lens power selected will be the spherical equivalent of the prescription. In this case +3.25 + (–1.00 ÷ 2) = +3.25 + (–0.50) = +2.75.

Bibliography

Jacob N. Answer to question #11378 submitted to "Ask the Experts." Website of Health Physics Society (HPS) Specialists in Radiation Protection. Published November 30, 2015. Accessed March 12, 2023. https://hps.org/publicinformation/ate/q11378.html

Wilkinson ME. Sharpen your subjective refraction technique. Review of Optometry Website. Published January 15, 2016. Accessed March 12, 2023. http://reviewofoptometry.com/article/sharpen-your-subjective-refraction-technique

Chapter 10

Biometry*

---

* Technically, the title "Biometry" is a bit of a misnomer. Biometry refers to measurement. Diagnostic/standardized ultrasound is not the same thing; it is used to evaluate, not measure.

Ledford JK.
Certified Ophthalmic Technician Exam
Review Manual, Third Edition (pp 167-172).
© 2023 Taylor & Francis Group.

> ### ABBREVIATIONS USED IN THIS CHAPTER
> - A/C   anterior chamber
> - mm   millimeter

1. **Essentially, every ultrasonic device will have the following components:**
    a) gate, gain control, spike amplifier, and Ganzfeld bowl
    b) gas electron source, power source, and transmitter
    c) pulse emitter, receiver, amplifier, processor, and display
    d) ray emitter, crystal probe, monitor, and keyboard

2. **Ophthalmic ultrasonic imaging is possible because an echo is produced as the sound waves encounter various tissues. This is known as:**
    a) refractive index
    b) echotivity
    c) prismatic effect
    d) acoustic impedance

3. **On an A- or B-scan, the gates or calipers refer to a:**
    a) wavelength
    b) spike height
    c) spike separation
    d) set of measurement markers

A-Scan

4. **Use of an A-scan to measure dimensions of the eye, including axial length and lens thickness, is referred to as:**
    a) biometric A-scan
    b) topographical A-scan
    c) optical A-scan
    d) diagnostic A-scan

5. **Which of the following is the most accurate when measuring axial length?**
    a) contact A-scan
    b) pachymetry
    c) immersion A-scan
    d) optical coherence tomography

6. **Diagnostic/standardized A-scan is used to:**
    a) evaluate the corneal surface
    b) evaluate characteristics of intraocular membranes
    c) measure the size of the optic disc
    d) evaluate the contour of the iris

7. **Which of the following represents a measurement of A/C depth?**
    a) tear film to anterior vitreous face
    b) anterior corneal surface to anterior lens surface
    c) anterior corneal surface to retina
    d) posterior corneal surface to anterior surface of iris

8. **Immersion A-scan axial length measurements are considered to be more accurate because:**
    a) optic nerve compression is not a factor
    b) corneal compression is not a factor
    c) decreased chance of corneal abrasion
    d) scleral rigidity is not a factor

9. **In immersion A-scan, what can happen if there are bubbles in the immersion fluid?**
    a) You will need to reset the calipers.
    b) The scan may have excessive high peaks.
    c) The scan may have excessive low peaks.
    d) The scan may be distorted and unreadable.

10. **The axial length of an average adult eye is:**
    a) 21 to 22 mm
    b) 23 to 24 mm
    c) 26 to 27 mm
    d) 29 to 30 mm

11. **Proper alignment of an A-scan probe is indicated by/when:**
    a) sharp spikes of roughly uniform height
    b) no blind spot is visible
    c) postoperative vision is 20/20
    d) spikes are close together

12. **In an axial length A-scan, if there is only one tall echo from the back of the eye with no other echoes behind it, this indicates:**
    a) the presence of a tumor and that an x-ray should be done
    b) that the sound beam is directed to the macula and the measurement is correct
    c) that the sound beam is directed to the optic disc and the measurement is incorrect
    d) that the sound beam is directed at the macula and the measurement is incorrect

13. **When comparing the axial lengths of a patient's left and right eye, how much of a difference between the eyes should signal you to repeat the measurement of both eyes?**
    a) 0.01 mm
    b) 0.03 mm
    c) 0.1 mm
    d) 0.3 mm

B-Scan

14. **A 2-dimensional image of the globe may be obtained by:**
    a) A-scan axial length ultrasonography
    b) diagnostic A-scan ultrasonography
    c) B-scan ultrasonography
    d) pachymetry

15. **The top of the B-scan display screen corresponds to:**
    a) the 12 o'clock position of the limbus
    b) the 12 o'clock position behind the equator
    c) the marker on the probe
    d) the position of the optic nerve in relation to the scan

16. **Changing the gain (sound intensity/amplification) settings on the B-scan is used to:**
    a) adjust probe reception
    b) adjust time-delay
    c) increase magnification
    d) move the calipers

17. **Label the following on the B-scan (Figure 10-1):**
    __ cornea
    __ iris
    __ lens
    __ macula
    __ optic nerve

Figure 10-1. B-scan. (Reproduced with permission from Kendall CJ. *Ophthalmic Echography.* SLACK Incorporated; 1990.)

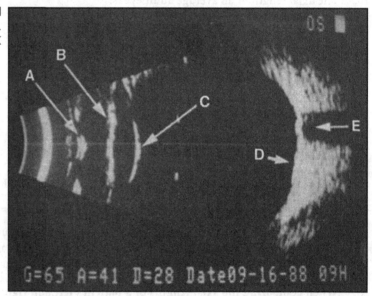

18. **The best method of evaluating B-scans is to:**
    a) view the scan in real time
    b) look at photos of the scan
    c) use a stereo viewer
    d) view them online where they can be enhanced

19. **During a B-scan, you see a quick, smooth movement of an apparent thin membrane. It is likely that the membrane is a(n):**
    a) vitreous detachment
    b) retinal detachment
    c) epiretinal membrane
    d) cloudy posterior capsule

20. **The patient has a dense traumatic cataract and count fingers vision with questionable pupillary response. The physician considering cataract surgery will often order a B-scan in this case in order to determine:**
    a) the patient's possible postoperative vision
    b) whether or not the retina is attached
    c) whether or not there is blood in the anterior chamber
    d) whether or not the eye is longer than normal

21. **Diagnostic/standardized A- and B-scan have a high accuracy in identifying:**
    a) floaters
    b) rod/cone dystrophy
    c) choroidal malignant melanoma
    d) cataracts

Study Note

Suggested reading in *Principles and Practice in Ophthalmic Assisting: A Comprehensive Textbook:*
    Chapter 17: Ophthalmic Ultrasound (pp 307-334)

Explanatory Answers

1. c) The pulse emitter sends the ultrasonic waves toward the tissue. The waves that are reflected back are picked up by the receiver and enlarged by the amplifier. The signal processor filters out the "noise" and reshapes the signal, sending it on to some type of display screen.

2. d) Acoustic impedance is the "resistance" of a substance to sound waves. Thus, when a sound wave encounters a new substance, an echo is created. You might consider this as analogous to how light waves are refracted as they travel through various media. "Echotivity" is a made-up word. Prismatic effect refers to a phenomenon of light, not sound.

3. d) The gates (calipers or over-lights) are measuring markers that tell the computer what part of the scan to measure (eg, the vertical or horizontal dimensions of a tumor). On an A-scan for axial length, most instruments have an "automatic" mode where the machine selects the appropriate-appearing spikes and measures those automatically.

4. a) The terminology alone should have given this answer away: bio- (life) and –metric (to measure). The A-scan is used, of course, for measuring the depth of the anterior chamber as well as the axial length of the eye, and the thickness of the crystalline lens. (A different type of A-scan [different probe, different amplitude, and other variations] can be used to measure and distinguish tumors in the eye.)

5. c) The immersion A-scan is the most accurate because it eliminates the potential of corneal compression; the question here was really contact vs immersion A-scan, because pachymetry and optical coherence tomography are not used to measure axial length.

6. b) Diagnostic/standardized A-scan is used when evaluating the reflective characteristics of elevated intraocular membranes and lesions. The probe used with this type of A-scan unit uses a calibrated gain setting called *tissue sensitivity*, which is not used in biometric A-scans.

7. b) A/C depth is measured from the anterior corneal surface to the anterior lens surface. Answer c) refers to the axial length of the entire eye. The tear film is not included in any A-scan measurement. The dimensions in Answer d) are not used.

8. b) Since the A-scan probe does not touch the cornea in immersion scanning, there is no chance of artificially shortening the axial length by pressing in on the cornea (possibly the most common error in contact A-scan). There is also decreased chance of corneal abrasion, since there is no

contact, but this does not render the results more accurate. The optic nerve is not compressed during any ultrasound testing. Scleral rigidity is a concern in measuring intraocular pressure.

9. d) Bubbles in the fluid bath can interfere with the sound waves, causing distortion and a poor display.

10. b) The average adult eye is 23 to 24 mm.

11. a) If the A-scan probe is properly directed onto the macula, the spikes will be sharply pointed and about the same height. There will be a gap (representing the vitreous cavity) between the anterior and posterior spikes. The blind spot is not imaged. Postoperative vision of 20/20 would be a good indication that the A-scan was accurate, but this is after the fact.

12. c) If the A-scan beam is falling on the optic disc, only one echo will appear from the back of the eye. Because the reading should be taken from the macula, this would be an inaccurate measurement.

13. d) A difference in axial length between the 2 eyes of *less* than 0.3 mm is considered a normal variation. A difference of 0.3 mm or more is just cause for repeat measurements.

14. c) Only B-scan ultrasound provides a 2-dimensional image of the globe. A-scan provides a one-dimensional measurement.

15. c) This fact is the basis for understanding orientation of B-scan displays. The B-scan probe has a mark on it (usually a white line). No matter which way you hold the probe, the area directly under the white line is always displayed at the top of the screen. This also shows why standardized technique and prompt documentation is necessary; no one but the ultrasonographer knows how the probe was oriented on a particular display.

16. a) Increasing the gain will allow display of the weaker echoes like vitreous opacities but will decrease resolution of the stronger echoes like the retina and optic nerve drusen. The opposite is also true. Most of the other controls on the unit, once set, are usually not changed. Gain does not increase magnification or move the calipers. There is no time-delay setting. *Note*: You may also see the term *brightness scan* associated with B-scan.

17. **Labeling**:
    A) cornea
    B) iris
    C) lens
    D) macula
    E) optic nerve

18. a) The best way to use a B-scan is in real time (ie, at the moment while the scan is being done). For one thing, real time offers the opportunity to detect the quality of any movement of structures in the eye that cannot be appreciated by looking at a photo (see Answer 19).

19. a) A vitreous detachment will be more "swishy"; a retinal detachment usually looks stiffer and the movement is not as pronounced.

20. b) If the patient cannot see out, then the physician cannot see in. If the retina is detached, there is little hope of visual improvement despite cataract surgery. If the retina is attached, the physician and patient may consider trying the surgery, hoping for visual improvement.

21. c) Choroidal melanoma is the most common type of cancerous intraocular tumor, and about half of these tumors will metastasize.[1] Accurate diagnosis with diagnostic/standardized A- and B-scan has been noted to be as high as 95%.[2]

References

1. Randolph J, Choi J, Miller K. Choroidal melanoma: treatment of metastatic disease. EyeWiki, Website of American Academy of Ophthalmology. Modified November 25, 2019. Accessed May 19, 2020. https://eyewiki.aao.org/Choroidal_Melanoma%3A_Treatment_of_Metastatic_Disease#cite_note-damato1-1

2. Garcia-Valenzuela E, Pons ME, Puklin JE, Davidson CA. What is the role of ultrasonography in the workup of choroidal melanoma? Medscape Website. Updated February 18,2020. Accessed May 19, 2020 www.medscape.com/answers/1190564-168446/what-is-the-role-of-ultrasonography-in-the-workup-of-choroidal-melanoma

Chapter 11

Supplemental Testing

Ledford JK.
*Certified Ophthalmic Technician Exam
Review Manual, Third Edition* (pp 173-197).
© 2023 Taylor & Francis Group.

ABBREVIATIONS USED IN THIS CHAPTER

- A/C — anterior chamber
- BAT — brightness acuity test(er)
- CCT — central corneal thickness
- CN — cranial nerve
- D — diopter
- EOG — electrooculogram
- ERG — electroretinogram
- FA — fluorescein angiography
- ICGA — indocyanine green angiography
- mm — millimeter
- PAM — potential acuity meter
- PSC — posterior supcapsular (cataract)
- RPE — retinal pigment epithelium
- TBUT — tear breakup time
- VEP — visually evoked potential

Part I*

Glare Testing/Brightness Acuity Tester

1. Your patient had a complete eye exam last year. Their diagnoses include blepharospasm, dry eye, PSC, and optic nerve drusen. Which condition warrants a BAT?
   a) blepharospasm
   b) dry eye
   c) PSC
   d) optic nerve drusen

2. Which BAT level simulates bright sun reflecting off sand or water?
   a) 1
   b) 2
   c) 3
   d) 4

3. The BAT can be used to perform/evaluate any of the following *except*:
   a) macular photostress test
   b) effectiveness of lens tints
   c) photosensitivity testing
   d) grading afferent pupillary defects

---

* Sections have been inserted into this lengthy chapter for ease of study, to allow for a logical "break" point.

Potential Acuity Meter

4. **The PAM is commonly used to evaluate macular function in the presence of:**
    a) glaucoma
    b) retinal disorders
    c) optic nerve disease
    d) media opacities

5. **Which of the following might warrant a PAM test?**
    a) preoperative posterior capsulotomy
    b) preoperative refractive surgery
    c) preoperative laser trabeculectomy
    d) preoperative laser iridotomy

6. **Before performing a PAM test, it is important to:**
    a) set the eyepiece
    b) enter the patient's refractive error
    c) calibrate the unit
    d) have the patient wear their best correction

7. **An alternate test to the PAM that uses multi-positioned grating to estimate acuity (by-passing imperfections in the ocular media) is:**
    a) contrast sensitivity
    b) laser interferometry
    c) optical coherence tomography
    d) Ishihara plates

Contrast Sensitivity Testing*

8. **The standard Snellen chart may not be adequate for evaluating how a patient really sees because:**
    a) it cannot be used in varying light conditions
    b) it does not measure macular function
    c) it is high contrast
    d) it is easy to memorize

9. **The test objects used in contrast sensitivity testing are:**
    a) graduated contrast
    b) Snellen equivalents
    c) laser-enhanced graphics
    d) various lighting conditions

10. **When testing the patient's contrast sensitivity, the following correction should be used:**
    a) none
    b) patient's habitual correction
    c) best correction
    d) spherical equivalent

* Contrast sensitivity is not listed anywhere in the criteria, but I thought it prudent to include.

11. **During contrast sensitivity testing, it is important that the patient:**
    a) be urged to guess even when not sure
    b) respond only when definitely sure of the answer
    c) maintain alignment
    d) stop when unsure of the answer

12. **During contrast sensitivity testing using gratings, the score sheet is marked to indicate the last correctly identified object in each row. This information is used to:**
    a) calculate potential acuity
    b) plot a contrast sensitivity curve
    c) calculate vision loss due to media opacities
    d) determine disability ratings

13. **Which of the following might benefit *least* from contrast sensitivity testing?**
    a) red/green color blindness
    b) diabetic
    c) pre- and postop LASIK
    d) traumatic brain injury

Proper Use of Slit Lamp

14. **The feature(s) that has made the slit lamp biomicroscope ideal for ocular examination is:**
    a) the optical section
    b) variable magnifications
    c) various filters
    d) binocularity

15. **Label the following parts of the slit lamp (Figure 11-1):**
    base ____
    base lock ____
    brightness control ____
    chin rest ____
    fixation light ____
    glide plate ____
    headrest ____
    headrest height marker ____
    joy stick ____
    lamp assembly ____
    magnification ____
    oculars ____
    slit height control ____
    slit width control ____
    stage ____
    viewing arm ____

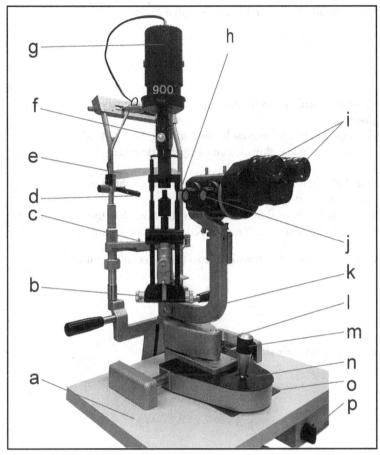

Figure 11-1.   Slit   lamp. (Reproduced with permission from Al Lens, COMT.)

16.   **When positioning the patient at the slit lamp:**
   a) shoulders should be aligned with the level of the chin rest
   b) the patient should clamp their teeth
   c) the patient should not have to strain to reach
   d) the patient should lean forward as far as possible

17.   **If positioning an infant at the slit lamp, the technique used is:**
   a) infant portability maneuver
   b) booster-seat mommy position
   c) high-five baby position
   d) flying baby position

18.   **When beginning the slit lamp exam, it is *least* advantageous to set the magnification on:**
   a) 6X
   b) 10X
   c) 16X
   d) 40X

19.   **Focusing the slit lamp on the patient's eye is accomplished by:**
   a) manipulating the joy stick
   b) manipulating the oculars
   c) manipulating the stage
   d) having the patient move forward and back

20. **All of the following features of the slit beam can be manipulated *except*:**
    a) intensity
    b) height/width
    c) depth of focus
    d) direction/angle

21. **Match the types of slit lamp illumination to its definition.**

    Term   <u>Definition</u>

    ___ diffuse   a) highlighting an area of interest by illuminating the structure behind it

    ___ direct   b) illumination source is shined at an oblique angle across the surface of a structure

    ___ indirect   c) a softer lighting that evenly illuminates the entire subject without highlighting any particular part

    ___ retroillumination d) illumination source is shined on another structure than the one of interest

    ___ tangential   e) the illumination source is shined directly on the area of interest

22. **The illumination technique used to observe cell and flare in the anterior chamber is:**
    a) retroillumination
    b) pinpoint illumination
    c) direct illumination
    d) diffuse illumination

23. **Number the following in order of a sensible slit lamp exam protocol:**
    ___ anterior chamber
    ___ conjunctiva/cornea
    ___ external/lids
    ___ iris/pupil
    ___ posterior chamber/lens

24. **To examine the temporal aspect of the patient's right eye, you would position the slit beam:**
    a) to your right and straight ahead
    b) to your right at about a 45-degree angle
    c) to your left at about a 45-degree angle
    d) to your left and at about a 180-degree angle

25. **A key step in maintaining the optics of the slit lamp is to:**
    a) polish lenses and mirrors daily
    b) replace bulb monthly
    c) lock the base after every use
    d) lubricate the glide plate weekly

26. **Which of the following would be the correct way to document a slit lamp finding?**
    a) WNL
    b) 3+ blepharitis
    c) 2+ lash crusting with 3+ lid edema
    d) 4+ viral conjunctivitis

Slit Lamp Lenses and Filters*

27. When evaluating the fit of a rigid contact lens using the slit lamp and fluorescein dye, in addition to the cobalt blue light, contrast can be improved by using a:
    a) red-free filter
    b) green filter
    c) Wratten filter
    d) diffuser

28. The slit lamp may be used to evaluate the posterior pole if one uses a(n):
    a) ophthalmoscope
    b) crosshair reticule
    c) scleral depressor
    d) Hruby lens

29. What is the dioptric power of a Hruby lens?
    a) –55 D
    b) –25 D
    c) +1.50 D
    d) +75 D

30. The physician wants to evaluate the patient's angles at the slit lamp. What device will be used?
    a) tonometer
    b) hypotenuse lens
    c) goniolens
    d) Hruby lens

31. Which of the following is a hand-held lens placed on the patient's cornea to view the retina using the slit lamp?
    a) contact fundus lens
    b) Posner lens
    c) slit lamp disc lens
    d) ophthalmometer

32. Which of the following is *not* a common feature of most slit lamps?
    a) cobalt blue filter
    b) red-free filter
    c) grid/reticule
    d) cylinder extender

Pen Light**

33. A disposable pen light might be most ideal in all of the following *except*:
    a) external exam
    b) pupil evaluation
    c) testing ocular versions/vergences
    d) Hirschberg test

* I have elected to discuss filters as well.
** For questions on the pupil exam itself, see Chapter 4: Pupil Assessment.

34. **When checking pupils, a transilluminator is preferred over a common pen light because:**
    a) the light intensity is more consistent
    b) it is more comfortable for the patient
    c) it is easier for the examiner to hold
    d) it projects an exact 40 lumens of light

Color Vision/Plates

35. **Normal color vision is referred to as trichromatic because of the 3 visual pigments that are sensitive to:**
    a) red, green, and blue
    b) red, yellow, and blue
    c) yellow, green, and blue
    d) red, green, and yellow

36. **If the patient is suspected of having an acquired color vision defect, all of the following apply except:**
    a) test color vision in each eye separately
    b) the defect tends to remain stable over time
    c) errors may be scattered all across the color wheel
    d) the defect can resolve

37. **If a woman is a carrier of the "red/green" color defect, the odds that any son she has will exhibit the color vision defect is:**
    a) 0.5%
    b) 5%
    c) 35%
    d) 50%

38. **Which of the following color vision tests uses pseudoisochromatic plates?**
    a) Farnsworth D-15
    b) Farnsworth-Munsell 100 hue
    c) Ishihara test
    d) anomaloscope

39. **Which of the following occupations can function well even with a color vision defect?**
    a) electrician
    b) bank teller
    c) public safety officer
    d) aviation

Pachymetry

40. **Measuring corneal thickness via non-optical pachymetry involves the use of:**
    a) specular microscopy
    b) ultrasound
    c) the slit lamp microscope
    d) contact mirrored lens

41. **One of the keys in accurate contact pachymetry is:**
    a) aiming the probe at the optic nerve
    b) aiming the probe at the macula
    c) maintaining contact with the coupling gel
    d) holding the probe perpendicular to the corneal surface

42. **Pachymetry readings are routinely taken prior to:**
    a) cataract surgery
    b) retinal surgery
    c) refractive surgery
    d) plastic surgery

43. **When performing pachymetry, it is generally best to begin:**
    a) with the corneal periphery at 12 o'clock
    b) with the central cornea
    c) with the mid-periphery at 12 o'clock
    d) a scleral reading for calibration

44. **CCT is an important factor in the interpretation of:**
    a) intraocular pressure
    b) visual fields
    c) optical coherence tomography
    d) fluorescein angiography

45. **Normal/average CCT is:**
    a) 480 to 500 µm
    b) 510 to 520 µm
    c) 540 to 560 µm
    d) 590 to 610 µm

Fusional Amplitudes*

Maddox Rod**

Corneal Sensitivity Testing

46. **A simple way to test gross corneal sensitivity is:**
    a) Schirmer's Test I
    b) red thread test
    c) Schiøtz tonometry
    d) cotton wisp test

* This topic also appears as a COMT® level item in *Ocular Motility Testing*. I have elected to cover it at the COT® level, in Chapter 7: Ocular Motility Testing, Questions 49-51.
** See same topic, Chapter 7: Ocular Motility Testing, Questions 84-91.

47. **The corneal esthesiometer is used to:**
    a) numb the cornea
    b) evaluate corneal sensation
    c) perform a basic Schirmer's test
    d) evaluate for perforations of the globe

48. **Before performing a corneal sensitivity test, one should:**
    a) anesthetize the cornea
    b) perform forced ductions
    c) explain the procedure to the patient
    d) measure intraocular pressure with a Goldmann tonometer

49. **The nerve that supplies sensation to the cornea is:**
    a) facial branch of the trigeminal
    b) ophthalmic branch of the trigeminal
    c) optic
    d) hypoglossal

50. **One might expect lower corneal sensitivity in all of the following *except*:**
    a) corneal abrasion
    b) herpes simplex or zoster of the eye
    c) long-term contact lens wearer
    d) patients who have had corneal refractive surgery

51. **Reduced corneal sensitivity might be associated with any of the following *except*:**
    a) diabetes
    b) multiple sclerosis
    c) cerebrovascular accident
    d) chronic obstructive pulmonary disease

52. **Persons with decreased corneal sensitivity are more prone to:**
    a) corneal injury
    b) keratoconus
    c) strabismus
    d) exophthalmos

Part II

Fluorescein Angiography Phases and Images*

53. **Number the following phases/steps of an FA:**
    ___ arterial phase
    ___ arteriovenous phase
    ___ choroidal flush
    ___ laminar flow
    ___ venous phase

* How-to instructions for FA is in Chapter 19: Ophthalmic Imaging.

54. **Match the photographs (Figure 11-2) to the correct FA phase:**
___ arterial phase
___ choroidal flush
___ full venous phase
___ laminar flow

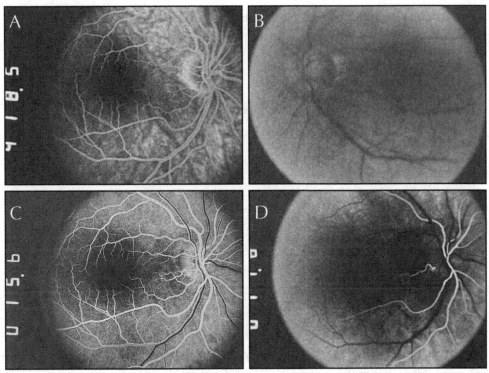

Figure 11-2. (Reproduced with permission from Cunningham D. *Clinical Ocular Photography*. SLACK Incorporated; 1998.)

55. **The "late shots" for FA are taken:**
a) 1 minute after injection
b) 2 minutes after injection
c) 10 minutes after injection
d) 60 minutes after injection

Indocyanine Green Angiography Phases and Images

56. **One of the main advantages in use of ICGA is the detection of:**
a) choroidal neovascularization
b) retinal vein blockage
c) diabetic retinopathy
d) macular edema

57. **During which phase of ICGA do the choroidal arteries fill?**
    a) early phase
    b) early mid-phase
    c) late mid-phase
    d) late phase

58. **At what point after injection does the late phase of ICGA occur?**
    a) 0 to 60 seconds after injection
    b) 1 to 15 minutes after injection
    c) 15 to 45 minutes after injection
    d) 60 to 75 minutes after injection

59. **At what point during ICGA are the choroidal vessels very faint or not seen?**
    a) early phase
    b) early mid-phase
    c) late mid-phase
    d) late phase

Electrophysiology Tests

60. **The full-field ERG evaluates:**
    a) macular cone activity
    b) both rod and cone activity
    c) rod activity only
    d) cone activity only

61. **Which of the following is *not* an indication for full-field ERG?**
    a) rule out the retina as the problem in suspected cortical blindness
    b) evaluate retinitis pigmentosa, night blindness, partial and total color blindness
    c) evaluate macular degeneration and cortical blindness
    d) evaluate central retinal artery or vein occlusion, carotid insufficiency, drug toxicity

62. **A flicker fusion ERG may be contraindicated in a patient with a history of:**
    a) angina
    b) epilepsy
    c) diabetes
    d) anxiety

63. **The VEP is an evaluation of the response to a visual stimulus by the:**
    a) cornea
    b) sclera
    c) occipital cortex
    d) extraocular muscles

64. **The stimulus most used in VEP testing is:**
    a) a set of flashing vertical lines
    b) optotypes
    c) horizontal and vertical rotating bars
    d) flashing light and alternating checkerboard pattern

65. **The indications for VEP testing include:**
    a) macular degeneration, retinal detachment
    b) media opacity
    c) unexplained vision loss, evaluating visual potential
    d) determining the cause of blindness

66. **The purpose of retinal EOG is to evaluate the:**
    a) rods
    b) cones
    c) retinal pigment epithelium
    d) retina as a whole

67. **Disorders where a retinal EOG might be useful include:**
    a) retinal detachment, central retinal artery occlusion, carotid artery insufficiency
    b) retinitis pigmentosa, juvenile macular degeneration, retinal toxicities
    c) identification of malingering patient, evaluation of cortical blindness
    d) nystagmus, nerve palsies

68. **Indications for an EOG to evaluate eye movements include:**
    a) nerve palsies and mechanical restrictions
    b) differentiate between a phoria and tropia
    c) cases of monocular diplopia
    d) none of the above

Patient Education Material

69. **"The degree to which individuals have the capacity to find, understand, and use information and services to inform health decisions and actions for themselves and others"[1] is known as:**
    a) learning style
    b) health literacy
    c) informed consent
    d) education level

70. **The ability of a patient to remember information given during an exam may depend on which of the following?**
    a) patient education level
    b) time lapse between instruction and recall
    c) patient's recall ability
    d) all of the above

71. **Each of the following is a standard learning style *except*:**
    a) automatic
    b) action-based
    c) hearing
    d) visual (verbal or nonverbal)

Assess Anterior Chamber Depth

72.   **When using a transilluminator to evaluate anterior chamber depth, one shines the light:**
a) vertically across the iris
b) horizontally (temporal to nasal) across the iris
c) at a 45-degree angle across the iris
d) horizontally (nasal to temporal) across the pupil

73.   **You are using a transilluminator to evaluate anterior chamber depth. The nasal iris is brightly lit. This means that:**
a) this patient is having an angle-closure glaucoma attack
b) the patient's pupils are normal
c) you should ask the practitioner before dilating
d) you may safely dilate this patient

74.   **When evaluating anterior chamber depth with the slit lamp, the illumination technique used is:**
a) diffuse
b) direct, narrow beam
c) direct, wide beam
d) proximal

75.   **You are evaluating anterior chamber depth with the slit lamp and cannot see any shadow between the cornea and iris. This means that:**
a) the angle is open
b) dilate with 2.5% phenylephrine only
c) the angle is narrow
d) an iridectomy is needed immediately

Ocular Coherence Tomography*

Tear Tests**

76.   **The layers of the tear film are:**
a) basal and reflex
b) mucus, aqueous, and lipid
c) mucus, aqueous, and vitreous
d) mucus, nutritive, aqueous, and oily

77.   **A tear test is appropriate in each of the following cases *except*:**
a) prior to eyelid surgery
b) prior to fitting contact lenses
c) chronic ocular irritation
d) evaluation for intraocular foreign body

---

* This topic is covered in Chapter 19: Ophthalmic Imaging, Questions 27-37.
** Rose bengal is covered in Chapter 13: Pharmacology, under *Diagnostic Agents*, Questions 156-157.

78. **If the Schirmer tear test is performed using an anesthetic, this means that you will *not* be testing:**
    a) emotional tearing
    b) basal tearing
    c) meibomian gland function
    d) reflex tearing

79. **Which of the following is *not* an element of the Schirmer tear test?**
    a) filter strip in lower cul-de-sac
    b) 5-minute timer
    c) patient looking down
    d) dimly lit room

80. **Which of the following indicates a normal Schirmer test after 5 minutes without using a topical anesthetic?**
    a) 1.5 mm
    b) 5 mm
    c) 10 mm
    d) 15 mm

81. **The normal TBUT is:**
    a) less than 5 seconds
    b) 5 to 10 seconds
    c) 10 seconds or more
    d) greater than 30 seconds

82. **Which of the following is *not* required for a TBUT test?**
    a) slit lamp
    b) rose bengal strip
    c) cobalt filter
    d) fluorescein dye

Study Notes

Suggested reading in *Principles and Practice in Ophthalmic Assisting: A Comprehensive Textbook:*
   Note: Since there are so many references, only page numbers are listed, in order of each topic's appearance in this chapter.
      BAT (*Glare Testing* pp 109-111)
      PAM (pp 111-112)
      Contrast sensitivity (pp 108-109)
      Slit lamp (p 127, Chapter 12 pp 213-232, *Slit Lamp Biomicroscope* p 388, *Slit Lamp Exam* pp 395-396, *Slit Lamp Evaluation* p 531)
      Slit lamp lenses (*Goniolens and Hruby Lens* and *90 Diopter Lens* pp 217-218)
      Transilluminator/pen light (*Transilluminator* p 67)
      Color vision plates (in *Color Vision* pp 129-130)
      Pachymetry (*Pachymeter* pp 60-61, *Central Corneal Thickness* p 533)
      FA phases (*Descriptive Interpretation* pp 286-287)
      ICG phases (*Descriptive Interpretation* pp 290-291)
      Electrophysiology tests (Chapter 18: Electrophysical Testing pp 335-343)
      A/C depth (*Angle Evaluation* p 127, *Estimation of Anterior Chamber Depth* pp 230-231)
      Tear tests (*Tear Testing* pp 131-132, Sidebar 12-1 p 228, *Dyes* pp 426-427)

Explanatory Answers

Part I

1.   c) PSC can drastically reduce a patient's vision in the presence of glare. You will want to find out if the patient experiences any visual disability in glare conditions. Dry eye can sometimes make a patient photosensitive, but c) is still the best answer. If the patient has PSC and the vision decrease is significant enough to meet insurance standards, cataract surgery may be indicated even though the patient's room-light Snellen acuity is excellent. To approve cataract surgery, insurance is generally looking for a loss of 2 lines of acuity on the "medium" BAT setting.

2.   c) The BAT has 3 levels, designated 1, 2, 3 (or low, medium, high). The highest level (3) simulates bright/direct overhead sun reflected off concrete, sand, or water, and is used to identify vision dysfunction in high-glare conditions. Level one represents a brightly/fluorescent lit room. The midlevel is meant to be like outdoor light on a cloudy day.

3.   d) The BAT cannot be used to grade afferent pupillary defects. The macular photostress test can be done by blocking the aperture with the instrument's occluder. The patient looks into the lit instrument for 10 seconds. Then the BAT is removed, and you time how long it takes until the patient can read 2 lines above their usual best acuity. Normal is 0 to 30 seconds. Thirty to 60 is "marginally prolonged" and over 60 seconds indicates the presence of maculopathy. The effectiveness of a tint or coating can be evaluated subjectively by showing the patient the different glare conditions while wearing the lenses. Photosensitivity can be evaluated in the same manner (eg, "Patient fairly comfortable at level 1, but level 2 is unbearable").

4.   d) The PAM transmits a tiny, bright eye chart to the back of the eye, bypassing media opacities. Its most common use is in evaluating macular function in the presence of cataracts (especially very dense ones where the physician has a hard time viewing the macula directly).

5.   a) The posterior capsulotomy is treatment for a cloudy lens capsule following cataract surgery. It is a media opacity and thus might warrant a PAM reading prior to the procedure.

6.   b) There is a knob on the side of the unit where you must dial in the spherical equivalent of the patient's refractive error. There is no eyepiece or calibration to set. The patient does not wear correction.

7.   b) Laser interferometry projects gratings directly onto the retina, much like the PAM. The patient is asked to identify the direction that the gratings are running until the distinction can no longer be made. The final grating that is correctly identified is translated into a Snellen equivalent, the prediction of acuity.

8.   c) The standard Snellen chart employs black letters on a bright, white background. In other words, it has high contrast. How much of our world is of such high contrast? Most of what we look at are shades and shadows. Therefore, the Snellen chart may give an exaggerated sense of the patient's acuity. Low-contrast situations that are difficult for a person with normal contrast sensitivity may be virtually debilitating to a person with low-contrast sensitivity.

9.   a) Various test objects have been used as targets for contrast sensitivity testing, including letters, objects, and gratings. The objects generally go gradually from high contrast to low contrast on a graduated scale. The patient is requested to identify the faintest object (ie, the one with the lowest contrast) possible. When gratings are used, not only is the contrast graduated, but the lines in the gratings are varied from wide to moderate to narrow. This gives more detailed information.

10.   c) The patient should be provided with best correction. If the "best" correction is their glasses, then the habitual correction may be worn... *provided that the lenses are not tinted* (which may reduce the patient's ability to discern subtle contrasts). If the glasses are tinted and/or do not provide the best acuity, then use a trial frame.

11.   a) The patient should be urged to guess when nearing their contrast threshold. If the patient is allowed to respond only when sure of the answers, the measurement will be artificially decreased. You must judge the patient's threshold by noting the point at which "guessed-at" answers begin to be consistently wrong.

12.   b) The *contrast* of the gratings vary and are assigned percentages (eg, 50% contrast or 30% contrast). The *width* of the bands also varies, known as spatial frequency. The higher the frequency, the more bars in the circle. Generally, the frequency gets *higher* as you go down the chart. The contrast goes *down* as you go from left to right. Once the test is done, the information is used to plot the patient's contrast sensitivity curve. Score sheets from one type of test may not be accurate when used with another type of test.

13.   a) Of those listed, contrast sensitivity would probably be of least benefit when examining a person with red/green color deficiency. The contrast sensitivity test can detect subtle changes that won't show up when using the standard Snellen-style charts. Contrast may be lowered in a person with ocular involvement of diabetes or someone who has had a traumatic brain injury. Macular degeneration, cataracts, glaucoma, and optic nerve disorders may also show contrast changes. The test may also be used to evaluate contrast sensitivity before and/or after refractive surgery. Persons in professions that have high-level vision requirements (eg, pilots, fire fighters, police, high-performance athletes) may need to be tested as well.

14.   a) The optical section of the light source is what makes the slit lamp so unique, and what specifically qualifies it for examination of the eye. The other items are nice, but without the optical section, examination of the eye (and especially of the cornea) would not be what it is today. You may see it written *slit-lamp*; this is also correct.

15.   **Labeling:**

base	n
base lock	l
brightness control	p
chin rest	c
fixation light	d
glide plate	o
headrest	e
headrest height marker	h
joy stick	m
lamp assembly	g
magnification	j
oculars	i
slit height control	f
slit width control	b
stage	a
viewing arm	k

16.   c) The patient should be as comfortable as possible at the slit lamp. This is especially important if you will be doing applanation tonometry, where straining can cause an artificial elevation in intraocular pressure.

17.   d) In this technique, the infant is held horizontally, belly down, with chin in the rest and forehead against the top. I made up the rest of the answers.

18.   d) At 40X, it will be difficult to orient yourself at first. In addition, even very tiny movements on the patient's part will be greatly magnified, causing the eye to "swoosh" in front of you. Start with a lower power. This will enable you to focus the instrument quickly and to locate the areas of specific interest. Once that is done, then you can increase the magnification as needed. Please refer to Table 11-1 for more examination information.

TABLE 11-1 SLIT LAMP EXAMINATION	
Suggested Power	
6X or 10X	External (lids, conjunctiva), contact lenses
16X	Angles, cornea, lens, foreign bodies, corneal abrasions
40X	Corneal endothelium
Beam Width	
1) Narrowest	Angles, cornea, anterior chamber
2) A bit wider	Cornea, lens, etc
3) A bit wider yet	External, contact lenses
4) Full width	External, applanation tension (with blue filter)
Beam Height	
Full	Most areas and structures
Short	Checking anterior chamber for cells and flare
Color/Filter	
White	Most areas and structures
Blue (with fluorescein dye)	Applanation tensions, corneal staining, tear film, staining patterns of rigid contact lenses
Green (red-free)	Evaluating blood vessels, iron lines
Diffuser	General viewing of the eye as a whole, orientation
Wratten filter	Contact lens evaluation (along with blue filter)
Adapted from Ledford JK, Sanders V. *The Slit Lamp Primer*. SLACK Incorporated; 1998.	

19. a) Once the patient and examiner are properly positioned, the slit lamp is pushed close to the patient so that the light beam focuses on the face, temporal to the eye. Then you can look through the slit-lamp oculars and use fine movements of the joy stick in/out and up/down to focus on the item of interest. It is easier if the patient is braced into the head and chin rests and not moving around.

20. c) Depth of focus is a photography term, referring to the range at which a given object of interest will stay in focus. Intensity is controlled with the voltage setting. Height/width of the beam (and slit tilt) are controlled with an adjustment knob. The observation system arm allows you to change the direction/angle of the beam.

21. **Matching**:
    diffuse   c)
    direct   e)
    indirect   d)
    retroillumination a)
    tangential   b)

22.   b) To check the anterior chamber for cells and flare, the slit lamp light is narrowed and the height reduced as much as possible (to a pinpoint) and the illumination increased. Then the light is positioned at 45 degrees and focused into the anterior chamber, in slight back and forth/left right movements, scanning the "empty space" in the A/C.

23.   **Order:**

anterior chamber	3
conjunctiva/cornea	2
external/lids	1
iris/pupil	4
posterior chamber/lens	5

Note: It is best to develop a protocol for your slit lamp examination, and to follow it on every patient. Having an established routine helps ensure that you don't miss anything. Most examiners start with the external (lids/skin) and work their way in systematically to the lens.

24.   c) To best view the temporal side of the patient's right eye, you would move the base to your left and swing the arm to your left at about a 45-degree angle.

25.   c) If the base is not locked, then every time the stage is moved there is the chance that the base will slide and "bang" when it reaches the end of the glide plate. This constant jarring is hard on the optics of the instrument. The other items are not appropriate measures.

26.   c) Puzzled? Answers b) and d) are diagnoses, not findings. Answer a) is an abbreviation that lawyers laugh at and say that it means "we never looked," although it is supposed to mean "within normal limits." Answer c) is best because it simply describes what is seen and does not make a diagnosis. (Remember, diagnosing is outside the legal realm of ophthalmic medical personnel at any certification level.)

27.   c) The Wratten filter is also called a #12 yellow filter. It enhances the color of the fluorescein by blocking out excess blue light. (By the way, the green filter *is* red-free. It is used when viewing blood vessels, among other things. See Table 11-1.)

28.   d) The Hruby lens is a slit lamp attachment that can be used to view a limited portion of the posterior pole (eg, for cup-to-disc ratios). A contact fundus lens can also be used. The ophthalmoscope is not used at the slit lamp. The reticule is a grid pattern or measuring line/cross that is in the eyepiece, used to indicate the size of a lesion or other entity. The scleral depressor is used to "push" the peripheral retina into view and is used with an ophthalmoscope.

29.   a) The Hruby lens is a –55-diopter lens used at the slit lamp to view the optic nerve.

30.   c) The lens used to evaluate the angle of the eye is the goniolens. There are several types. Generally, the eye is anesthetized, a thick coupling fluid is placed on the lens, then the lens applied to the eye itself. The examiner looks through the slit lamp and through the goniolens in order to see the angle structures. I made up the term hypotenuse lens. The Hruby lens is used to evaluate the retina/optic nerve. The tonometer measures intraocular pressure.

31.   a) The retina can also be viewed at the slit lamp with a contact fundus lens. Generally, the eye is anesthetized, a thick coupling fluid is placed on the lens, then the lens applied to the eye itself. The examiner looks through the slit lamp and through the fundus lens to see the retina. The Posner is a type of goniolens. I made up the term slit lamp disc lens. Ophthalmometer is another term for the keratometer.

32.   d) The cylinder extender is an attachment for the phoropter, if the refractive cylinder is over 6 diopters. In addition to the other items listed, other common slit lamp accessories are a diffuser filter, tonometer, and Hruby lens.

33.   b) A disposable pen light is great for examining the external eye. It is also useful for muscle testing such as versions and vergences, as well as Hirschberg and Krimsky tests. That's because, for these tests, all you need is light; the light doesn't have to have a consistent level of illumination. Not so with pupil evaluation (see Answer 34).

34. a) Modern transilluminators have halogen bulbs and rechargeable batteries, making the intensity of light more consistent than your average pen light. You may have heard it said that the most common cause of a Marcus Gunn (afferent pupillary defect) is weak pen light batteries! I found several references that mentioned a pen light being too weak to use for identifying APDs. *Note:* You may also see the transilluminator referred to as a *Finoff transilluminator* or a *muscle light*. In the UK a pen light might be called a *pen torch*. The comment about 40 lumens of light is something I made up.

35. a) The colors that the cones specifically respond to are red, green, and blue. This sensitivity comes from the cone cell's pigment. Cones that are sensitive to red contain the pigment erythrolabe. Cones that absorb green contain chlorolabe. The blue-absorbing cones contain cyanolabe. Color vision is not totally a matter of the cones, however; some interpretation takes place in the brain.

36. b) An acquired color vision defect (as opposed to a congenital defect) tends to gradually worsen unless the cause is treated. Because an acquired defect may affect the eyes differently, each eye should be tested separately. (Congenital color vision defects can be tested with both eyes together.) Instead of making matching errors in a specific color range, as with a congenital defect, those with acquired defects tend to make matching errors scattered all across the color wheel. (There are, of course, exceptions.)

37. d) There is at least 50% chance that any son she has will test as color deficient. This is true whether the father is color-blind or not. The mother is genetically XX and can contribute only an X chromosome to *any* offspring; a male is genetically XY. The carrier-mother has the color-deficient gene on only one of the Xs. With each pregnancy there is basically a 50% chance that the child will be male. For every male child, there is a 50% chance that he will get the mother's color-deficient X chromosome. (For purposes of this question and certification level, only very basic genetics are being explained. If you're interested in dominant/recessive genes, see Chapter 24: Genetics in *Principles and Practice in Ophthalmic Assisting: A Comprehensive Textbook* or some other equally reputable reference.)

38. c) The Ishihara pseudoisochromatic color plates are probably the most commonly used color vision test. Tests in Answers a) and b) are arrangement tests, where the patient must line up small caps with tips of various colors. The anomaloscope is an instrument where the patient turns a dial attempting to match the color of a test slide.

39. b) Intact color vision is not considered essential to work as a bank teller but is required for the other occupations listed. The electrician must be able to identify wire colors. The public safety officer must discern road signals and the color of vehicles and clothing. An aviator must also be able to accurately identify colors of lights and other objects.

40. b) Pachymetry is usually performed with an ultrasonic measurement. There is an optical pachymeter that uses the slit lamp, but in general the ultrasonic instrument is easier to use and more portable.

41. d) The probe must be held perpendicular to the portion of the corneal surface being measured. When measuring central cornea, this is not too difficult. The hard part is measuring the periphery, where the cornea is more curved.

42. c) The thickness of the cornea is vital information in refractive surgery, where instruments are used to alter the shape of the cornea in order to change the patient's refractive error. An error could result in a perforation or inaccurate correction.

43. b) The central cornea should be the easiest to measure since it is easier to maintain proper alignment in this position. It is also the thinnest part of the cornea, providing a number with which to compare subsequent readings. Therefore, it is best to start the measurements with the central cornea.

44. a) CCT has been implicated in the interpretation of intraocular pressure, thus becoming an issue in patients with glaucoma as well as glaucoma suspects. A thicker CCT may generate a falsely higher intraocular pressure than actually exists, meaning these patients are at less risk for developing glaucoma.

45. c) The average corneal thickness in a human is 540 to 560 micrometers (μm).

46. d) In the cotton wisp test, fibers of a cotton-tipped applicator are teased out from the tip. The cotton-tipped applicator is held at the side of the eye, and the wisp allowed to contact the cornea. If corneal sensation is present, the patient will respond (recoil, verbalize, gasp, blink, etc). The response is then recorded as normal, reduced, or absent. Each of 4 quadrants of the cornea is evaluated and rated.

The Schirmer's Test I and the red thread test are tear tests that do not involve using a topic anesthetic. These 2 tests may thus cause irritation, but they do not evaluate corneal sensitivity per se. Schiøtz tonometry (which uses a topical anesthetic) measures intraocular pressure.

47. b) The combining form *esthesio-* refers to sensation, thus an esthesiometer is an instrument used to measure sensation. *Anesthetic* (*an-* meaning without and *-esthesia* denoting sensation) logically means "without feeling," and refers to an agent used to numb tissue. A Schirmer's test is used to evaluate tear function.

48. c) Explaining any procedure to the patient prior to any testing is always advised. Evaluating corneal sensitivity must be done prior to any instillation of topical anesthetic, as in Answers a), b), and d). (Forced ductions involve using forceps to pull an eye to a specific position/duction. Topical anesthetic is required.)

49. b) The trigeminal has 3 branches: the ophthalmic (which supplies sensation to the eye [including the cornea], lids, face, and forehead), the maxillary, and the mandibular. There is no "facial branch" of the trigeminal; the facial nerve (CN VII) is a mixed nerve that affects blinking and reflex tearing. The optic nerve (CN II) transmits light and images from the retina to the brain. The hypoglossal supplies the tongue.

50. a) Believe me, a person with a corneal abrasion could wish for lowered sensation! A lower sensitivity might be found in patients who have had herpetic keratitis, long-time contact lens wearers, and patients with a history of corneal trauma (even if it is intentionally, surgically induced).[2]

51. d) Of those listed, a lower corneal sensitivity is not usually seen in chronic obstructive pulmonary disease.[2]

52. a) A person with reduced corneal sensation has a higher tolerance for ocular irritation, whether it's caused by dryness, foreign body, or infection. Because of this, they may delay seeking treatment until the case is more advanced and more damage has occurred. Patients with more severe keratoconus have been shown to have decreased sensitivity, but not that the sensitivity issue caused the keratoconus.[3]

Part II

53. **Numbering:**

arterial phase	2
arteriovenous phase	4
choroidal flush	1
laminar flow	3
venous phase	5

Note: For further study, see Table 11-2.

54. **Matching:**

arterial phase	Figure 11-2D
choroidal flush	Figure 11-2B
full venous phase	Figure 11-2A
laminar flow	Figure 11-2C

TABLE 11-2

PHASES OF FLUORESCEIN ANGIOGRAPHY

Step/Phase	Features	Time*
Injection of dye		Set to zero at beginning of push
Prearterial	Choroidal flush	10 seconds
Arterial Note: Early phase runs from beginning of injection to filling of arteries	Arteries fill	10 to 12 seconds
Capillary	Capillaries fill	13 seconds
Laminar flow	Dye begins to move from capillaries to enter veins, visible as if lining the vessel walls	14 to 15 seconds
Arteriovenous	Dye in all vessels	15 to 16 seconds
Venous Note: The Transit phase runs from beginning of injection to the point that the dye has gone through the ocular vasculature once (ie, before recirculation begins)	Dye fills veins, drains from arteries May now take photos of the other eye	16 to 25 seconds
Recirculation Note: Mid-phase runs from arteriovenous through recirculation		60 seconds
Elimination Note: Also called Late phase	Dye fading, optic nerve may be "stained"	5 to 20 minutes

55.   c) After the full venous phase (about 24 seconds after injection), the dye slowly moves out of the eye. The "late shots" are taken about 10 minutes after the dye was injected and includes photos of both eyes. Late shots on certain patients may be taken as late as 30 minutes after the injection.

56.   a) Because of the molecular structure of ICG, it penetrates the retinal pigment epithelium (RPE) better than fluorescein. It thus gives a better image of the blood system of the choroid. Other entities well seen with ICGA are choroidal tumors, inflammatory disease affecting the choroid, exudative macular degeneration (which may involve choroidal neovascularization), and central serous chorioretinopathy. The disorders listed in the other answers are better evaluated with fluorescein angiography.

* Times are estimated and vary somewhat from one reference source to another.

57.   a) The choroidal arteries fill in the early phase of ICGA (sometimes referred to as ICG *choroidal angiography*) and occurs in the first 60 seconds following injection. *Note:* The mid-phase is broken into early mid-phase and late mid-phase.

58.   c) The early phase occurs in the first minute after injection. The early mid-phase is at 1 to 3 minutes, the late mid-phase at 3 to 15 minutes, and the late phase from minutes 15 to 45. *Note:* Timing of the phases may be slightly different depending on what reference you consult.

59.   d) By the time 15 minutes have passed since injection (late phase), the choroidal vessels are either barely seen or not seen at all.

60.   b) The ERG is a test of the entire retina, including rods and cones. The test can also be modified to test rods or cones alone. During the test, the patient is exposed to a flash of light. This causes all the rods and cones to fire at the same time (a mass retinal response). The mass retinal response is recorded and evaluated. There is a specialized ERG known as a focal ERG that tests only a small area of the retina (usually the macula), but this test is not in common use. There is also a pattern ERG used to test the function of the ganglion cells. However, the full-field ERG (described first) is the one generally referred to when one speaks of an ERG. A Ganzfeld globe, which is similar to a Goldmann perimeter in appearance, is used for the test.

61.   c) All are true except evaluating macular degeneration (in situations where the ERG is not sensitive enough to pick it up). Cortical blindness is better evaluated by running a VEP; however, one might run an ERG to rule out the retina as a factor in suspected cortical blindness. An ERG might also be used to evaluate chorioretinal degenerations or inflammations, giant-cell arteritis, hypothyroidism, and hypervitaminosis. Finally, ruling out the retina as a problem in dyslexia and disproving visual loss in the hysterical and malingering patient can also be done via ERG.

62.   b) Because seizures can sometimes be triggered by flashing lights, a patient with epilepsy (or other seizure disorder) should be tested with a single flash and fewer times. The light should be covered with a red filter as well so that only cones are stimulated.

63.   c) The VEP is the response of the occipital cortex (also called the visual cortex) of the brain to a specific visual stimulus. It "provides excellent information about the functional integrity of the visual system..."[4] Unfortunately, it does not tell you which part of the visual system is at fault if an abnormal result is obtained. The VEP *does* let you know whether or not the signal is getting through all the way to the brain, and whether or not it is getting through well, poorly, or not at all. The rods and cones, as well as the ganglion cells and optic nerve, all contribute to the VEP.

64.   d) For most settings, a flashing light and an alternating checkerboard pattern are used in VEP testing. The light flash test gives information about whether or not the visual system as a whole is intact. The alternating checkerboard is an indicator of visual acuity (the examiner varies the size of the grid). It takes about half a second for information to get from the eye to the brain (if all is normal); the VEP represents the brain's response to the visual stimulus. The patient is tested many times (maybe 200) and the results are averaged.

65.   c) Because the VEP is objective, it can be used where there is a question about whether or not the patient's apparently decreased visual acuity is, in fact, due to a disorder within the visual system. It is used to evaluate optic nerve disease and visual cortex abnormalities. When combined with information from an ERG and/or EOG, the VEP can help differentiate between retinal problems and problems with the visual pathway. *Note:* As with the flicker-fusion ERG, the flash-VEP may precipitate seizures in patients with epilepsy.

66.   c) The EOG is a test of RPE function used when the physician suspects some type of retinal abnormality (especially degenerative disorders). The rods also contribute to the EOG, but it is used primarily to test RPE function.

67.   b) The RPE (as well as the photoreceptor cells) is involved in retinitis pigmentosa. In Best's disease (a juvenile-onset type of macular degeneration), the ERG is normal but the EOG will be abnormal. Retinal toxicities affecting the RPE may be due to medications (or other substances) or intraocular metallic foreign bodies. The EOG is used to evaluate nystagmus and nerve palsies (see Answer 68), but this would not be a *retinal* EOG evaluation.

68.   a) The EOG can also be used to evaluate eye muscles. An EOG might be indicated to evaluate a third, fourth, or sixth nerve palsy. The test may also be used in cases of mechanical restriction (as in an orbital floor fracture or severe scarring following strabismus surgery), neurological diseases (such as myasthenia gravis), and Duane's syndrome.

69.   b) The health literacy of a patient or guardian is an indication of how able they are to get, comprehend, and use needed health information and then to use it to make informed and sensible decisions about their health.

70.   d) All of the factors listed affect the patient's ability to recall information given during an exam. Education level affects the terms that the patient understands; they will not remember what they didn't understand. The longer the period of time between "learning" and recall, the less accurate the recall is likely to be. And some patients lack the cognitive ability to remember and process what was said. Additional factors include how much information is presented (only 1 or 2 items is ideal, but not very practical), as well as whether the patient was able to understand what the instructor is telling them. Use medical terms sparingly unless you are certain that the patient knows what you're talking about. Written patient education material should likewise use laymen's terms.

71.   a) Everyone has a way they learn best. Many students learn best if they are physically and actively involved (known as *kinetic* learning). Others are auditory learners, who need to hear the information in order to process it best. Visual learning (this is where printed and video patient education materials fall) can be verbal (reading the printed word while also hearing it or watching a video) or nonverbal (reading silently). We could certainly wish that learning was automatic! Most of us have to work at it.

72.   b) The transilluminator is held temporally and shined horizontally across the iris, temporal to nasal. You may see this referred to as the *oblique flashlight test*.

73.   d) If the nasal iris has no shadow, then the angle is open, and you may safely dilate. Conversely, if the temporal side of the iris casts a shadow on the nasal side, the angle is suspect, and you should ask the practitioner to double-check before you dilate. The shadow occurs because the iris is "bunched up" into the angle. When you shine the light across it, the bunched-up iris casts a shadow. (This would be like the rising sun shining on a hill, creating a shadow on the opposite side.)

74.   b) A direct, narrow beam (the narrowest available) directed at the limbus from about 60 degrees is used to evaluate chamber depth. This method puts a sharply focused beam of light on the cornea and an unfocused beam on the iris. The dark band in between these 2 is the object of your interest, because it represents the depth of the anterior chamber (ie, the space between the cornea and iris). See also Answer 75.

75.   c) Compare the width of the shadow to the width of the corneal band. If the shadow is one-fourth to one half as wide as the corneal band, then the angle is open (or the chamber is deep). If the shadow is less than one-fourth that of the corneal band, then the angle is narrow (or the chamber is shallow). If the shadow is missing, then the cornea and iris are so close together that the angle is closed or nearly closed (or the chamber is flat).

76.   b) The tear film has 3 layers. The mucus layer lies directly on the corneal epithelium; it serves to create a smooth surface. The aqueous (watery) layer is the bulk of the tear film; it is the middle layer. The outer layer is the lipid (oil); it helps prevent evaporation of the tears, keeping the tears on the eye longer. *Note:* There is a difference between mucus and mucous. Mucus is a noun and refers to the goopy stuff itself. Mucous is an adjective, and describes an object (eg, mucous membrane).

77.   d) If there is any suspicion of an intraocular foreign body, fluorescein (or any other drops) or tear strips should NOT be applied because the globe may have been penetrated. This scenario would be considered an ocular emergency, so tear testing would not be indicated. It is common practice to evaluate for dry eye prior to eyelid surgery because the procedure may make dry eye worse. When considering contact lenses, you need to know if the patient's tear film can support the lens. Chronic irritation is often a symptom of dry eye, and the test is appropriate.

78.   d) An anesthetic means that the tear strip will not be felt, so *reflex tearing* (or tearing caused by irritation) will not be part of the result. *Basal tearing*, which is considered to be the tearing that occurs normally, without irritation or emotional tearing, will be measured this way. The Schirmer test does not directly evaluate meibomian gland function.

79.   c) The patient is directed to close the eyes or blink normally. The patient should avoid looking down so that the filter strip does not contact the cornea. The filter strip is placed in the lower cul-de-sac for 5 minutes in a dimly lit room.

80.   d) Without anesthetic, 15 mm of wetting on the filter strip is considered normal. Anything less is indicative of dry eye.

81.   c) A tear breakup time of 10 seconds or more indicates a normal tear film. Five to 10 seconds is generally classified as marginal and less than 5 seconds as low.

82.   b) Rose bengal dye is used to evaluate the ocular tissues but is not used for a TBUT. To conduct a TBUT, fluorescein dye is instilled, and the eye is examined under a slit lamp with cobalt blue filter. The patient blinks, and the examiner begins to count the seconds, watching for the dyed tear film to start to break up. When this happens, time is called; this is the TBUT.

References

1.   Health Resources & Services Administration. Health Literacy. Health Resources & Services Administration Web site. Last reviewed October 2022. Accessed March 14, 2023. www.hrsa.gov/about/organization/bureaus/ohe/health-literacy

2.   Bernfeld E, Legault GL. Corneal esthesiometry. EyeWiki. American Academy of Ophthalmology Web site. Updated July 10, 2022. Accessed March 14, 2023. http://eyewiki.aao.org/Corneal_Esthesiometry

3.   Spadea L, Salvatore S, Vingolo EM. Corneal sensitivity in keratoconus: a review of the literature. *Sci World J*. doi:10.1155/2013/683090

4.   van Boemel G. *Special Skills and Techniques*. SLACK Incorporated; 1999.

Bibliography

Bennett TJ. Descriptive interpretation. Ophthalmic Photographers' Society Web site. Accessed March 14, 2023. www.opsweb.org/page/FAinterpretation

Chapter 12

Microbiology

Ledford JK.
*Certified Ophthalmic Technician Exam
Review Manual, Third Edition* (pp 199-210).
© 2023 Taylor & Francis Group.

```
╭─────────────────────────────────────────────────────────╮
│          ABBREVIATIONS USED IN THIS CHAPTER               │
│   • ANSI       American National Standards Institute      │
│   • OSHA       Occupational Safety and Health             │
│                Administration                             │
│   • PPE        personal protective equipment              │
╰─────────────────────────────────────────────────────────╯
```

1.   **Microbiology is the study of:**
      a) tiny organisms
      b) viral diseases
      c) how disease is spread
      d) the prevalence of an illness in the population

2.   **The microbes that live in and on our bodies but don't normally harm us are called:**
      a) pathogens
      b) normal flora
      c) infectious
      d) hosts

3.   **Microbes that can cause infection are called:**
      a) bacteria
      b) lethal
      c) single-celled
      d) pathogens

4.   **Which of the following regarding bacteria is *false*?**
      a) Most are a single cell.
      b) Most are pathogens.
      c) They are considered nonplant and nonanimal.
      d) They have no nucleus.

5.   **Bacteria are identified and classified based on:**
      a) whether or not the disorder is fatal
      b) shape and staining characteristics
      c) epidemiology
      d) disorder characteristics and species

6.   **The key feature of viruses is:**
      a) they must feed on nonorganic material
      b) they are all pathogens
      c) they have a complex structure
      d) they must have a host in order to replicate

7.   **Which of the following regarding fungi is *true*?**
      a) They are all multicelled organisms.
      b) They are considered plants.
      c) They include yeasts and molds.
      d) They have no environmental purpose.

Types of Organisms

8.   **Which of the following regarding protozoa is *false*?**
      a) Not all are microbes.
      b) They are more complex than bacteria.
      c) They are more complex than viruses.
      d) They are considered plants.

9.   **Matching. Designate each organism/disorder as:**
      a) bacteria
      b) protozoa
      c) virus
      d) fungus

      Note: Answers will be used more than once.

      __ *Acanthamoeba*
      __ *Candida albicans*
      __ Chlamydia (trachoma)
      __ *Clostridium botulinum*
      __ Epidemic keratoconjunctivitis
      __ herpes
      __ Histoplasmosis
      __ HIV
      __ *Pseudomonas aeruginosa*
      __ Rabies
      __ Staph infection
      __ Strep infection
      __ Toxoplasmosis
      __ Zoster/shingles

Pathways of Disease Transmission

10.   **The method by which contagious disease is spread is known as:**
      a) pathogen
      b) carrier
      c) direct contact
      d) chain of infection

11.   **In order for infection to occur, there must be a(n):**
      a) direct contact with the host
      b) pathogen
      c) bacterial source
      d) allergic reaction

12.   **Which of the following could be a source of pathogens in the clinic?**
      a) a mosquito
      b) the damp area behind the faucet
      c) a sandwich forgotten in a drawer
      d) all of the above

13.   **Any of the items listed in the previous question is an example of a(n):**
      a) reservoir
      b) allergen
      c) immunity
      d) inoculation

14.   **A "carrier" is an infected person:**
      a) with symptoms who cannot pass the germs along
      b) without symptoms who can pass the germs along
      c) without symptoms who cannot pass the germs along
      d) with symptoms who can pass the germs along

15.   **In order for a pathogen to find a new host, there must be a(n):**
      a) direct contact
      b) indirect contact
      c) mode of transmission
      d) contaminated surface

16.   **The most basic method to break the transmission of pathogens is to:**
      a) avoid persons with symptoms
      b) wash your hands
      c) stay home during flu season
      d) avoid touching other people

17.   **Which of the following would be most likely to transmit ocular disease in the eye clinic?**
      a) applanation tonometer tip
      b) noncontact tonometer
      c) single-use eye drop container
      d) properly used Tono-Pen

18.   **In order to infect the next potential host, a pathogen must have a:**
      a) portal of entry
      b) secondary infection
      c) primary opportunity
      d) nucleus

19.   **The best defense against external ocular infection is a(n):**
      a) clean lid margin
      b) properly fit bandage contact lenses
      c) antibiotic
      d) intact corneal surface

20.   **To complete the chain of infection, the pathogen must:**
      a) avoid the digestive system
      b) enter the respiratory system
      c) cause illness in the new host
      d) invade and infect a new host

21. Which statement regarding the chain of infection is *true*?
     a) It can be broken only if the host is treated.
     b) It can be broken at any stage.
     c) It can only be broken at certain stages.
     d) It must simply run its course.

Collection of Specimens

22. A culture is used to:
     a) identify cancer
     b) grow microorganisms
     c) treat infection
     d) identify tissue type

23. A smear is:
     a) a sample of tissue sent for biopsy
     b) a sample of tissue sent for growth in the lab
     c) a sample of material to look at under the microscope
     d) a small amount of ointment to treat ocular infection

24. Which of the following is the study of cells?
     a) biology
     b) microbiology
     c) cytology
     d) physiology

25. When the body's immune system has been activated, this triggers the response of:
     a) red blood cells
     b) white blood cells
     c) hemoglobin
     d) Golgi bodies

26. You are examining a smear on a microscope slide from a patient suspected of having allergic conjunctivitis. What cell type would you expect to be the most dominant?
     a) monocytes
     b) erythrocytes
     c) neutrophils
     d) eosinophils

27. When obtaining material for a conjunctival culture it is important to:
     a) use topical anesthesia before taking the smear
     b) avoid any discharge that is present
     c) swab both the conjunctiva and lid margin
     d) use a sterile swab moistened with sterile saline solution

28. A corneal scraping might be indicated in cases of:
     a) corneal ulcer
     b) corneal dystrophy
     c) contact lens over-wear
     d) corneal abrasion of unknown origin

29.   When taking a corneal scraping, it is important to:
       a) use a topical anesthetic prior to the scraping
       b) apply the spatula while it is hot
       c) obtain material from the center of the ulcer
       d) rub the spatula back and forth across the ulcer

30.   When obtaining material from the lid margin for a culture or smear, one should first:
       a) cleanse the area with iodine
       b) remove crusts and scales from the lid margin
       c) trim the lashes to avoid contamination
       d) apply antibacterial ointment

31.   In addition to traditional lid margin, conjunctival, and corneal smears, material may be taken
       for smears or cultures from:
       a) the anterior chamber via a tap
       b) any excised tissue
       c) the meibomian glands, canaliculi, and lacrimal sac
       d) all of the above

32.   If a test tube of broth is used as a medium, one may obtain the swab with a cotton-tipped
       applicator. The applicator is then:
       a) broken off and left in the broth
       b) flamed to sterilize it
       c) reapplied to the eye to obtain another sample
       d) squeezed to remove all traces of the broth

33.   The patient is having a small growth removed, and the surgeon is not sure if it is cancerous. In
       addition to the excision, the doctor will also prepare a:
       a) bacterial culture
       b) biopsy specimen
       c) photograph of the site
       d) transplant tissue

Clinical Asepsis

34.   The purpose of aseptic technique is to:
       a) reduce the number of chemicals present
       b) ensure proper safety measures
       c) reduce the chances of infection
       d) ensure proper ventilation

35.   To test the effectiveness of any sterilization method, one may:
       a) attempt to culture bacteria from "sterilized" instruments
       b) visually inspect the "sterilized" instruments
       c) use heat-activated testing tape
       d) keep records of any ensuing patient infections

36.   Which of the following items in the exam room is *least* likely to be contaminated?
a) phoropter
b) chin rest of slit lamp
c) chair arm rests
d) properly used Tono-Pen

37.   Surfaces should be cleansed between each patient. This is known as:
a) cleaning
b) sterilizing
c) disinfecting
d) contaminating

38.   The organism that may contaminate ophthalmic solutions, including fluorescein, and can destroy an eye in 48 hours is:
a) herpes simplex
b) *Haemophilus influenzae*
c) *Mycobacterium tuberculosis*
d) *Pseudomonas aeruginosa*

39.   Which of the following is *not* true regarding epidemic keratoconjunctivitis?
a) It can live on a surface for 30 days.
b) It can be spread via contact tonometry.
c) It is caused by the herpes virus.
d) There is no treatment.

Universal (Standard) Precautions

40.   Universal precautions are:
a) a method of infection control regulated by OSHA
b) a set of standards regulated by ANSI
c) a set of safety standards set by each clinic
d) a method of evaluating infection control

41.   The purpose of universal precautions is to:
a) maintain cleanliness
b) break the chain of infection
c) prevent contamination
d) protect the patient

42.   Universal precautions would include all of the following *except*:
a) use of PPE
b) method of cleaning contaminated spills
c) method of disposing contaminated materials
d) regarding some body fluids as always "safe"

43.   In order to comply with health and safety guidelines, one should:
a) wear gloves when collecting conjunctival specimens
b) dispose of contaminated materials in a biohazard waste receptacle
c) dispose of used needles in a sharps container
d) all of the above

Study Note

Suggested reading in *Principles and Practice in Ophthalmic Assisting: A Comprehensive Textbook:*
       Chapter 23: Microbiology (pp 439-457)

Explanatory Answers

1.   a) If you break the word down, *micro-* means small and *-biology* refers to the study of life. Thus, microbiology is the study of tiny organisms, or microbes. Most are single cells, visible only with a microscope, and include bacteria, fungi, and protozoa. Many biologists do not consider viruses to be microbes (the debate seems to center around the definition of "living"). Of course, the large fungi, such as mushrooms, are not considered microbes.

2.   b) Also called resident microbes, our normal flora consist of microbes that are normally found on our skin and in various places of our bodies. Some are actually beneficial to us. Others are potentially infectious (capable of causing infection) but only if they get the opportunity to gain entrance into the tissues (via a wound, for example). But until then, they just enjoy a benign life on the outside. We play host to them. Regarding pathogens, see Answer 3.

3.   d) Also called "germs," pathogens (Latin *patho-* meaning illness and *-gen* meaning beginning) are the originators of infection. Not all are bacteria, not all are lethal, not all are single-celled. However, just because a microbe is pathogenic doesn't mean it *will* cause illness. Some are opportunistic, and cause disease if they're in the wrong place at the wrong time. For example, the bacteria in your normal flora on your skin usually won't hurt you. But if it isn't removed prior to surgery (by disinfecting the skin during a presurgical cleansing), it can enter the wound and cause infection.

4.   b) All are true except that most bacteria do *not* cause disease. They are mainly single-celled organisms with a simple structure that does not include a nucleus. They don't qualify as either plants or animals.

5.   b) Bacteria are identified by their shape (rods, chains, etc), staining characteristics (most notably whether they are gram-positive or -negative), and culture characteristics (shape, color, smell, etc). Other identifying characteristics include size, presence or absence of a capsule, grouping or arrangement, food requirements, and oxygen requirements.

6.   d) All viruses must have host in order to reproduce. This means that they are all infectious, but not all are pathogens. There is a debate as to whether or not they are actually living things. Their structure is simple: mainly genetic material inside a protein coat. They do not "eat," but get their energy from the host cell. Technically, they don't even replicate themselves; they convince the host cell to do it for them.

7.   c) Fungi include yeast, molds, and mushrooms. Thus they can be uni- or multicellular. They are actually nonplant and nonanimal. Their function in the universe is as decomposers.

8.   d) There is debate about whether protozoa are plants or animals; the best term might be "animal-like." With lots of organelles and a nucleus, they are more complex than bacteria (and viruses) to the point where some protozoa can live independently. Not all are microbes, however. The largest is up to 20 cm... you could run away from this one! (Well, technically, you'd have to swim. It's found in the ocean.)

9.   **Matching:**

Acanthamoeba	b)
Candida albicans	d)
Chlamydia (trachoma)	a)
Clostridium botulinum	a)
Epidemic keratoconjunctivitis	c)
herpes	c)
Histoplasmosis	d)
HIV	c)
Pseudomonas aeruginosa	a)
Rabies	c)
Staph infection	a)
Strep infection	a)
Toxoplasmosis	b)
Zoster/shingles	c)

10.   d) The chain of infection is the pathway by which diseases are spread. If you break the chain, you can interfere with transmission (ie, the spread of disease). That is what universal (standard) precautions and office asepsis are all about. The pathogen is the microbe ("germ") that causes the disease. A carrier is an infected person in whom the pathogen is living, but who does not exhibit symptoms of the disease. Direct contact is only one method by which disease can be spread. The chain of infection involves:

- Presence of a pathogen
- Environment that supports the pathogen (reservoir)
- Portal of exit
- Method of transmission
- Portal of entry
- Susceptible host

These will be explained further in Answers 11 through 21.

11.   b) In order for there to be an infection, there must be a pathogen (or disease-causing microbe). Thank goodness, every direct contact does not result in disease! Bacteria are not the only potential disease-causing microbes. While an allergic reaction may occur, it is not an infectious disease in itself.

12.   d) Any of the items mentioned can serve as a place where pathogens can be living and multiplying. Such an item is a necessary part of the chain of infection.

13.   a) A reservoir implies a holding pen where the pathogens grow and build up. This could be an animal/insect, water, food, organic waste products, plant, or inanimate objects. An allergen causes an allergic response, not a disease (although some pathogens may also cause an allergic response in addition to disease). Immunity (which may be granted via an inoculation) would render a potential host immune to a particular pathogen.

14.   b) A carrier is a person who is a reservoir of the pathogen (ie, the pathogen is in their body) but does not have symptoms of the disease. Without symptoms, the person does not realize they are infected and trots happily about town spreading the pathogen. (Think of "Typhoid Mary," an historical woman who had typhus without symptoms and thus unknowingly spread the disease from one household to another.)

15.   c) Once the pathogen has exited its original host, there must be a way for it to travel to the next. This is known as the mode of transmission. Direct contact with the current host and indirect contact (as with an inanimate surface) are both methods of transmission.

16.   b) It cannot be stressed enough: Wash Your Hands! Avoiding others and staying home might be helpful but are not the first line of basic defense.

17.   a) An improperly sanitized applanation tonometer tip can harbor pathogens and spread them to the next patient. Epidemic keratoconjunctivitis, which is highly contagious, is just one example. Probably THE most likely route of transmission, however, are human hands. Wash them!

18.   a) There must be a way for the pathogen to enter the next host, which requires a portal of entry. Secondary infection occurs when a first pathogen has rendered the host susceptible (weakened), and a second pathogen uses this opportunity to invade. Not all pathogens (bacteria, for example) have a nucleus.

19.   d) An intact corneal surface is a barrier to pathogens on the surface of the eye. Once the cornea is compromised (via an abrasion, for example), pathogens have an easy way in as there is now an available portal of entry.

20.   d) The pathogen has not found a new host unless the pathogen can gain entry and then invade. For this to happen, the potential host must be susceptible. However, even if the next person has a strong immune system and can resist illness, they may still serve as a carrier to infect yet another person. Some pathogens can survive the digestive system, and the respiratory system is only one possible portal of entry.

21.   b) The chain of infection can be broken at *any* link in the process:
    • eliminated (via sterilization of instruments, for example)
    • eliminate the reservoir (perhaps by using disposable items)
    • control portal of exit (proper use of PPE)
    • eliminate transmission (WASH YOUR HANDS, cover coughs/sneezes, proper use of PPE)
    • remove portal of entry (proper use of PPE)
    • prevent infection of next host (reduce susceptibility by immunizations, healthy lifestyle, etc)
    Standard (universal) precautions are designed to break the chain pretty much at all levels. See Answers 40 through 43 for more on that.

22.   b) By definition, a culture is a method of attempting to grow microorganisms from material taken from the site (usually collected by swabbing) of a presumed infection. The swabbed substance is introduced (or inoculated) onto or into a culture medium, which is a sterile gel or broth of nutrients designed to encourage growth of microorganisms. The inoculated medium is then incubated, or given time to grow at specific controlled temperature.

23.   c) When a sample of material is collected and thinly spread on a microscope slide for viewing, this is a smear. The intent is to evaluate the material for pathogens as well as other cells that may indicate the presence/cause of a disorder. Samples of actual tissue (a biopsy) are usually sent off for evaluation by a pathologist.

24.   c) Cytology is the study of cells, which is what you're looking for under the microscope when you take a smear. Biology is the study of living things, and microbiology of small living things. Physiology studies "how things work" as applied to living things.

25.   b) White blood cells (leukocytes) are the "fighter" cells that are released any time there is an infection or allergic reaction in the body. There are several different kinds (some of which have subtypes), each with its own specific job. Even when the specific antigen, virus, or bacteria cannot be seen, the presence of a specific type of leukocyte on a microscope slide strongly suggests what is causing the infection/inflammation.
    For example, lymphocytes detect and seek to remove anything identified as "foreign" to the body; they are the most numerous white blood cells (40% to 70%). Polymorphonuclear cells (ie, granulocytes) include basophils (mast cells), which increase blood flow to an inflamed area; eosinophils (associated with allergies), which engulf foreign material; and neutrophils (associated with bacterial and fungal infections). Monocytes (single nucleus) are commonly seen in viral infections.
    As to the other answers, red blood cells carry hemoglobin to oxygenate the blood. Golgi bodies are organelles in a cell that are involved with protein synthesis.

26.   d) The presence of eosinophils suggests that an allergic response is in progress (see Answer 25). Erythrocyte is another name for red blood cell.

27. d) To obtain a conjunctival culture, do not instill anesthetic. For one thing, the procedure is only mildly uncomfortable at worst. For another, the anesthetic may be contaminated (introducing a false microbe into the study), may dilute the culture sample, or may have an antiseptic effect. Rub a moistened swab across the conjunctiva of the lower fornix, obtaining any exudate present. Avoid the lid margin (if the lid margin needs to be cultured, it would be done separately). Note that this procedure is different from a *scraping*.

28. a) A corneal ulcer can be sight-threatening and may be scraped to evaluate under the microscope for microorganisms and cells. An abrasion, even from an unknown source, would not generally be cultured unless and until there was an obvious infection or ulcer.

29. a) The patient would hardly be able to tolerate a corneal scraping without topical anesthetic. The spatula is heated to sterilize it but allowed to cool before use. Material is obtained by passing the spatula across the base or edges of the ulcer in one direction only.

30. b) Debris should be removed from the lid prior to obtaining material for a smear or culture. Use a swab moistened (but not dripping) with sterile saline.

31. d) An anterior chamber tap may be used to remove material from the chamber for culturing. Any excised tissue might be cultured. Material from any of the meibomian glands, etc, may be obtained by first cleansing the area (with a swab moistened with sterile saline) then expressing any secretions or concretions from the structures.

32. a) The rim of the tube is flamed, the swab inserted and broken off, then the rim is flamed again. A sterile swab and sterile gloves should be used. Ideally, the stick is broken off below the point where it was handled but long enough to remain above the broth. The cotton-tipped applicator is immersed in the broth.

33. b) If tissue is to be removed and there is some question as to whether or not it's cancer, the physician will do a biopsy. This involves sending the removed lesion (or a piece of it) to the lab for analysis.

34. c) The purpose of aseptic technique is to eliminate microorganisms that could potentially cause infection both for the patient and the examiner/assistant.

35. a) If bacteria can be cultured from instruments that have supposedly been sterilized, the method of sterilization is ineffective. The indicator tape or bags only testify that the required temperature occurred, not that sterilization has necessarily been achieved.

36. d) A properly used Tono-Pen has the tip covered with a disposable sheath, fresh for each patient. The other items can easily be contaminated with disease-causing pathogens (not necessarily ocular).

37. c) Inanimate surfaces that are points of patient contact (slit lamp forehead and chin rest, exam chair, back of phoropter, etc) should be disinfected between each patient. Disinfection, remember, is for inanimate surfaces. *Cleaning* is an ambiguous term, and generally refers to the removal of surface grime (eg, wiping makeup off the back of the phoroptor with a tissue). Sterilization is the total destruction of pathogens from an inanimate object, accomplished by autoclaving, etc. The surfaces in the exam room cannot be sterilized. Contamination is the introduction of pathogens to a surface.

38. d) *Pseudomonas aeruginosa* is a bacterium known to contaminate eye drops. It is particularly destructive.

39. c) Epidemic keratoconjunctivitis is caused by the adenovirus. The remaining statements are true. Contact tonometry is always suspect when there is an outbreak from a clinic, so universal precautions are paramount (see next section). There is no specific treatment for the virus itself, which is usually cleared up in about 2 weeks. Medication may be given to help alleviate symptoms.

40. a) Universal precautions (previously known as *standard precautions*) were developed and are regulated by OSHA. The universal precautions mindset considers body fluids (notably blood, semen, vaginal secretions, vitreous, and wound exudates) as potentially infectious.

41. b) The purpose and intent of universal precautions is to break the chain of infection (see Answers 10 to 21). "Cleanliness" is an ambiguous term that might mean anything from removal of visible debris to sterilization. Contamination is only one part of the chain. While there is no infection without contamination, proper handling of contaminated material/surfaces breaks the chain. And while the patient must, of course, be protected, so should you. Answer b) is the best.

42. d) The word "always" should have helped clue you in that this was the correct answer. Universal precautions calls for considering *any* body fluid as contaminated and potentially pathogenic.

43. d) All of the above procedures apply. Material obtained from the eye for cultures or smears is potentially hazardous, so you must wear gloves. Contaminated materials (gauze used during surgery, for example) and used sharps must be disposed of properly to avoid transmission of pathogens.

Chapter 13

Pharmacology*

* Drugs discussed in this chapter are those available in the United States.

Ledford JK.
*Certified Ophthalmic Technician Exam
Review Manual, Third Edition* (pp 211-252).
© 2023 Taylor & Francis Group.

ABBREVIATIONS USED IN THIS CHAPTER

- CAI   carbonic anhydrase inhibitor
- Disp   dispense
- i   one
- LASA   look alike/sound alike (drugs, abbreviations)
- NSAID   nonsteroidal anti-inflammatory drug
- PDT   photodynamic therapy
- PF   preservative-free
- Rf   refill
- RKI   Rho kinase inhibitors
- Rx   prescription (medicinal)
- Sig   signatura (how to use a medication)
- TM   trabecular meshwork
- VEGF   vascular endothelial growth factor

Note: See also Question 12.

Part I*

Drug Delivery

1. **Your patient is being treated with intravitreal anti-VEGF. This is an example of:**
   a) systemic injection
   b) topical injection
   c) local injection
   d) sustained-release injection

2. **Your patient has been given an Rx for doxycycline tablets for acne rosacea. This is an example of:**
   a) topical medication
   b) systemic medication
   c) local medication
   d) intravenous medication

3. **Your patient has been prescribed brinzolamide suspension. What key information should you give the patient?**
   a) shake the bottle well before using
   b) keep the bottle in the refrigerator
   c) rinse the bottle tip after using
   d) transfer it to a glass bottle after opening

---

* Sections have been inserted into this lengthy chapter for ease of study, to allow for a logical "break" point.

4.   **Restasis is an emulsion. This means that it:**
     a) is preservative free
     b) contains lipids
     c) is an ointment
     d) contains antibiotics

5.   **The unique feature of Timoptic XE is that it:**
     a) is preservative free
     b) is time-released
     c) forms a gel once it's on the eye
     d) has no side effects

6.   **Most preservative-free eye medications are supplied:**
     a) by Rx only
     b) as ointments
     c) for short-term use
     d) in single-dose units

7.   **Currently one of the most common preservatives used in ophthalmic preparations is:**
     a) thimerosal
     b) 5% sodium chloride
     c) 10% sodium hypochlorite
     d) benzalkonium chloride

Medicinal Prescriptions

8.   **Your physician has written the following Rx. What does it mean?**
     Rx: timolol 0.5% oph drops
     Sig: i gt bid OD
     Disp: 2 (two) 15 ml bottles
     Rf: six
     a) two 15-ml bottles of timolol 0.5% eye drops, used twice daily in the right eye, 6 refills
     b) 30-ml bottle of timolol 5%, used twice daily in the right eye, 6 refusals
     c) two 1.5-ml bottles of timolol 0.5% eye drops, used twice daily in the right eye, 6 refills
     d) 215-ml bottle of timolol 0.5%, 2 drops daily in right eye, 6 refills

9.   **Regarding medicinal Rx's, what is the NPI?**
     a) National Practitioner Identification
     b) Neuro-Pathologist Indicator
     c) National Provider Identifier
     d) National Prescribing Identifier

10. **Of what purpose is a "do not use" abbreviation list?**
     a) to make sure that everyone in the clinic uses the same notation
     b) to prevent confusion and medication mistakes
     c) to prevent the prescribing of certain drugs
     d) to monitor compliance

11.   The doctor asks you to write the patient a Rx for Tobradex drops. It is clinic policy to write it as TobraDEX in order to:
    a) make sure there is no generic substitute
    b) make sure the pharmacist spells it correctly
    c) avoid possible confusion
    d) make sure the patient can read it

12.   Match the abbreviations* to their meaning.

Abbreviation	Meaning
bid	__ as needed
d	__ at bedtime
gt	__ by mouth
gtt	__ daily
h	__ drop
mg	__ drops
ml	__ every
po	__ every day
prn	__ 4 times daily
q	__ hour
qd	__ milligram
qhs	__ milliliter
qid	__ 3 times daily
tid	__ twice daily

Instilling Drops and Ointments

13.   To prevent passage of a drug from the eye into the system as a whole and thereby decreasing the chances of systemic side effects, one should utilize:
    a) medications that are cold
    b) medications that are room temperature
    c) more than one drop
    d) punctal occlusion

Ophthalmic Drugs and the Nervous System**

14.   Pupillary dilation, rapid pulse, increased respirations, and other "fight or flight" responses are generated by:
    a) the voluntary nervous system
    b) the cranial nerves
    c) the parasympathetic system
    d) the sympathetic system

* Some of these may be on your clinic's "do not use" abbreviation list.
** Not a specific criteria topic.

15. The branch of the autonomic nervous system that is responsible for *balancing* the sympathetic system is the:
     a) peripheral system
     b) parasympathetic system
     c) antisympathetic system
     d) adrenergic system

16. The principal neurotransmitter(s) of the sympathetic nervous system is/are:
     a) acetylcholine
     b) epinephrine (adrenaline) and norepinephrine
     c) cholinesterase
     d) insulin

17. A cholinergic drug exerts its effect by impacting:
     a) blood flow
     b) spinal nerves
     c) the sympathetic system
     d) the parasympathetic system

18. A drug that copies the effect of the sympathetic system is known as:
     a) sympathomimetic
     b) sympatholytic
     c) antagonistic
     d) cholinergic

19. One example of a sympathomimetic drug is:
     a) betaxolol
     b) dapiprazole
     c) pilocarpine
     d) phenylephrine

20. The vasoconstrictors naphazoline and tetrahydrozoline fall into which group of drugs?
     a) sympatholytic
     b) sympathomimetic
     c) parasympatholytic
     d) parasympathomimetic

21. The glaucoma drug brimonidine is classified as:
     a) sympathomimetic
     b) sympatholytic
     c) parasympathomimetic
     d) a beta blocker

22. A sympatholytic drug exerts its effect by:
     a) inhibiting the parasympathetic pathway
     b) inhibiting cholinesterase
     c) enhancing the sympathetic pathway
     d) blocking the sympathetic pathway

23. **Timolol is an example of a:**
    a) parasympatholytic agent
    b) parasympathomimetic agent
    c) sympathomimetic agent
    d) sympatholytic agent

24. **Pupil dilation reversal via the topical drugs dapiprazole and thymoxamine is accomplished via:**
    a) enhancing the sympathetic system
    b) blocking of the sympathetic system
    c) destroying cholinesterase
    d) enhancing adrenaline

25. **An example of a parasympathomimetic drug is:**
    a) cocaine
    b) atropine
    c) pilocarpine
    d) carteolol

26. **The parasympathomimetic used in glaucoma treatment decrease intraocular pressure by means of:**
    a) increasing aqueous outflow
    b) decreasing aqueous production
    c) pupillary dilation
    d) increased blood flow to the eye

27. **An undesirable side effect of the miotics is brow ache, which is caused by the parasympathetic action of:**
    a) mydriasis
    b) iris sphincter contraction
    c) increased blood flow
    d) accommodative spasms

28. **A cholinergic-blocking drug (such as cyclopentolate) is an example of a:**
    a) parasympathomimetic drug
    b) parasympatholytic drug
    c) cholinesterase inhibitor
    d) sympatholytic drug

29. **An example of a parasympatholytic drug that is sometimes used to treat severe blepharospasm is:**
    a) edrophonium
    b) botulinum A toxin
    c) dapiprazole
    d) acetazolamide

30. **As a group, the following are parasympatholytic:**
    a) mydriatics
    b) cycloplegics
    c) miotics
    d) vasoconstrictors

31.   **The biochemical cholinesterase acts on:**
a) acetylcholine
b) epinephrine
c) norepinephrine
d) aqueous

32.   **Drugs that are cholinesterase inhibitors (anti-cholinesterases) will affect the:**
a) levels of epinephrine
b) voluntary nervous system
c) sympathetic system
d) parasympathetic system

33.   **As a group, the cholinesterase inhibitors include:**
a) the direct-acting miotics
b) the indirect-acting miotics
c) the beta blockers
d) the cycloplegics

34.   **A cholinesterase inhibitor used in the differential diagnosis of ptosis is:**
a) cocaine
b) edrophonium
c) tetrahydrozoline
d) botulinum A toxin

Mydriatics and Cycloplegics

35.   **Of the following drug groups, which are used in the clinic for pupil dilation?**
a) nonsteroidal anti-inflammatories
b) antibiotics
c) miotics
d) mydriatics

36.   **Number these cycloplegics and mydriatics from 1 to 6 in order from *shortest* lasting to *longest* lasting.**
atropine   ____
cyclopentolate   ____
homatropine   ____
phenylephrine   ____
scopolomine   ____
tropicamide   ____

37.   **Which of the following is most appropriate for use on an 8-year-old patient needing a refraction?**
a) phenylephrine
b) atropine
c) phospholine iodide
d) cyclopentolate

38. If an adult patient is unintentionally dilated with atropine for a routine eye exam, they will probably call the office in a few days complaining of:
   a) redness
   b) itching
   c) persistent dilation
   d) anaphylactic shock

39. Which of the following is appropriate for a 65-year-old patient with painful iritis to use at home?
   a) homatropine
   b) tropicamide
   c) phenylephrine
   d) tetracaine

40. Which of the following is the most potent cycloplegic?
   a) tropicamide
   b) cyclopentolate
   c) atropine
   d) scopolomine

Part II

Glaucoma Medications

41. The most ideal drug for treatment of chronic open-angle glaucoma:
   a) effectively lowers intraocular pressure
   b) has no side effects
   c) requires once-a-day dosing
   d) all of the above

42. Medical use of marijuana for glaucoma is not advocated because:
   a) the intraocular pressure lowering is brief and small
   b) medical marijuana is illegal in all 50 states
   c) the side effects are unpleasant
   d) it can lead to use of illegal drugs

Beta Blockers

43. Which of the following is *not* a beta blocker?
   a) timolol
   b) soperonol
   c) levobunolol
   d) betaxolol

44.   **Which of the following is *not* a beta blocker?**
a) Timoptic
b) OptiPranolol
c) Betagan
d) Iopidine

45.   **Beta blockers are identified by:**
a) purple caps
b) green or red caps
c) blue or yellow caps
d) brown bottles

46.   **Which of the following is *not* true regarding beta blockers?**
a) They can be used in addition to miotics.
b) They act by reducing aqueous production.
c) They are safe to use even in cases of chronic obstructive pulmonary disease.
d) They are convenient because they usually are administered twice daily.

47.   **Before beginning a patient on a beta blocker for glaucoma, the physician may request:**
a) complete blood work
b) a baseline blood pressure
c) a chest X-ray
d) oxygen saturation

48.   **The unique feature of the beta blocker Timoptic XE is:**
a) it comes in unit-dose capsules
b) it is available over the counter
c) it has the least side effects
d) it forms a gel when applied

49.   **Systemically, beta blockers are used to treat:**
a) congestive heart failure and hypertension
b) fluid retention and insomnia
c) asthma
d) inflammatory conditions

50.   **Which of the following would be safer to use in a patient with a history of lung problems?**
a) Timoptic
b) Betagan
c) Betoptic
d) OptiPranolol

51.   **Possible side effects of beta blockers include:**
a) decreased heart rate and decreased respiration rate
b) decreased heart rate and increased respiration rate
c) increased heart and increased respiration rate
d) increased heart rate and decreased respiration rate

52. **Other side effects of beta blockers can include:**
    a) miosis and ciliary spasms
    b) depression, insomnia, and impotence
    c) increased need of insulin in diabetics
    d) depression of the immune system

Alpha-2 Agonists

53. **Topical ophthalmic alpha-2 agonists are used to:**
    a) reduce inflammation
    b) lower intraocular pressure
    c) clear the cornea
    d) reduce allergy symptoms

54. **Alpha-2 agonists reduce intraocular pressure by:**
    a) reducing aqueous production
    b) increasing trabecular outflow
    c) increasing uveoscleral outflow
    d) both a) and b)

55. **Which of the following is an alpha-2 agonist used short-term to prevent intraocular pressure spikes following some laser procedures?**
    a) iopidine
    b) brimonidine
    c) pilocarpine
    d) tetracaine

56. **Alpha-2 agonist eye drops have a high rate of causing:**
    a) eye color change
    b) skin discoloration
    c) an allergic reaction
    d) eyelash growth

Prostaglandin Analogs

57. **In ophthalmology, prostaglandin analogs are used to treat:**
    a) glaucoma
    b) allergy symptoms
    c) infection
    d) inflammation

58. **Prostaglandin analogs work by:**
    a) decreasing inflammation
    b) increasing aqueous production
    c) preventing infection
    d) increasing aqueous outflow

59. Patient compliance using prostaglandins may be better than other treatments because:
     a) they can be used at home
     b) they are administered once every week
     c) they are used once daily
     d) they have no side effects

60. Possible side effects of prostaglandin analogs include all of the following *except*:
     a) lash growth
     b) change in iris color
     c) breakdown of ocular fat
     d) bleached sclera

61. Examples of prostaglandin analogs include:
     a) Xalatan, Lumigan
     b) Betagan, Betoptic
     c) Diamox, Trusopt
     d) Pred Forte, Inflamase

62. Which of the following is a contraindication for treatment with prostaglandin analogs?
     a) choroidal nevus
     b) active uveitis
     c) corneal dystrophy
     d) diabetic retinopathy

Carbonic Anhydrase Inhibitors

63. CAIs have what effect on the eye?
     a) reduce corneal edema
     b) lower intraocular pressure
     c) stimulate accommodation
     d) reduce inflammation

64. CAIs are used in the treatment of glaucoma because they:
     a) increase aqueous outflow
     b) decrease aqueous outflow
     c) increase aqueous production
     d) reduce aqueous production

65. All of the following are topical medications containing CAIs for glaucoma treatment *except*:
     a) Lumigan
     b) Trusopt
     c) Azopt
     d) CoSopt

66. The *most* common side effect of oral CAIs is:
     a) development of kidney stones
     b) tingling of the extremities
     c) metallic taste in the mouth
     d) depression and fatigue

67. **CAIs should not be given to patients who are allergic to:**
    a) penicillin
    b) sulfa drugs
    c) sulfur drugs
    d) erythromycin

Rho Kinase Inhibitors

68. **RKIs lower intraocular pressure by:**
    a) reducing aqueous production
    b) increasing trabecular outflow
    c) increasing uveoscleral outflow
    d) both a) and b)

69. **Which of the following are RKIs?**
    a) Rhopressa and Rocklatan
    b) Azopt and Trusopt
    c) Lotemax and Durezol
    d) Viagmox and Ocuflox

70. **In addition to redness and stinging, which of the following can be a side effect of RKIs that the patient might notice?**
    a) subconjunctival hemorrhage
    b) corneal whorls
    c) decreased night vision
    d) metallic taste

71. **The action of RKIs has been shown to be enhanced by the addition of:**
    a) betaxolol
    b) epinephrine
    c) latanoprost
    d) brimonidine

Miotics

72. **Miotics exert their effect by:**
    a) stimulating the TM
    b) stimulating the dilator muscle of the iris
    c) stimulating the sphincter muscle of the iris
    d) stimulating the ciliary body

73. **Miotics may be used in all of the following *except*:**
    a) open- and closed-angle glaucoma
    b) overcorrection following refractive surgery
    c) convergent strabismus
    d) posterior subcapsular cataracts

74. **Miotics act to lower intraocular pressure by:**
    a) increasing aqueous outflow
    b) decreasing aqueous production
    c) providing a new outlet for aqueous drainage
    d) dilating the pupil

75. **Which of the following is the most commonly used miotic for intraocular pressure control?**
    a) carbachol
    b) dapiprazole
    c) echothiophate
    d) pilocarpine

76. **Which of the following is part of the patient education information regarding use of miotics?**
    a) Call the office immediately if you experience headaches.
    b) Discontinue the medication if you experience headaches.
    c) Any drug-related headaches usually go away with continued use.
    d) This medication frequently causes headaches during the entire time it is used.

Epinephrine

77. **The most common use of topical ocular medications containing epinephrine is:**
    a) dilation
    b) glaucoma treatment
    c) decrease wound bleeding
    d) dry eye treatment

78. **Epinephrine acts to lower the intraocular pressure by:**
    a) preventing mast cells from releasing histamine
    b) facilitating aqueous production
    c) decreasing aqueous formation and facilitating outflow
    d) binding to specific receptor cells

79. **Epinephrine stimulates the "fight or flight" (sympathetic) division of the nervous system. Therefore, its side effects may include:**
    a) rapid pulse and respiration, stomach upset
    b) muscle cramps, dry mouth
    c) headache, accommodative spasms
    d) slow pulse and respiration, increased digestion

Osmotics*

80. **Oral and intravenous osmotics are used in the treatment of:**
    a) corneal edema
    b) angle-closure glaucoma
    c) open-angle glaucoma
    d) iritis

81. **Osmotics exert their effect by:**
    a) drawing water out of the tissues
    b) drawing water out of the blood stream
    c) causing blood vessels to constrict
    d) causing blood vessels to dilate

82. **Oral glycerin is best administered:**
    a) diluted with water
    b) straight from the bottle so it can be drunk quickly
    c) followed by 32 ounces of water
    d) over ice and sipped slowly with a straw

83. **If a patient who is being given an oral osmotic for rapid intraocular pressure reduction complains of thirst, they should:**
    a) be given more osmotic
    b) be given a drink of water
    c) not be given anything to drink
    d) be told to lie down

84. **Possible side effects of oral or intravenous osmotics include:**
    a) tearing, excess salivation, and insomnia
    b) dehydration, headache, and disorientation
    c) tissue edema, metallic taste, and tingling of extremities
    d) ringing in the ears, kidney stones, and back pain

Part III

Anti-Infective Agents

Antibiotics

85. **Antibiotics are used in ophthalmology in cases of:**
    a) fungal infections
    b) bacterial infections
    c) viral infections
    d) allergic reactions

* This particular treatment of osmotics is regarding intraocular pressure control only.

86. **Antibiotics that kill microorganisms are called:**
    a) sulfonamides
    b) bacteriocidal
    c) bacteriostatic
    d) antiseptics

87. **Antibiotics that inhibit the reproduction and growth of microorganisms are called:**
    a) penicillins
    b) bacteriocidal
    c) bacteriostatic
    d) germicidal

88. **In order to select an antibiotic that will kill a specific microorganism, the physician might order:**
    a) a biopsy
    b) a slit lamp exam
    c) a culture
    d) a fluorescein angiogram

89. **An antibiotic that will kill many different types of microorganisms would be referred to as:**
    a) broad spectrum
    b) narrow spectrum
    c) bacteriostatic
    d) hyper-effective

90. **What should patients be told regarding the use of oral antibiotics?**
    a) Take it until you feel better, then discontinue.
    b) Take several days' worth, then discontinue even if you have medication left.
    c) Take all but 2 days' worth, in order to save some in case you relapse later.
    d) Take all of the medication until it is gone, even if you feel well.

91. **Which topical antibiotic is most likely to cause a local allergic reaction?**
    a) tobramycin
    b) gentamicin
    c) neomycin
    d) erythromycin

92. **Systemic effects of antibiotics, especially oral antibiotics, can include all of the following *except*:**
    a) development of resistant bacteria
    b) allergic and anaphylactic reactions
    c) gastrointestinal disturbance
    d) increased blood glucose levels

93. **What percentage of the population is reported to be allergic to penicillin?**
    a) 10%
    b) 15%
    c) 20%
    d) 30%

Antivirals

94. **Vidarabine is used specifically to treat:**
    a) herpes zoster
    b) herpes simplex
    c) bacterial conjunctivitis with allergic response
    d) lice living on the lash line

95. **Which of the following is *not* an indication for use of a topical antiviral medication if the eye is affected?**
    a) cytomegalovirus
    b) shingles
    c) chicken pox
    d) acanthamoebiasis

96. **On slit lamp exam, the physician has found a corneal dendrite. This will most likely be treated with:**
    a) neomycin
    b) sulfonamide
    c) acyclovir
    d) natamycin

Antifungals

97. **Which of the following is a topical ophthalmic antifungal drug?**
    a) natamycin
    b) mycomycin
    c) prednisolone
    d) viderabine

98. **Topical natamycin is used in which of these ocular infections?**
    a) mycotic endophthalmitis
    b) mycotic keratitis
    c) chalazion
    d) chlamydia keratitis

Anti-Parasitics

99. **Which of the following is *true* regarding treatment of ocular parasites?**
    a) Treatment always involves removal of the specific parasite.
    b) Treatment must be specific to the type of invading parasite.
    c) First-line treatment is antibiotics to prevent secondary infection.
    d) Steroids are used because they are toxic to parasites.

Allergy Medications

100. **Vasoconstrictors act by:**
    a) constricting blood vessels
    b) constricting the heart
    c) constricting the dilator muscle
    d) constricting the crystalline lens

101. **Vasoconstrictors are used to:**
    a) lower intraocular pressure
    b) enhance drug absorption
    c) "whiten" the eye
    d) reduce itching and watering

102. **Vasoconstrictors also are known by the term:**
    a) antibiotics
    b) antihistamines
    c) decongestants
    d) lubricators

103. **Which of the following is *not* commonly used as a decongestant?**
    a) phenylephrine
    b) scopolamine
    c) tetrahydrozoline
    d) naphazoline

104. **Use of topical vasoconstrictors is contraindicated in the patient with:**
    a) dry eye
    b) hay fever
    c) subconjunctival hemorrhage
    d) tired, red eyes

105. **A possible side effect of ocular vasoconstrictors is:**
    a) miosis
    b) inflammation
    c) angle closure
    d) cataract formation

Antihistamines

106. **The purpose of antihistamines is to block the release of histamine, thus:**
    a) lowering intraocular pressur
    b) reversing pupil dilation
    c) blocking some symptoms of the allergic response
    d) stopping the allergic response

107. **Each of the following contains a topical antihistamine *except*:**
    a) epinastine (Elestat)
    b) naphazoline (Naphcon A)
    c) cromolyn (Crolom)
    d) olopatadine (Patanol)

108. **Topical antihistamines are combined frequently with:**
    a) antivirals
    b) decongestants
    c) steroids
    d) nonsteroidal anti-inflammatories

109. **All of the following are *false* regarding antihistamines *except*:**
    a) They are available only by Rx.
    b) Topical preparations have no systemic side effects.
    c) Some oral preparations may cause drowsiness.
    d) They are used to treat infection.

110. **A patient taking oral antihistamines may notice:**
    a) dry eye symptoms
    b) increased vision
    c) decreased night vision
    d) floaters in the eyes

Mast Cell Stabilizers

111. **Drugs designed to prevent the allergic response by blocking histamine release are:**
    a) beta blockers
    b) mast cell stabilizers
    c) anesthetics
    d) steroids

112. **Which of the following is a mast cell stabilizer?**
    a) cromolyn
    b) pilocarpine
    c) atropine
    d) ketorolac

113. **Allergies affecting the eyes are most often treated with:**
    a) mast cell stabilizers
    b) antihistamines
    c) combination mast cell stabilizer and antihistamine
    d) combination vasoconstrictor and antihistamine

Steroids

114. **Steroids are used to treat:**
    a) bacterial infections
    b) viral infections
    c) inflammatory conditions
    d) glaucoma

115. **All of the following might logically be treated with topical steroids *except*:**
    a) iritis
    b) scleritis and episcleritis
    c) herpes zoster ophthalmicus
    d) herpes simplex keratitis

116. **In ophthalmology, oral steroids are usually used in cases of:**
    a) disorders involving the conjunctiva and cornea
    b) secondary glaucoma
    c) disorders involving the anterior segment
    d) disorders involving the posterior segment

117. **All of the following are examples of steroids *except*:**
    a) prednisolone
    b) diazepam
    c) dexamethasone
    d) hydrocortisone

118. **Which of the following are topical steroid drops?**
    a) Durezol, FML, PredForte
    b) Blephamide, Cortisporin, Maxitrol, TobraDex
    c) Ocufen, Voltaren, Acular PF
    d) Tobrex, Ciloxin, Vigamox

119. **Your patient has been using topical steroids 4 times per day for iritis. There are no longer signs of inflammation in the anterior chamber. Most likely the physician will have the patient:**
    a) stop the medication
    b) increase the drops to 6 times per day
    c) gradually decrease the drops
    d) switch to an antibiotic to ward off secondary infection

120. **A patient who had successful cataract surgery one-and-a-half weeks ago calls with onset of redness and mild pain. You ask how they are using their drops, and they have stopped using them all. The patient may be experiencing:**
    a) elevated intraocular pressure
    b) rebound inflammation
    c) subcapsular opacity
    d) displaced intraocular lens

121. **Your patient is taking topical steroid drops for keratitis. Which of the following tests is *most* important?**
    a) tonometry
    b) color vision test
    c) glare test
    d) keratometry

122. **Your patient is taking oral steroids for posterior uveitis. Which of the following tests or exams is *most* important?**
    a) fundus exam
    b) slit lamp exam
    c) Schirmer's tear test
    d) extraocular muscle function tests

123. **The systemic side effects of steroids include:**
    a) dizziness, dehydration, elevated blood pressure, and insomnia
    b) headaches, sleeplessness, hallucinations, and increased pulse
    c) dehydration, lowered blood pressure, excitability, and confusion
    d) sweating, elevated blood pressure, weakness, and delayed wound healing

124. **A serious drawback of oral or topical steroids is that they can:**
    a) boost the immune system
    b) depress the immune system
    c) cause strokes
    d) decrease blood glucose levels

125. **Ocular side effects of topical steroids can include:**
    a) development of subcapsular cataracts
    b) subnormal intraocular pressure
    c) miotic pupil
    d) accommodative spasms

126. **Topical steroids are frequently combined with which of the following?**
    a) timolol to lower intraocular pressure
    b) NSAIDs to decrease inflammation
    c) antivirals to combat infection
    d) antibiotics to combat infection

Nonsteroidal Anti-Inflammatory Drugs

127. **Topical NSAIDs might be indicated in all of the following *except*:**
    a) reducing postoperative inflammation
    b) elimination of most ocular allergic symptoms
    c) relief of allergic itching
    d) preventing pupillary miosis during surgery

128. **Topical NSAIDs are sometimes preferred over steroids because:**
    a) they do not significantly elevate intraocular pressure with long-term use
    b) they control inflammation better
    c) they can be combined with antibiotics
    d) they do not sting on instillation

129. **All of the following are topical NSAIDs *except*:**
    a) Nevanac
    b) FML
    c) Voltaren
    d) Acular PF

130. **In which situation is use of topical NSAIDs contraindicated?**
    a) mild uveitis
    b) acute infection
    c) postoperative refractive surgery
    d) allergic conjunctivitis

131. **Which of the following is an NSAID that may be used following cataract or corneal refractive surgery?**
     a) pilocarpine
     b) Patanol
     c) ketotifen
     d) ketorolac

Part IV

Ocular Lubricants

132. **Patients who use nonpreserved artificial tears supplied in "bullets" should be told to:**
     a) use them only once per day
     b) discard the leftover solution at the end of the day
     c) use them only at night
     d) make their own saline because it is cheaper

133. **Dry eye patients should be told to use artificial tears:**
     a) morning and night
     b) only when the eyes water
     c) 4 times daily
     d) as often as needed to control symptoms

134. **Which of the following lubricant types would stay on the eye longest?**
     a) liquid drop
     b) liquid drop with emulsifier
     c) gel
     d) ointment

135. **Which of the following is *not* a disadvantage of a thicker ocular lubricant?**
     a) it blurs vision
     b) the adhesion of allergens
     c) it may mat the lashes
     d) it has a long contact time

Anesthetics

136. **Anesthesia used to induce sleep is known as:**
     a) topical anesthesia
     b) regional anesthesia
     c) local anesthesia
     d) general anesthesia

137. **An example of a procedure that would use local anesthetic is:**
     a) cataract extraction on an infant
     b) chalazion excision on an adult
     c) noncontact tonometry
     d) corneal topography studies

138. **Local anesthetic can be injected into the area of the nerve that supplies sensation to the surgical site. This is known as:**
    a) a regional block
    b) a site-specific local
    c) general
    d) topical

139. **The type of anesthesia named in the previous question might be used for which surgical situation?**
    a) chalazion excision
    b) corneal transplant
    c) cataract surgery
    d) laser trabeculoplasty

140. **In addition to eliminating sensation, local anesthetic is sometimes required to:**
    a) temporarily block vision
    b) prevent movement
    c) calm the patient
    d) irrigate the surgical site

141. **Which of the following are commonly used local anesthetics?**
    a) lidocaine, procaine
    b) cocaine, proparacaine
    c) butane, tetracaine
    d) benoxinate, butacaine

142. **The most common side effect of local anesthetic is:**
    a) cardiac arrest
    b) respiratory arrest
    c) increased blood pressure
    d) dizziness and nausea

143. **Other side effects of *local* anesthetics include:**
    a) lowered blood pressure, slowing of respiration
    b) lowered blood pressure, rapid heartbeat
    c) increased blood pressure, rapid respiration
    d) increased blood pressure, respiratory collapse

144. **Which of the following drugs is an anesthetic?**
    a) mannitol
    b) cortisone
    c) cocaine
    d) betaxolol

145. **All of the following procedures are routinely performed using topical anesthetic *except*:**
    a) specular microscopy
    b) pachymetry
    c) initial contact lens fitting
    d) applanation tonometry

146. **The most common side effect of topical anesthetics is:**
    a) contact allergic reaction
    b) fainting
    c) increased blood pressure
    d) dizziness

147. **Which of the following are commonly used topical anesthetics?**
    a) cocaine, lidocaine
    b) proparacaine, tetracaine
    c) procaine, bupivacaine
    d) prilocaine, epinephrine

148. **After instilling a topical anesthetic into the eye, the patient should be warned:**
    a) to keep the eyes dry
    b) to keep the eyes closed
    c) to be careful driving
    d) not to rub the eye

149. **Epinephrine might be added to a local anesthetic in order to:**
    a) decrease pain further
    b) make the anesthetic last longer
    c) make the anesthetic metabolize faster
    d) promote healing

Diagnostic Agents

150. **Your patient may have a corneal abrasion, so you have instilled topical fluorescein. What else must you do to view the cornea most clearly?**
    a) use a cobalt blue light
    b) use an ultraviolet light
    c) use polarized light
    d) use a red-free light

151. **When appropriately applied and viewed, a fluorescein stain is:**
    a) reddish purple
    b) orange/yellow
    c) greenish yellow
    d) colorless

152. **Your patient has glaucoma and also wears soft contact lenses. You have removed the contact lens, instilled fluorescein, and performed applanation tonometry. What is your next step?**
    a) irrigate the eyes
    b) re-insert the contacts
    c) apply a drop of artificial tears
    d) throw the contact away

153. **Because of possible microbial contamination, topical fluorescein dye is available as:**
    a) multi-use containers
    b) intravenous liquid
    c) impregnated filter strips
    d) pellets to insert into the cul-de-sac

154. **The aggressive bacterium that can contaminate fluorescein drops is:**
    a) *Staphylococcus aureus*
    b) *Pseudomonas aeruginosa*
    c) *Treponema pallidum*
    d) *E. coli*

155. **The side effects or complications of fluorescein dye injection include:**
    a) yellowish skin and urine
    b) nausea and vomiting
    c) infiltration
    d) all of the above

156. **In which condition would using rose bengal be of most benefit?**
    a) glaucoma
    b) severe dry eye
    c) conjunctival injection
    d) corneal foreign body

157. **Lissamine green dye may be preferred to rose bengal because:**
    a) it is less irritating
    b) the dye disappears faster
    c) no cobalt blue light is needed
    d) it does not require a diffusing filter

158. **Which of the following might be used to image the deeper layers of the choroid?**
    a) indocyanine green dye
    b) fluorescein dye
    c) trypan blue dye
    d) methylene blue dye

159. **Which of the following might be used to stain the anterior capsule during cataract surgery?**
    a) methylene blue dye
    b) lissamine green dye
    c) Gram stain
    d) trypan blue dye

Nutritional Supplements

160. **Vitamins and minerals that have been indicated in treatment of macular degeneration are:**
    a) Vitamins B, B_{12}, and D, and magnesium
    b) Vitamin C, calcium, and iron
    c) Vitamin D, fluoride, and manganese
    d) Vitamins C and E, beta-carotene, and zinc

161. **Smokers who take "eye vitamins" should avoid those containing:**
    a) Vitamin A
    b) Vitamin C
    c) beta-carotene
    d) lutein

162. **Nutrients that have been cited to be of especial help in patients with dry eye:**
    a) iron
    b) omega-3 fatty acids
    c) free radicals
    d) cinnamon

163. **Your physician is recommending that a patient begin taking "eye vitamins" for macular degeneration. The doctor asks the patient if they are taking any vitamins already. This question is pertinent because:**
    a) high levels of some vitamins are toxic
    b) the more, the better
    c) only name-brand vitamins are helpful
    d) "eye" vitamins can counteract regular vitamins

164. **Some patients believe that eating carrots can help them see better, especially at night. While this is not true, it is based on the fact that Vitamin A is needed to form:**
    a) red blood cells
    b) aqueous
    c) vitreous
    d) rhodopsin

Antineovascular Drugs

165. **VEGF stands for:**
    a) vascular epithelial germination factor
    b) vascular endothelial growth factor
    c) vasoendotrachial growth faction
    d) vasotubular endothelial ganglion factor

166. **Currently, retinal neovascularization may be treated with:**
    a) steroidal drugs
    b) NSAIDs
    c) anti-VEGF drugs
    d) miotics

167. **Which of the following conditions might be treated with anti-VEGF?**
    a) Christmas tree cataract
    b) xanthelasma
    c) wet macular degeneration
    d) retinal detachment

168. **The majority of patients treated with anti-VEGF drugs experience:**
    a) stabilization of vision
    b) vision improvement
    c) loss of central vision
    d) floaters and flashes

169. Which of the following is *not* an anti-VEGF medication for retinal neovascularization?
    a) pegaptanib (Macugen)
    b) ranibizumab (Lucentis)
    c) verteporfin (Visudyne)
    d) aflibercept (Eylea)

Miscellaneous*

170. A commonly used topical osmotic for the long-term treatment of corneal edema is:
    a) mannitol
    b) rose bengal
    c) sodium chloride drops or ointment
    d) fluorescein sodium solution

171. A disadvantage to use of topical osmotic agents is:
    a) ocular discomfort
    b) ciliary spasm
    c) brow ache
    d) blurred vision

172. A patient calls in, complaining of coughing, wheezing, and shortness of breath. They had cataract surgery 2 weeks ago. They are using the usual postop ketorolac and Vigamox drops. Their intraocular pressure was elevated on their day one postop appointment, and they were prescribed Betoptic. Which could be associated with the patient's pulmonary symptoms?
    a) ketorolac
    b) Vigamox
    c) Betoptic
    d) none of the above

173. A patient calls in complaining of a funny taste in their mouth and tingling in their fingers. This is most likely a side effect of which medication?
    a) ketorolac
    b) erythromycin
    c) ketotifen
    d) latanaprost

174. A patient calls in complaining of blurred vision and dilation in the right eye since the second day of a 2-week cruise. They got home yesterday, and the problem persists. A list of medications they used during the cruise include the following. Which is the most likely to have caused the problem?
    a) artificial tears
    b) antinausea patch
    c) ocular decongestant
    d) oral antihistamine

*Note to the student: While these topics are not specifically on the official COT® criteria list, they are things I believe a COT® should know.

175. A patient requires a topical eye medication that is not commercially available. The physician has contacted a pharmacist who will hand-make the medication. This is known as:
   a) standardizing
   b) compounding
   c) prepackaging
   d) concocting

176. A medication has been FDA-approved for a specific use. It is, however, commonly used for other treatments that are not specified. This is known as:
   a) off-label use
   b) illegal use
   c) preapproval use
   d) banned usage

Study Notes

Suggested reading in *Principles and Practice in Ophthalmic Assisting: A Comprehensive Textbook*:
   Chapter 9: Basic Eye Exam (*Dilation* pp 127-128)
   Chapter 22: Pharmacology (pp 419-438)
   Chapter 29: Glaucoma (*Treatment*, Medication pp 527-528)

Explanatory Answers

Part I

1. c) Intravitreal means within the vitreous, so the medication must be delivered via a local injection. Systemic injection would mean that the medication be dispersed throughout the entire body (eg, intravenous or oral). Topical means on the surface, which would not require an injection at all. Work is being done regarding sustained delivery of anti-VEGF (including use of microparticles, nanoparticles, gene therapy, and refillable implants), but at publication these are experimental.

2. b) Oral medications, such as tablets and capsules, are considered systemic medications. They enter the blood stream via the digestive system and are then carried throughout the body.

3. a) Any suspension such as brinzolamide (Pred Forte is another common example) consists of particles in a liquid. The bottle must be shaken in order to make sure that the drop will actually contain medication. Brinzolamide is stable at 39° F to 86° F, so it is not necessary to store it in the refrigerator. One should not rinse the tip, as this may dilute and/or contaminate the medication.

4. b) An emulsion by definition contains lipids, making the medication "oily." This helps restore the lipid layer of the tears and keeps the medication on the eye a little longer. Some brands of tear drops are an emulsion as well.

5. c) Timoptic XE is actually considered a semi-solid. Once applied, the body heat of the eye melts it a little, turning it into a gel. This keeps the medication on the eye longer, although it is not time-released. Some tear drops use this form as well. Timoptic XE is preserved with benzododecinium bromide. The timolol without preservative is Timoptic Ocudose, which is supplied in single-dose units. Any drug can have side effects.

6. d) Because there is no preservative to prevent contamination, most preservative-free (PF) eye drops come in single-use bullets. The most common preservative free eye drop is over-the-counter artificial tears. Some Rx drops, however, are also available in a PF formulation, including Timoptic Ocudose and Alphagan P, both of which are used long term.

7.   d) Benzalkonium chloride is a very common preservative used in eye drops and other eye preparations. Thimerosal is also a preservative, but because so many people developed a reaction to it, it
is rarely used any more. Five percent sodium chloride is salt (think Muro 128). Sodium hypochlo-
rite is household bleach.

8.   a) Rx is the recipe, indicating what medication in what form in what concentration is to be dis-
pensed. Sig stands for *signatura*, which tells the patient how to use the medication. It is often written in abbreviated Latin, which the pharmacist translates to English (or other native tongue) on the
label for the patient. Any additional information for the patient is included here as well (eg, take
with food, take at bedtime). In this example, only the right eye is to receive the drop. If the medication is to be taken as needed ("prn"), the Rx should describe under what conditions the patient is
to use it (eg, prn itching). Disp is the dispensing instructions to the pharmacist, telling how many
and what size to give the patient. Rf stands for refills, where the physician indicates how many
times the patient can get more medication. This number should be written out as a word, rather
than as an Arabic number. In the example given, the practitioner has prescribed timolol (drug
name) 0.5% (strength) ophthalmic drops (medication form). The patient is to instill one (i) drop
(gt) twice daily (bid). The pharmacist is to give the patient two 15 ml (milliliter) bottles to the
patient, who may refill it 6 times. Not mentioned in this example are the prescriber's information,
the patient's information, and the prescriber's signature.

9.   c) The prescriber's National Provider Identifier is unique to each practitioner who communicates
with federal health programs electronically and must often be added at the bottom of a Rx along
with their signature. Failure to include it will create hassles when filing federal health care claims.

10.   b) The purpose of a "do not use" abbreviation list is to prevent confusion and mistakes in prescrib-
ing medications. For example, the use of qd and qod may be prohibited because they can be confused with each other. But qd means every day and qod means every other day, which could make
a big difference to the patient's well-being. Instead, write the instructions out longhand. Every
clinic should have such a list.

11.   c) You want to make sure that the pharmacist notices that the doctor has ordered Tobradex and not
plain Tobrex. This is a case of a look-alike/sound-alike (LASA) medication. Writing part of the Rx
in capital letters like this is called using "tall man lettering." (I'm serious!) LASA can be important
in the patient's general medical history as well, where you might write glyburide when the patient
said (or meant) glipizide. Another LASA of note in ophthalmic circles is where the dyes trypan
blue and methylene blue have been confused and swapped, much to the patient's detriment (see
Answer 159).

12.   **Matching:**

bid	twice daily
d	daily
gt	drop
gtt	drops
h	hour
mg	milligram
ml	milliliter
po	by mouth
prn	as needed
q	every
qd	every day
qhs	at bedtime
qid	4 times daily
tid	3 times daily

13.   d) Blocking off the puncta prevents the drug from traveling through the nasolacrimal system and
into the throat, where it can be swallowed and absorbed systemically. It also keeps the drop on the
eye a bit longer, increasing potential benefits. (It is estimated that somewhere from 50% to 90% loss

TABLE 13-1

TERMS AND COMBINING FORMS FOR SPEAKING ABOUT THE AUTONOMIC NERVOUS SYSTEM

lytic/lysis	Refers to the decomposition of something
mimetic	To "mime" is to mimic or copy or to be like something else
sympathomimetic	Mimicking (having the same action as, or causing the same reaction as, or stimulating of) the sympathetic (nervous system)
sympatholytic	Causing the decomposition (break down) of the sympathetic (nervous system), thus having a parasympathetic effect
parasympathomimetic	Mimicking (having the same action as, or causing the same reaction as, or stimulating of) the parasympathetic (nervous system)
parasympatholytic	Causing the decomposition (break down) of the parasympathetic (nervous system), thus having a sympathetic effect

Reproduced with permission from Anderson PD, Bokor G. Pharmacology. In: Ledford JK, Lens A, eds. *Principles and Practice in Ophthalmic Assisting: A Comprehensive Textbook.* SLACK Incorporated; 2018.

of the medication occurs after instillation, and that normally the drop spends less than 5 minutes in the tear film!) Punctal occlusion is accomplished by gently pressing the fingers into the nasal corners of the closed eyes.

14.   d) The "fight or flight" response (including all the details listed) results from stimulation to the sympathetic branch of the autonomic nervous system. By way of review, the autonomic nervous system controls "automatic" functions such as pulse and respiration rates, blood flow, digestion, etc. Refer to Table 13-1 as a reference while you go through these questions regarding the nervous system and various types of drugs.

15.   b) The other branch of the autonomic nervous system is the parasympathetic system. It has essentially the opposite effect of the sympathetic system. (You should especially note that pupil constriction is a product of the parasympathetic system.)

16.   b) A neurotransmitter is a biochemical released by the neurons (nerve cells) that take a message of action or inaction to the target organ or tissue. Once a neurotransmitter is released, it attaches itself to specific receptor sites. When the neurotransmitter is connected to a receptor (which might be in the heart, organs, glands, or blood vessels), then the specific action is carried out. (You might think of this as a key that fits into a lock.) The neurotransmitters for the sympathetic nervous system are epinephrine (also called adrenaline) and norepinephrine. Drugs that have their effect on the sympathetic system are also known as adrenergic drugs. (*Note:* The prefix *adren-* appears in adrenaline and adrenergic.) The sympathetic system has several types of receptors: alpha and beta. You will sometimes see drugs listed as alpha or beta blockers; this is a reference to the specific types of receptors of the sympathetic system.

17.   d) Acetylcholine is the major neurotransmitter of the parasympathetic system. Thus, a cholinergic drug affects the parasympathetic system. It is especially important to understand that the drugs in these 2 groups are classified according to the system that they affect, and *not* by the effects they have on the body. Please refer to Table 13-2 as you go through this set of questions.

18.   a) Something that copies could also be said to mime. The word mime is your clue to help you remember that sympathomimetic drugs mime, copy, or imitate the sympathetic system.

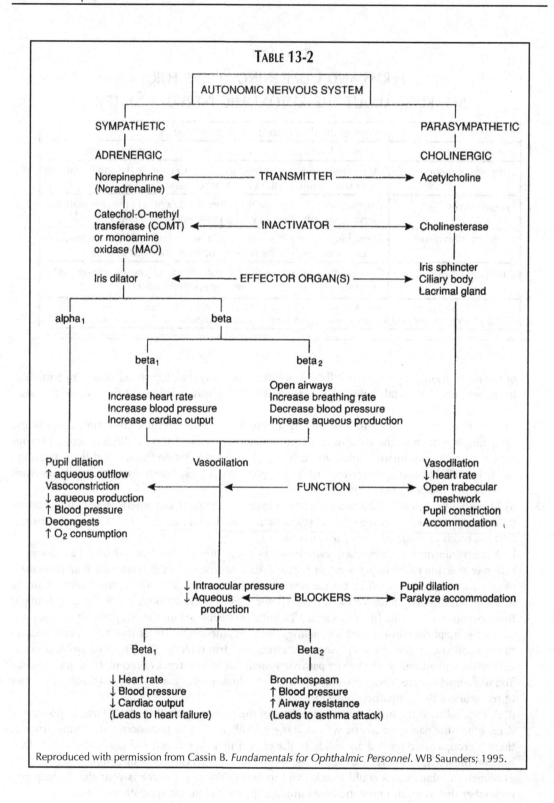

TABLE 13-2

AUTONOMIC NERVOUS SYSTEM

SYMPATHETIC		PARASYMPATHETIC
ADRENERGIC		CHOLINERGIC

Norepinephrine (Noradrenaline)	◄── TRANSMITTER ──►	Acetylcholine
Catechol-O-methyl transferase (COMT) or monoamine oxidase (MAO)	◄── INACTIVATOR ──►	Cholinesterase
Iris dilator	◄── EFFECTOR ORGAN(S) ──►	Iris sphincter Ciliary body Lacrimal gland

alpha₁ | beta

beta₁ | beta₂

beta₂
Open airways
Increase breathing rate
Decrease blood pressure
Increase aqueous production

beta₁
Increase heart rate
Increase blood pressure
Increase cardiac output

Pupil dilation ↑ aqueous outflow Vasoconstriction ↓ aqueous production ↑ Blood pressure Decongests ↑ O₂ consumption	Vasodilation ◄──── ◄── FUNCTION ──►	Vasodilation ↓ heart rate Open trabecular meshwork Pupil constriction Accommodation

↓ Intraocular pressure ↓ Aqueous production	◄── BLOCKERS ──►	Pupil dilation Paralyze accommodation

Beta₁
↓ Heart rate
↓ Blood pressure
↓ Cardiac output
(Leads to heart failure)

Beta₂
Bronchospasm
↑ Blood pressure
↑ Airway resistance
(Leads to asthma attack)

Reproduced with permission from Cassin B. *Fundamentals for Ophthalmic Personnel.* WB Saunders; 1995.

TABLE 13-3
DRUG CATEGORIES

I. Adrenergic drugs (sympathetic system)
   a. Mydriatics (sympathomimetics)
       phenylephrine
       hydroxyamphetamine
       cocaine
   b. Decrease aqueous formation
       1. Sympathomimetics (alpha receptor agonists)
          apraclonidine
          brimonidine
       2. Sympatholytics (beta receptor blockers/antagonists)
          betaxolol
          levobunolol
          metipranolol
          timolol
          carteolol
   c. Increase aqueous outflow (sympathomimetics)
       epinephrine
       dipivefrin
   d. Vasoconstrictors (sympathomimetics)
       phenylephrine
       naphazoline
       oxymetazoline
       tetrahydrozoline
   e. Dilation reversal (sympatholytic)
       dapiprazole
       thymoxamine

(continued)

19. d) Phenylephrine, used for pupil mydriasis, is sympathomimetic. It mimics the sympathetic response of pupil dilation by causing the iris dilator muscle to contract. It has no effect on the ciliary muscle, so accommodation is not affected. Please refer to Table 13-3 for more study information on adrenergic (sympathetic) and cholinergic (parasympathetic) drugs as you answer the remaining questions. *Note:* Some references call the iris muscles the *circular* and *radial* muscles. These are the sphincter and dilator muscles, respectively.

20. b) Vasoconstriction is an effect of the sympathetic system. Thus these sympathomimetic drugs (in addition to phenylephrine and oxymetazoline) are used to whiten the eye.

21. a) Brimonidine acts to decrease aqueous formation by assisting specific receptor sites (alpha receptors, thus it is an alpha-2 agonist) in the sympathetic system. Thus it is sympathomimetic.

22. d) A sympatholytic drug blocks the pathway required for a response in the sympathetic system. (*Note:* The suffix *-lysis* means to destroy something. A sympatholytic drug "destroys" the effect of the sympathetic system.)

23. d) Beta blockers (which include timolol, betaxolol, levobunolol, carteolol, and metipranolol) are sympatholytic agents used to decrease the formation of aqueous. Their action is on the sympathetic system (they block the beta receptors in the sympathetic system), so they are adrenergic drugs.

```
┌──────────────────────────────────────────────────────┐
│                TABLE 13-3 (CONTINUED)                  │
│                  DRUG CATEGORIES                       │
│                                                        │
│  II.  Cholinergic drugs (parasympathetic system)      │
│        a.  Miotics (parasympathomimetics)             │
│            1. Direct-acting                            │
│               pilocarpine                              │
│               carbachol                                │
│            2. Indirect-acting (cholinesterase inhibitors)│
│               physostigmine                            │
│               echothiophate                            │
│               isoflurophate                            │
│               demarcarium                              │
│               bromide                                  │
│        b.  Cycloplegics (parasympatholytics)          │
│            atropine                                    │
│            scopalomine (hyoscine)                      │
│            homatropine                                 │
│            cyclopentolate                              │
│            tropicamide                                 │
│        c.  Diagnostic (cholinesterase inhibitor)      │
│            edrophonium                                 │
│        d.  Muscle paralysis (parasympatholytic)       │
│            botulinum A toxin                           │
└──────────────────────────────────────────────────────┘
```

24.   b) The drugs dapiprazole and thymoxamine are sympatholytic drugs that are adrenergic (sympathetic) blockers (they block the alpha receptors). Thus they can be used to reverse mydriasis.

25.   c) Pilocarpine, which is used to control glaucoma, is a parasympathomimetic drug. In other words, it mimics the action of the parasympathetic system and causes pupillary miosis. All of the miotics are parasympathetic agonists (agonists are good guys who want to help!). There are 2 groups of miotics: direct acting (pilocarpine and carbachol), which act directly on the end-organ, and indirect acting. The indirect-acting miotics are cholinesterase inhibitors, which are explained in Answers 31 through 34. Carteolol is a beta blocker.

26.   a) The parasympathomimetics cause the iris sphincter and ciliary body to contract. This pulls on the scleral spur, which opens up the TM and increases the outflow of aqueous.

27.   d) Accommodative spasms, associated with the parasympathomimetics, can cause a brow ache when the patient first begins using them. This tends to decrease with time.

28.   b) This question was packed with info! First, if the drug is cholinergic-*blocking*, this is telling you that acetylcholine (the neurotransmitter for the parasympathetic system) has been blocked. Thus, the parasympathetic effect has been destroyed or lysed (parasympatholytic). This dilates the pupil and freezes accommodation. *Note:* A drug that enhances or stimulates acetylcholine would be *parasympathomimetic*.

29.   b) Botulinum A toxin is a parasympatholytic drug that blocks acetylcholine and has the effect of paralyzing muscles. In tiny amounts, it can be used to treat blepharospasm if injected into the eyelid muscles, or to treat strabismus if injected into the proper extraocular muscle. Edrophonium is used to help diagnose myasthenia gravis-related ptosis. Dapiprazole is a dilation-reversal drug. Acetazolamide is an oral carbonic anhydrase inhibitor used to lower eye pressure.

30.   b) The cycloplegics act to block acetylcholine from acting on the muscles. This paralyzes the iris sphincter and ciliary muscle, resulting in dilation and loss of accommodation. The cycloplegics include atropine, scopolomine, homatropine, cyclopentolate, and tropicamide.

31.   a) Cholinesterase is a biochemical that act as a "clean up man" for acetylcholine. Once a neurotransmitter is released, it attaches itself to specific receptor sites. When the neurotransmitter is connected to a receptor (which might be in the heart, organs, glands, or blood vessels), then the specific action is carried out. (You might think of this as a key that fits into a lock.) Cholinesterase removes acetylcholine from the receptor sites. This has the effect of reducing the parasympathetic effect.

32.   d) Cholinesterase removes acetylcholine from the receptor sites. This has the effect of reducing the parasympathetic reaction. If you are inhibiting cholinesterase, then you are allowing acetylcholine to accumulate. This has the effect of a continued stimulation of the parasympathetic system, enhancing that system.

33.   b) The indirect-acting miotics exert their effect by blocking cholinesterase, thus allowing acetylcholine to act freely. These miotics include physostigmine, echothiophate, isoflurophate, and demecarium bromide.

34.   b) Edrophonium (Tensilon) is a cholinesterase inhibitor (also known as anticholinesterase drug) used to differentiate ptosis due to myasthenia gravis from that due to other causes. (If the ptosis is due to myasthenia, an IV injection of edrophonium will cause a temporary elevation of the lid.)

35.   d) Mydriatics (such as tropicamide) are routinely used in the clinic to dilate the pupils. Nonsteroidal anti-inflammatories are used to treat inflammation, antibiotics are used to treat infections, and miotics make the pupil smaller.

36.   **Order:**

atropine	7 to 14 days	6
cyclopentolate	6 to 24 hours	3
homatropine	3 days	4
phenylephrine	3 to 5 hours	1
scopolomine	4 to 7 days	5
tropicamide	4 to 6 hours	2

37.   d) For refracting a young child, accommodation needs to be disabled using a cycloplegic. Of the drugs listed, cyclopentolate is the most appropriate, with peak effect at about 25 to 60 minutes. It wears off in 6 to 24 hours. Phenylephrine is a mydriatic and has little effect on accommodation. Atropine is a cycloplegic, but the effects can last for 1 to 2 weeks. Phospholine iodide is a miotic.

38.   c) Dilation with atropine can last 7 to 14 days; the patient will complain of blurred vision and light sensitivity. Any allergic reaction (redness, itching) would likely occur right away, as would life-threatening anaphylactic shock.

39.   a) The pain in iritis is basically caused by spasms of the ciliary muscle. A cycloplegic will "freeze" the ciliary muscle, increasing patient comfort. Homatropine, which lasts around 3 days, is the best choice of those listed. Tropicamide, also a cycloplegic, has a duration of action that is too short (4 to 6 hours) for this use. Phenylephrine will dilate but have little effect on the ciliary muscle. Tetracaine is a topical anesthetic, which will not be effective on ciliary spasms; it numbs the external eye and is never prescribed for home use because of its corneal toxicity.

40.   c) Of the cycloplegics listed, atropine is the longest lasting, with the effects lasting from 7 to 14 days. See also Answer 36.

Part II

41.   d) Another factor is expense of the drug. However, no medication perfectly fits each of these criteria. The physician will select the best one for each patient, often after a trial to find the most ideal.

42.   a) Marijuana does have some intraocular pressure–lowering effects, but this does not last long enough or lower the intraocular pressure enough to make it a good choice for glaucoma treatment. Some states have legalized medical marijuana.

43.   b) Soperonol is not a real medication. Answers a), c), and d) are generic names for various beta blockers.

44.   d) Iopidine is an alpha-2 agonist, not a beta blocker.

45.   c) Beta blockers have blue or yellow caps. (Blue is 0.25% and yellow is 0.5%.)

46.   c) The beta blockers classically have been contraindicated in patients with chronic obstructive pulmonary disease because the drugs can cause bronchospasms and decreased respiratory rate. The other statements are true. One or 2 beta blockers are approved for use once daily, but as a group they usually are given twice a day.

47.   b) Because beta blockers (even topical, ocular ones) can affect the heart, many physicians will require a baseline blood pressure and heart rate reading prior to beginning therapy, and on regular intervals thereafter.

48.   d) Timoptic-XE is currently the only beta blocker gel that actually forms the gel when it is applied to the eye. See also Answer 5. Dosage is once daily, making it convenient.

49.   a) Systemic beta blockers are used to treat congestive heart failure and hypertension. Examples are Tenormin, Lopressor, Toprol, and Inderal. They are not used for the other conditions listed, and are contraindicated in asthma.

50.   c) Of the drugs listed, Betoptic is a selective beta blocker. Selective beta blockers block only specific receptors and are thus less likely to have respiratory side effects.

51.   a) Side effects of beta blockers (systemic or topical/ocular), as indicated previously, can include decreased heart rate and decreased respiratory rate.

52.   b) Other possible side effects of beta blockers include depression, insomnia, and impotence. Topical ocular beta blockers have minimal, if any, ocular side effects; over half of the people using them say they don't even sting. This contributes to their popularity.

53.   b) Alpha-2 agonists are used to lower intraocular pressure. Examples are Iopidine (alpraclonidine) and Alphagan (brimonidine).

54.   d) The dual nature of the alpha-1 agonists make them a useful tool in controlling intraocular pressure. *Note*: Most (an estimated 85%) of the aqueous leaves the eye via the TM. However, a small amount exits the eye via uveoscleral outflow, which involves resorption and drainage of aqueous via portions of the eye's vascular system.[1] Toris and Kiel have an excellent, short video demonstrating this phenomenon, as well as how it is affected by various antiglaucoma agents (see References).

55.   a) Of the drugs listed, Iopidine is an alpha-2-agonist that is more prone to cause an allergic reaction, so it is not used long term. Pilocarpine is a miotic, and tetracaine is a topical anesthetic.

56.   c) There is a high rate of allergic reaction (irritation, redness) to the alpha-2 agonists. Iopidine is the worst, so is used only short term. If long term use is desired, the drug of choice is brimonidine.

57.   a) Prostaglandin analogs are substances that act like prostaglandins (which can either raise or lower intraocular pressure). They seem to be more effective and have fewer side effects than beta blockers. You may also see them referred to as simply prostaglandins.

58.   d) In glaucoma treatment, prostaglandin analogs cause increased uveoscleral outflow (see Answer 54).

59.   c) Because prostaglandin analogs are only used once a day, many patients are more compliant than with twice-daily treatments. All eye drops for glaucoma are for use at home. And every medication can potentially have side effects.

60.   d) In contrast, prostaglandins may cause *redness*. If the orbital fat begins to break down, the eye may sink into the socket.

61.   a) Currently marketed prostaglandin analogs are latanaprost (Xalatan), bimatoprost (Lumigan), travoprost (TravatanZ), and tafluprost (Zioptan, which is preservative-free). Drugs in Answer b) are beta blockers, in c) are CAIs, and in d) are prednisolones.

62.   b) Prostaglandin analogs are contraindicated if there is active inflammation (such as iritis, uveitis, etc) in the eye because they may make it worse. It is also not used if the patient has cystoid macular edema.

63.   b) CAIs have the effect of lowering intraocular pressure.

64.   d) CAIs act by reducing the amount of aqueous that is formed, thereby lowering intraocular pressure.

65.   a) Lumigan is a prostaglandin. The rest are either a CAI (Trusopt and Azopt) or have a CAI in combination with another drug (CoSopt, which has timolol in it as well).

66.   b) All of the items listed can occur as side effects of CAIs. However, tingling in the hands, feet, and tongue is so common that it has been suggested you can judge a patient's compliance by the presence (or absence) of this symptom.

67.   b) Patients who are allergic to sulfa drugs should not take CAIs. Sulfa is an anti-infective. Sulfur is a chemical element, otherwise known as brimstone.

68.   b) RKIs lower intraocular pressure by increasing aqueous outflow via the TM, which accounts for approximately 85% of aqueous drainage.[1] They are thought to do this by "relaxing" the meshwork, opening it more. *Note:* You may also see them referred to as ROC inhibitors or ROCK inhibitors.

69.   a) The generic name of the currently available RKI is netarsudil (Rhopressa). If combined with latanoprost, the trade name is Rocklatan. Azopt and Trusopt are CAIs. Lotemax and Durezol are steroids. Viagmox and Ocuflox are antibiotics.

70.   a) Incidents of subconjunctival hemorrhage have been reported. Also noted have been corneal verticillata ("whorls"), but they are not something that the patient would be aware of. (Did you notice that Answers a), c), and d) were symptoms? Answer b) is a sign.)

71.   c) The RKI netarsudil has been combined with the prostaglandin analog latanoprost. In this form, there is an increase of outflow through both the trabecular and uveoscleral routes. The patient may experience side effects of both drugs, however.

72.   c) Miotics stimulate the sphincter muscle of the iris, causing the pupil to close (miosis). This is suspected to pull on the TM (opening it) but does not directly stimulate the TM. Stimulating the dilator muscle would cause dilation. Stimulating the ciliary body would cause increased aqueous production.

73.   d) Miotics are not used in patients with posterior subcapsular cataracts because decreasing the pupil size would force the patient's visual axis straight through the cataract, drastically reducing vision. Miotics are used in open-angle glaucoma to lower intraocular pressure and in closed-angle glaucoma to open the iris blockade. They are used in overcorrection (too much plus) following corneal refractive surgery. In addition, they reduce accommodative effort in convergent strabismus.

74.   a) Miotics act to increase aqueous outflow (see Answer 72). They constrict the pupil, not dilate it.

75.   d) Although miotics are rarely used anymore for intraocular pressure control, pilocarpine is the most often used. All 4 drugs listed, are miotics, however. Dapiprazole is the "dilation reversal" drug sometimes used in clinics. Echothiophate (phospholine iodide) is sometimes used in treating accommodative esotropia. It was unavailable for a while, but the supply has reportedly resumed by a different company.

76.   c) Patients should be warned that they may experience a headache or brow ache when first starting a miotic. They should be encouraged to stick with treatment, as this side effect diminishes with use.

77.   b) While topical epinephrine can cause pupil dilation, this is a secondary action. The primary use of topical epinephrine is in glaucoma treatment. Epinephrine is used in injectable (not topical) anesthetic to decrease wound bleeding. It is not used in treatment of dry eye.

78.   c) Epinephrine act to both decrease the production of aqueous as well as increasing outflow. Because of its action to dilate the pupil, it is not used in narrow angles or angle-closure glaucoma.

79.   a) Side effects of epinephrine can include rapid pulse and respiration, stomach upset, pupil dilation, headache, fainting, increased blood pressure, and heart palpitations.

80.   b) Oral and intravenous osmotics are used to lower the intraocular pressure rapidly in cases of angle-closure glaucoma. *Topical* osmotics are used in corneal edema. They are not indicated in open-angle glaucoma or iritis.

81.   a) If there is a permeable membrane separating 2 areas, then fluid will cross the system to equalize the fluid content on both sides of the membrane. If the membrane will allow fluids through but not particles, then the fluid will cross the membrane from the side with the least particles to the side with the most. Thus, the influx of fluid dilutes the particle concentration. This process is called *osmosis*. Osmotics raise the concentration of particles in the blood, which lowers the fluid content. Fluid (aqueous) then leaves the tissues (in the anterior chamber) and enters the blood stream in an attempt to equalize or dilute the concentration of particles.

82.   d) Glycerin is sickly sweet and may cause nausea and vomiting if ingested quickly. Pour the liquid over ice and tell the patient to sip it slowly through a straw. If you dilute or follow the dose with water, you are adding water to the system and less fluid will be drawn out of the tissues.

83.   c) If a patient in angle-closure attack is being given oral osmotics and complains of thirst, they should be told that this means the medicine is working. The patient should not be given a drink, as this would reduce the amount of fluid being drawn out of the tissues. Giving more medication is done on doctor's orders only. Lying down won't help thirst.

84.   b) Dehydration, headache, and disorientation are other side effects of systemic osmotics.

Part III

85.   b) Antibiotics are used to treat bacterial infections.

86.   b) Bacteriocidal antibiotics are those that actually kill bacteria. (Your hint of death is the suffix "-cidal.") Antibiotics that inhibit bacteria are called bacteriostatic, which includes the sulfonamides. An antiseptic inhibits germs and is used on surfaces.

87.   c) See Answer 86. Penicillins are bacteriocidal. A germicide is used to kill bacteria on inanimate objects.

88.   c) One can determine the sensitivity of a germ to a particular antibiotic by taking a culture. Material from the infected tissue is spread on the culture plate. Tiny paper disks that have been impregnated with an antibiotic are spaced out on the plate. If the bacteria is sensitive to the antibiotic on a specific disk, there will be a zone of no growth around that disk. (A biopsy evaluates excised tissue. One cannot identify an antibiotic sensitivity by slit lamp or fluorescein angiogram.)

89.   a) If an antibiotic has an effect on many different kinds of bacteria, it is called a broad-spectrum drug. These are very useful when the infecting organism is not known, because chances are good that it will be sensitive to the drug.

90.   d) An oral antibiotic should be taken until all the pills are gone.

91.   c) The use of topical neomycin has largely been phased out (except in combination drugs) because of its high rate of allergic reaction.

92.   d) In general, antibiotics do not affect the blood glucose level. Any of the other answers are possible.

93.   a) Approximately 10% of the population is reportedly allergic to penicillin.

94.   b) Vidarabine (Vira-A) seems to be effective only on the herpes simplex virus.

95.   d) Acanthamoebiasis is an amoebic infection, so an antiviral will not have any effect. Shingles and chicken pox are caused by the same virus, *herpes varicella zoster*. The cytomegalovirus is also a type of herpes. Along with *herpes simplex*, they are the most common type of virus that affects the eye.

96.   c) Corneal dendrites are classic for infection with herpes virus, so an antiviral would be prescribed. Acyclovir is an antiviral drug. Neomycin and sulfonamide are antibacterial; natamycin is antifungal.

97. a) Natamycin is the only antifungal currently available for topical use in the eye. Mycomycin is a nonophthalmic antibiotic used to treat tuberculosis. Prednisolone is a steroid, and viderabine is an antiviral.

98. b) Natamycin does not penetrate well so is mainly used for fungal infections of the corneal surface (ie, mycotic or fungal keratitis). Other ocular infections associated with fungi (such as a mycotic endophthalmitis) may be treated with local (intraocular) injections or systemically. A chalazion is not caused by fungi, nor is chlamydial keratitis (caused by a bacterium).

99. b) Treatment of ocular parasites can be very complicated and must be specific to the type of parasite encountered. Removal may be a treatment, as in lice, but this is not always the case. (One cannot "remove" *Acanthamoeba*!) It is not a given that there will be a secondary infection, so antibiotics are not given as a matter of course unless warranted. Besides, a secondary infection could be caused by a virus, against which antibiotics are ineffective. Steroids offer no particular toxic effect and may exacerbate any secondary viral infection or cause elevated intraocular pressure.

100. a) Vasoconstrictors cause constriction of blood vessels.

101. c) Vasoconstrictors make the conjunctival vessels smaller, thus whitening (getting the red out of) the eye. They do not have the effects listed in Answers a), b), or d).

102. c) Another term for vasoconstrictors is decongestants.

103. b) Scopolamine is a cycloplegic agent. True, phenylephrine *is* a mydriatic drug, but it is also used in weaker concentrations as a decongestant.

104. a) Patients with dry eye should be discouraged from using vasoconstrictors, as these chemicals tend to dry the eye further. Hay fever and tired, red eyes can indicate the need for a decongestant. Using a decongestant in case of a subconjunctival hemorrhage won't really help the red to go away any faster but is not contraindicated.

105. c) Because vasoconstrictors can dilate the pupil, it is possible that this could precipitate angle closure, bringing on an angle-closure glaucoma attack.

106. c) When an allergic reaction takes place, special cells (mast cells) respond to the allergen by releasing histamine. Histamine is the chemical responsible for the redness, itching, watering, and rash seen in the typical allergic response. Antihistamines block the release of histamine. They cannot block the reaction but do block some of the symptoms.

107. c) Cromolyn is a mast cell stabilizer only. Elestat and Patanol are combination antihistamine and mast cell stabilizers. Naphcon A contains an antihistamine and decongestant.

108. b) Decongestants to reduce redness are frequently combined with antihistamines to alleviate allergy symptoms. Naphcon A and Vasocon-A are examples of such combinations.

109. c) Many oral antihistamines cause drowsiness. Many are available over the counter. Any drug can have systemic side effects. (In addition, a patient might be allergic to a preservative or other additive in such a medication.) Antihistamines are used to treat symptoms of allergies, not infections.

110. a) Antihistamines dry everything up, including the tear film.

111. b) The mast cells are stimulated to release histamine in response to allergens. This happens when histamine-containing granules in the mast cell are released in a process known as degranulation. Mast cell stabilizers prevent degranulation.

112. a) The mast cell stabilizer in the list is cromolyn. Pilocarpine is a miotic. Atropine dilates the pupil, and ketorolac is a NSAID.

113. c) Drops that contain both a mast cell stabilizer and an antihistamine are very effective for ocular allergies. They contain the faster-acting antihistamine to block the histamine that has been released, as well as the more preventative action of the mast cell stabilizer (which blocks release of histamine but takes longer to have effect, due to the histamine that has been released prior to treatment). Ketotifen is an example.

114. c) Steroids are anti-inflammatory drugs, not anti-infectives. In fact, they can reduce the immune system and thus allow infections to occur. Steroids act to reduce swelling, redness, drainage, and scarring. They do not have an effect on bacteria or viruses. They can elevate the intraocular pressure and reduce immunity.

115. d) Steroid use in *herpes simplex* keratitis can prolong the disorder. This sometimes occurs when a red eye is not thoroughly evaluated, and topical steroids are given to relieve the symptoms. Steroids are used in *herpes zoster* to treat resulting keratitis, conjunctivitis, and iritis. Iritis, scleritis, and episcleritis are all inflammatory conditions well treated by steroids. *Note:* topical steroids may sometimes be used (carefully) if there is uveitis in diagnosed *herpes simplex* where antivirals have been started.

116. d) Topical steroids usually are used for surface and anterior segment inflammation. Oral steroids are used for deeper ocular inflammations, such as posterior uveitis and optic neuritis. In some cases, scleritis might be treated with both topical and systemic steroids. Steroids can *cause* secondary glaucoma, so they are not used to treat it.

117. b) Diazepam is the generic term for Valium. All of the others are steroids. Betamethasone and cortisone acetate are 2 other steroids. Often, drug names ending in *–one* are steroids.

118. a) Drugs in Answer b) are combination steroid-antibiotics. Answer c) lists NSAIDs, and Answer d) is a list of antibiotics.

119. c) Steroids, whether topical or oral, are not discontinued suddenly. Instead, the dosage is tapered off gradually.

120. b) If a steroid drop is discontinued suddenly, inflammation may recur. This is known as *rebound.* Elevated intraocular pressure (except in angle closure) does not cause redness or pain. Neither does a subcapsular opacity. The main thing a patient with a displaced intraocular lens will notice is a change in vision, sometimes drastic.

121. a) Because steroids can cause secondary glaucoma, tonometry is important to monitor intraocular pressure.

122. b) Steroids also can cause formation of posterior subcapsular cataracts. Hence the importance of the slit lamp exam.

123. d) Systemic side effects of steroids include sweating, elevated blood pressure, weakness, and delayed wound healing. They also can cause fluid retention, muscle wasting, bone demineralization, growth retardation, immunity suppression, and diabetes.

124. b) Steroids can lower the immune system, opening the tissues or system to opportunistic infection. They *can* increase blood glucose levels, and do *not* cause strokes.

125. a) Prolonged use of topical steroids (6 months or more) can cause the development of subcapsular cataracts. After 2 to 6 weeks of use, some patients will experience a rise in ocular pressure. Other possible side effects include ptosis, mydriasis, and increased corneal thickness.

126. d) Steroids are often combined with antibiotics to fight both bacterial infection and inflammation. Examples are TobraDex, Blephamide, NeoPolyDex, and Maxitrol.

127. b) NSAIDs can offer relief of itching, but not other ocular allergic symptoms such as redness and watering. Items in Answers a), c), and d) are indications for topical NSAID use.

128. a) NSAIDs do not appreciably elevate intraocular pressure, a significant problem in long-term use of steroids. The NSAIDs do not do a better job, are not combined with antibiotics, and do sting when instilled.

129. b) FML is a steroid eye drop. Answers a), c), and d) are all topical NSAIDs.

130. b) NSAIDs are not indicated in an acute infection because in reducing the inflammation they may mask the advancement of the infection itself.

131. d) Ketorolac is an NSAID that may be used after cataract or corneal refractive surgery to help control pain; it has FDA approval for this use. Other NSAIDs may be used in the same manner, but as of this writing, this is an off-label use. Pilocarpine is a miotic, Patanol and ketotifen are antihistamines (ketotifen also has some mast cell–stabilizing effects).

Part IV

132. b) Because there is no preservative to retard bacterial growth, any solution remaining in the bullet at the end of the day should be discarded. These drops may be used many times throughout the day. No one should use homemade saline in the eye because of the risk of contamination. *Note:* some do not advise retaining an opened bullet throughout the day, but opening a fresh one for every use.

133. d) Dry eye is a condition that cannot be cured, only controlled. Thus, patients are advised to use the drops as often as needed.

134. d) Of those listed, the ointment will stay on the eye the longest. The liquid drop would be gone from the eye first. An emulsifier is a lipid, added to some tear drops and Restasis to make it more "oily." The gels are considered a semi-solid that are "melted" by body temperature once they are on the eye. But the ointment (also a "melting" semi-solid) lasts longest.

135. d) The thicker the preparation, the more likely it is to cause a film over the cornea, causing blurred vision. The thicker drops and ointment can also trap allergens (think pollen) on the eye, and stick to the lashes.

136. d) Anesthesia that puts the patient to sleep is known as general anesthesia. Topical anesthetic is applied to the skin (or eye), and local or regional is injected into a specific area.

137. b) Local anesthesia would be used in the chalazion excision. A baby cannot be relied upon not to move, so it needs to be totally asleep. Noncontact tonometry and topography are performed without any anesthetic.

138. a) In a regional block, anesthetic is injected into the area of the nerve (or nerves) that supplies the surgical site. An example would be a retrobulbar block, where the anesthetic is injected behind the eye to block sensation and to paralyze the muscles. Local anesthetic can also be injected into the tissues at the surgical site. "Site-specific local" is a bogus term.

139. b) A corneal transplant requires a regional block. The chalazion uses local, and topical is enough for cataract surgery and laser trabeculoplasty.

140. b) It often is necessary for the patient's eye to be immobilized, which can be accomplished with local anesthetic.

141. a) Lidocaine and procaine are commonly used local anesthetics. Answers b) and d) and tetracaine are *topical* anesthetics. Butane, in Answer c), is cigarette lighter fluid.

142. d) The most common side effects of local anesthetics are dizziness and nausea. Answers a) and b) can occur but are not common. Blood pressure may be *reduced*, not increased; see also Answer 143.

143. a) Local anesthetics also may cause depression of both blood pressure and respiration.

144. c) The suffix *-caine* usually indicates that the drug is an anesthetic. Mannitol is an osmotic, cortisone is a steroid, and betaxolol is a beta blocker.

145. c) The initial contact lens fitting is not usually done with topical anesthetic. Lens fitters often use the patient's reaction to having lenses in the eye to help determine the patient's level of motivation.

146. a) The most common reaction to topical anesthetics is a contact allergic response. Some patients might experience dizziness and fainting, but this is not common. A decrease in blood pressure might occur on very rare occasions.

147. b) Proparacaine and tetracaine are the most commonly used topical anesthetics in ophthalmology. Drugs in Answer a) also are topical anesthetics, but not used very often. Procaine, bupivacaine, and prilocaine are local anesthetics, and epinephrine is sometimes an additive to local anesthetics.

148. d) The patient should be warned not to rub eyes after the topical anesthetic has been instilled. Without corneal sensation, the patient might rub hard enough to cause a corneal abrasion.

149. b) Epinephrine, as a neurotransmitter of the sympathetic nervous system, causes blood vessel constriction so that the anesthetic will remain at the site longer. This makes the numbness last, giving the surgeon more time to do the procedure before the patient's sensation returns. (Roughly speaking, when something is *metabolized*, it means that it has entered the system, has had its effect, and is being broken down and eliminated from the system.)

150. a) Fluorescein dye pools in corneal defects and glows in a cobalt blue light. You may use a blue filter on a pen light or on the slit lamp.

151. c) When instilled onto the eye and lit with a cobalt blue light, fluorescein dye glows a bright green/yellow.

152. a) Fluorescein will stain a contact lens, so you must irrigate the patient's eyes prior to re-inserting the lenses. A drop of artificial tears is not enough. (There is a form of fluorescein drops with a larger molecule that does not permanently stain contact lenses; this is used mainly for contact lens fitting, not intraocular pressure checks. But even that can stain a contact after a few minutes.)

153. c) The dye is released from the strip when moistened.

154. b) *Pseudomonas aeruginosa* contamination of fluorescein has long been documented. This aggressive bacterium can liquefy the cornea, leading to perforation; destruction of the eye can occur within a matter of days. The infection is more common in soft contact lens wearers and following trauma. It is difficult to treat. The other bacteria listed can infect the eye, although it is uncommon for *E. coli* to do so.

155. d) The patient should be informed that the skin and urine may be discolored for several hours after injection. Side effects of the dye can include nausea and vomiting (always have an emesis basin available). Infiltration (extravasation) occurs if the dye is injected into the tissues instead of into the vein; ice may help. Allergic reaction (including rash, itching, shortness of breath, and anaphylaxis) can also occur, so it is essential to have a properly equipped crash cart handy.

156. b) Rose bengal stains dead (necrotic) tissue and would be of most use in a case of severe dry eye. It is of no use in glaucoma or conjunctival injection. Fluorescein dye would be more useful in the case of a corneal foreign body.

157. a) Lissamine green dye also stains dead and damaged tissue, as well as mucus. The stain usually lasts longer than rose bengal. But it is less irritating, and many practitioners now prefer it. The fact that no filters or special lights are needed is neither here nor there.

158. a) An angiography using indocyanine green allows imaging of deeper layers of the choroid than does fluorescein angiography. Trypan blue and methylene blue dyes are not used in imaging studies.

159. d) Trypan blue is a dye sometimes used to stain the anterior lens capsule during cataract surgery. Methylene blue may be used externally to mark skin or sclera. This is a crucial difference; accidental intraocular use of methylene blue can be catastrophic. This is a case of LASA where everyone must be extremely careful that steps are taken to avoid the mistake. Lissamine green is an external dye (used much the same way as rose bengal), and Gram stain is used to colorize samples on microscope slides.

160. d) The National Eye Institute's Age-Related Eye Disease Study shows that Vitamins C, E, beta-carotene (which converts to Vitamin A), and zinc can help slow down the progression of macular degeneration. (The NEI added copper and some antioxidants as well.) Hence the popularity of "eye vitamins" such as Ocuvite and ICaps.

161. c) Beta-carotene use in smokers can raise the risk of lung cancer. "Smokers formula" eye vitamins remove the beta-carotene and substitute other nutrients.

162. b) Omega-3 fatty acids improve the lipid (oil) layer of the tears, helping to prevent evaporation and keeping the tears on the eye longer. Free radicals are unstable atoms that damage tissues.

163. a) Some vitamins are toxic if taken at high levels (hypervitaminosis). Examples are Vitamin D, Vitamin A, Vitamin K, Vitamin E, Vitamin B_6, Vitamin B_{12}, folate, and niacin. Patients should check with their pharmacist and/or primary care physician to evaluate, because in some cases the amount taken required for toxicity is almost higher than it's possible for one person to take. However, even a normal dose can cause side effects. Niacin is a good example where the common side effects include itching, warm/red/tingly skin, mild dizziness, sweats/chills, nausea, diarrhea, muscle cramps, and insomnia.

164. d) Vitamin A is key in the formation of rhodopsin (also called visual purple), the photochemical present in the dark-activated rod cells. Severe Vitamin A deficiency can cause "night blindness," but this is rare in developed countries.

165. b) VEGF is the acronym for vascular endothelial growth factor. The other answers are bogus.

166. c) Because VEGF stimulates neovascularization, a drug used to block it is known as an anti-("against") VEGF.

167. c) Wet macular degeneration is the only one of the entities listed that might involve neovascularization. The lens (and cataracts) are not related to vascular disease. Xanthelasma is a cholesterol-related growth on the lids. Retinal detachments may be treated with laser or surgery.

168. a) According to one source, "Anti-VEGF treatment improves vision in about one-third (1 out of 3) people who take it. For a vast majority (9 out of 10), it at least stabilizes vision."[2]

169. c) Verteporfin (Visudyne) is used to treat neovascularization, but it is not an anti-VEGF; it is used in photodynamic therapy (PDT). The photo-sensitive agent is nontoxic until activated by light. In this case an infrared laser is used to activate the agent in very specific locations. When thus activated, the chemical releases free radicals (unstable atoms) that destroy the abnormal blood vessels. PDT has largely been replaced by intravitreal injections of anti-VEGF (see Answers 165 to 168). *Note:* Macugen is an anti-VEGF that is no longer available in the United States.

170. c) Two percent or 5% sodium chloride (salt) drops or ointment (such as Muro 128) are frequently prescribed for home use in cases of long-term corneal edema.

171. a) Topical osmotics usually sting. They clear vision temporarily (as long as the corneal edema stays "dried up").

172. c) Betoptic is a beta blocker, which can cause these types of pulmonary problems. This is probably an emergency, where the patient should be sent to the emergency room.

173. d) Latanaprost is a carbonic anhydrase inhibitor, which collectively are known to cause a metallic taste, as well as tingling/numbness in the extremities. Ketorolac is an NSAID, erythromycin is an antibiotic, and ketotifen is combination antihistamine/mast cell stabilizer, none of which cause these side effects.

174. b) With the information given, the anti-nausea patch is the most likely culprit, as these often contain scopolamine, which is a cycloplegic drug. Most likely the patient (who is probably right-handed, given this scenario) rubbed their eye after applying the patch. An ocular decongestant might cause a slight dilation but probably not enough to notice and certainly not lasting this long.

175. b) Sometimes a topical eye medication is needed but is not available commercially. For example, natamycin is currently the only antifungal eye drop that is commercially available. It is not effective against *Candida*, so the practitioner may ask a pharmacist to "mix up" (compound) an eye drop containing miconazole. The creation of such medications is a strict science, only performed by authorized compounding pharmacists.

176. a) Off-label use denotes that a medication is used for a purpose other than the one(s) specified by the FDA. An example is verteporfin, approved for use in PDT for treating age-related macular degeneration. Off label, it might also be used for pathologic myopia and choroidal rupture.

References

1. Toris C, Kiel J. Aqueous outflow and glaucoma drug mechanisms of action. The David E. I. Pyott Glaucoma Education Center, American Academy of Ophthalmology Website. Accessed March 17, 2023. www.aao.org/basic-skills/animation-of-aqueous-flow
2. Turbert D. Anti-VEGF treatments. American Academy of Ophthalmology Website. Accessed March 17, 2023. www.aao.org/eye-health/drugs/anti-vegf-treatments

Bibliography

Haynes J, Huddleson S, Rafieetary M. Anti-VGF in 2022: innovation and ambition. Review of Optometry Website. Published March 15, 2022. Accessed March 17, 2022. Reviewofoptometry.com/article/antivegf-in-2022-innovation-and-ambition

Simons M. Angiogeneses: where do we stand now? *Circulation*. 2005;111:1556-1566. doi:10.1161/01.CIR.0000159345.00591.8F

Chapter 14

Surgical Assisting*

* Some topics in this chapter overlap.

Ledford JK.
*Certified Ophthalmic Technician Exam
Review Manual, Third Edition* (pp 253-274).
© 2023 Taylor & Francis Group.

ABBREVIATIONS USED IN THIS CHAPTER

- AK   arcuate keratotomy
- BSS   basic salt solution
- CK   conductive keratoplasty
- CO_2 carbon dioxide (laser)
- DLK   diffuse lamellar keratitis
- FS   femtosecond (laser)
- IOL   intraocular lens
- IOP   intraocular pressure
- K   cornea/corneal
- LASEK   laser-assisted subepithelial keratectomy
- LASIK   laser-assisted in situ keratomileusis
- MMC   mitomycin C
- OR   operating room
- OSHA   Occupational Safety and Health Administration
- PRK   photorefractive keratectomy
- psi   pounds per square inch
- RK   radial keratotomy
- SMILE   small incision lenticule extraction
- YAG   yttrium aluminum garnet (laser)

Instrument Preparation

1.   **Instruments are generally laid out on the sterile tray:**
   a) from most sterile to least
   b) in the order in which they will be used
   c) largest on left, smallest on right
   d) as preferred by the circulator

2. Match the surgical instrument(s) to the procedure(s) it is associated with. Answers may be used more than once, with some instruments having more than one answer.

Procedure
a) cataract surgery
b) chalazion
c) corneal transplant
d) laceration repair
e) destruction of hair follicle
f) pterygium removal
g) strabismus surgery
h) stretch punctum
i) tear duct obstruction
j) tissue excision
k) trichiasis

Instrument
___ cannula
___ clamp
___ curette
___ dilator
___ electrolysis unit
___ forceps
___ lacrimal cannula
___ needle holder
___ phacoemulsification unit
___ probe
___ scalpel
___ scissors
___ speculum
___ trephine
___ vitrector

3. Match each instrument to its use. Answers may be used more than once.

Use/Purpose
a) cutting
b) delivering fluid
c) grasping
d) measuring
e) opens/isolates/separates
f) uses cold
g) uses electric pulses
h) uses heat
i) uses ultrasound

Instrument
___ calipers
___ cannula
___ cautery unit
___ clamp
___ cryosurgery unit
___ curette
___ dilator
___ electrolysis unit
___ forceps
___ needle holder
___ phacoemulsification unit
___ probe
___ scalpel
___ scissors
___ speculum
___ trephine
___ vitrector

Surgical Site Identification

4. Which of the following is an acceptable way to mark a surgical site?
a) speculum
b) grease pen
c) gentian violet skin marker
d) eye liner

5.   **When is the appropriate time to mark a surgical site?**
   a) once the patient is sedated
   b) when the patient is on the table
   c) once the site has been prepped
   d) prior to any medications being administered

6.   **Which of the following is *not* a part of a surgical time out?**
   a) verify patient
   b) verify instrumentation
   c) verify procedure
   d) verify surgical site

Aseptic and Sterile Technique*

7.   **Which of the following is *false*?**
   a) Sterile means free of organisms; aseptic means free of infection.
   b) Aseptic technique is used for major surgery.
   c) Skin is disinfected in both sterile and aseptic technique.
   d) Gloves may be used in both sterile and aseptic technique.

8.   **The purpose of aseptic and sterile techniques is to:**
   a) reduce the chances of infection
   b) reduce or eliminate the presence of microbes on objects
   c) reduce or eliminate the presence of infective agents in areas
   d) all of the above

9.   **If a sterile object is touched by another sterile object:**
   a) both are considered contaminated
   b) it should be replaced on the tray
   c) neither are contaminated
   d) both should be sterilized

10.   **What item may be placed on a sterile field during a procedure?**
   a) sterile gauze dumped out of packaging
   b) a glove that's been removed
   c) a premium intraocular lens that fell on the floor
   d) suture material in its package

11.   **The scrub assistant has been holding a clamp for a very long time, and their hand drifts down below their waist. This means that:**
   a) the clamp is now contaminated
   b) the surgeon needs to hurry up
   c) they need to pay more attention
   d) the clamp should be returned to the tray

* The criteria lists only aseptic technique; I have included sterile technique as well. See also the note on Answer 7.

12. **You are today's circulator. Mid-procedure, the surgeon wants the Mayo stand moved. How is this done, and by whom?**
    a) You can do it; push the stand below the sterile drape.
    b) You can do it; push the edge of the tray.
    c) You can do it; nudge the base of the stand with your foot.
    d) It is too late; no one may touch the tray or stand.

13. **The morning's 8 a.m. blepharoplasty, for which the tray is already prepared, has to be put off until 3:30 p.m. Which of the following should be done?**
    a) A sterile towel may be laid over the tray.
    b) Nothing; this tray will still be sterile.
    c) Reschedule the surgery for another day.
    d) A new tray should be prepared when it's time for the procedure.

14. **Who is responsible for monitoring the sterile field?**
    a) the circulator
    b) the surgeon
    c) all surgical staff
    d) the first assistant

15. **What part(s) of a sterile surgery gown is actually considered sterile?**
    a) the entire gown
    b) between the waist and armpits, and the sleeves up to 3 inches above the elbows
    c) the gown front
    d) between the waist and neck, and sleeves up to 3 inches below the elbows

16. **Which of the following is *not* acceptable on the sterile tray?**
    a) separating any fluids from the instruments on the tray
    b) fluids of any kind
    c) empty syringe with end extending off edge of tray, ready to grab
    d) sterile instruments that have been "dumped"

17. **How far away must a nonscrubbing assistant be from the sterile field?**
    a) 20 inches
    b) 12 inches
    c) 2 feet
    d) 3 feet

18. **You are circulating today. The first assistant dropped a clamp and needs a sterile replacement. You can do this by:**
    a) opening a sterile one and handing it to them
    b) opening a sterile one and dumping it on the Mayo stand
    c) opening a sterile one and holding the package so they can reach in and get it
    d) opening a sterile one and handing it to them over the Mayo stand

19. Which of the following, if practiced or used by a surgical assistant, carries a risk of transmitting a fungus to the patient?
    a) cologne
    b) artificial fingernails
    c) dentures
    d) hair extensions

Refractive Surgery

20. Laser refractive surgery is always considered:
    a) a sterile procedure
    b) a successful procedure
    c) an aseptic procedure
    d) an urgent procedure

21. The procedure where a laser is used to carve a lens-shaped piece of tissue inside the cornea, which is then extracted is known as:
    a) lenticular corneal extraction
    b) small-incision lenticule extraction
    c) lenticular capsulorrhexis
    d) lenticulo-canalis procedure

22. Which of the following regarding the femtosecond laser is *false*?
    a) It takes longer than other lasers.
    b) It has less collateral tissue damage than other lasers.
    c) It creates very precise incisions.
    d) It can be used in several types of refractive laser surgery.

23. You are screening a patient prior to LASIK. They say that sometimes they awaken in the morning with a moderate foreign body sensation. Their corneal topography is irregular. They may not be a good LASIK candidate because these are indications of:
    a) Fuchs' corneal dystrophy
    b) keratoconus
    c) corneal hydrops
    d) anterior basement membrane dystrophy

24. Match the modality(ies) used to each procedure. Answers may be used more than once, with some procedures having more than one answer.

Modality	Procedure
a) alcohol	__ AK
b) excimer laser	__ clear lensectomy/refractive lens exchange
c) femtosecond laser	__ corneal inlay
d) gem blade	__ LASEK
e) intrastromal insert	__ LASIK
f) IOL	__ phakic IOL/refractive lens implant
g) keratome	__ PRK
h) Mitomycin C	__ relaxing incisions
i) rotating brush	__ RK
	__ SMILE

Nonrefractive Laser Therapy

25. A laser beam is created by exposing a chemical substance to a power source and amplification system in order to:
    a) excite protons to emit polarized photons
    b) excite electrons to emit monochromatic photons
    c) excite neutrons to emit collimated photons
    d) slow down electrons to emit an intense photon stream

26. Which of the following ophthalmic lasers has the longest wavelength?
    a) YAG
    b) krypton
    c) carbon dioxide
    d) excimer

27. The argon and krypton are examples of laser action via:
    a) thermal photocoagulation
    b) ionizing (photodisruptive) reaction
    c) photochemical reaction
    d) photo-evaporation

28. The argon laser is especially useful for procedures involving:
    a) skin
    b) malignant tumors
    c) the macula
    d) blood vessels

29. If the patient's intraocular pressure has been checked via Goldmann tonometry, before treatment with the argon laser one should:
    a) irrigate the fluorescein dye from the eye
    b) use a laser lens to bypass the tear film
    c) abort the procedure if the intraocular pressure is low
    d) proceed as usual

30. The krypton laser might be used to:
    a) trim sutures following trabeculectomy
    b) remove benign skin lesions
    c) remove malignant skin lesions
    d) lyse vitreous adhesions

31. In comparison to the argon laser, the krypton laser is used to treat:
    a) superficial blood vessels
    b) retinal blood vessels
    c) synechiae
    d) deep choroid, outer retina, and macula

32. **The excimer laser has been approved for use in:**
    a) refractive surgery
    b) tumor treatment
    c) removal of skin cancers
    d) iridotomy

33. **The carbon dioxide laser is used to treat tissues that have a:**
    a) high melanin content
    b) high xanthophyll content
    c) high water content
    d) high hemoglobin content

34. **The carbon dioxide laser is used to:**
    a) sculpt the cornea in refractive surgery
    b) remove skin lesions and in eyelid surgery
    c) lyse vitreous adhesions
    d) perform iridotomies

35. **The advantage of tunable dye lasers is that:**
    a) various ultraviolet wavelengths can be selected
    b) various wavelengths from green to red can be selected
    c) various infrared wavelengths can be selected
    d) common fluorescein dye may be used

36. **The femtosecond laser is being evaluated for use during cataract surgery. In this case, the laser may be used for which of the following?**
    a) initial incision
    b) capsulorhexis
    c) cataract breakup
    d) all of the above

YAG Laser

37. **The ionizing YAG laser exerts its effect on tissues via:**
    a) thermal photocoagulation
    b) photodisruption
    c) photochemical reaction
    d) photoablation

38. **The YAG laser would likely be used for which of the following procedures?**
    a) treatment of diabetic retinopathy
    b) correcting refractive errors
    c) removal of skin lesions
    d) laser iridotomy

39.   YAG laser might be used in any of the following procedures *except*:
    a) trabeculectomy in open-angle glaucoma
    b) goniotomy in congenital glaucoma
    c) vitreolysis to break up floaters
    d) iridotomy for narrow angles

Laser Safety

40.   The laser has been moved from your old office across town to your new office. Recommended procedure is to:
    a) check beam alignment
    b) replace the dilithium crystals
    c) recalculate the wattage
    d) do a manual density calibration

41.   Which of the following is *not* an element of laser safety?
    a) remove reflective surfaces from the room
    b) post warning signs/lights
    c) appropriate ventilation/air filtering
    d) use only latex-free implements

42.   Which of the following is *not* required for laser safety?
    a) goggles of proper optical density
    b) appropriate patient education
    c) proper maintenance
    d) donning protective outerwear

Intraocular Injections

43.   Which of the following is *not* an advantage of intraocular injection?
    a) more precise medication delivery
    b) decreased systemic reaction to medication
    c) decreased toxicity to ocular tissues
    d) medication delivered to area where it's needed

44.   Introducing a substance into the eye via intravitreal injection might be used for any of the following *except*:
    a) diabetic macular edema
    b) retinal detachment
    c) antibiotic therapy
    d) angle-closure glaucoma

45.   A patient taking blood thinners may have a greater chance of developing which of the following after an intravitreal injection?
    a) decreased vision
    b) subconjunctival hemorrhage
    c) endophthalmitis
    d) pain/discomfort

46.   Which of the following is *not* a complication of intravitreal injections?
a) traumatic cataract
b) strabismus
c) retinal detachment
d) endophthalmitis

47.   Which of the following should be observed during administration of intravitreal injections?
a) limit povidone application to once
b) use the same speculum if both eyes are to be treated
c) limit talking
d) patch the eye tightly after the injection

48.   In addition to 5% povidone iodine, anesthetic, and syringe/needles, the tray set up for an intra-vitreal injection usually includes:
a) curette, clamp, scalpel, and eye patch
b) dilator, probe, and fluorescein
c) lid speculum, calipers, pledgets, and gauze
d) Wescott scissors, capsulorhexis forceps, and trypan blue

Procedures*

49.   Match the surgical procedure to the problem it is intended to correct. Answers may be used more than once, with some procedures having more than one answer.

Procedure	Disorder/Problem
__ blepharoplasty	a) blocked tear duct
__ corneal scraping	b) cataract
__ electrolysis	c) chalazion
__ entropion/ectropion repair	d) cyst
__ excision	e) dermatochalasis
__ extraocular muscle recession/resection	f) epiphora
__ incise and drain	g) eyelid malposition
__ intraocular air/gas bubble	h) narrow angles
__ iridotomy	i) recurrent corneal erosion
__ lacrimal irrigation and probing	j) retinal detachment
__ phacoemulsification and IOL	k) skin lesion(s)
__ ptosis repair	l) strabismus
__ retrobulbar injection	m) trichiasis
__ scleral buckle	n) vitreal hemorrhage
__vitrectomy	o) wet macular degeneration
	p) xanthelasma

* While not listed as a category, the flash cards have questions on procedures for specific conditions and instruments for specific procedures.

Sterilization

50. Instrument cleaning solutions sometimes contain enzymes in order to:
    a) dissolve organic debris
    b) kill bacteria
    c) lubricate moving parts
    d) kill spores

51. When preparing surgical scissors and forceps for the ultrasonic cleaner or autoclave, one should:
    a) package as many items together as possible
    b) wrap in a damp paper towel
    c) sharpen them first
    d) place instrument in most open position possible

52. Only instruments that are free of debris are ready to be sterilized. This is because:
    a) an autoclave cannot sterilize debris
    b) debris will contaminate any sterilization chemicals
    c) surfaces under debris will not get sterilized
    d) debris will contaminate sterile wrappings

53. The proper detergent for manual cleaning of surgical instruments is:
    a) acidic
    b) pH neutral
    c) basic
    d) saline

54. A devastating complication of anterior segment surgery caused by noninfective sources is:
    a) toxic shock syndrome
    b) Acanthamoeba syndrome
    c) toxic anterior segment syndrome
    d) Duane's syndrome

55. Diffuse lamellar keratitis following LASIK can be largely prevented by using which method of instrument sterilization?
    a) moist heat
    b) dry heat
    c) cold sterilization
    d) disinfectant spray

56. Which of the following is *not* a standard method of sterilizing surgical equipment?
    a) dry heat
    b) steam under pressure
    c) incineration
    d) chemicals

57. Which of the following is the most commonly used method of sterilizing instruments?
    a) dry heat
    b) autoclave
    c) chemicals
    d) ultrasound

58. Which of the following is *not* a commonly used germicide?
   a) ethylene oxide
   b) hydrogen peroxide
   c) bleach
   d) alcohol

59. Using chemicals as sterilizing agents is referred to as:
   a) chemotherapy
   b) liquid antiseptic
   c) ultrasonic cleaning
   d) cold sterilization

60. Which of the following is *not* used for chemical sterilization?
   a) hydrogen peroxide
   b) bleach
   c) glutaraldehyde
   d) isopropyl alcohol

61. Which of the following would be *most* reliable in indicating that an autoclaved instrument is, indeed, sterile?
   a) mechanical indicators
   b) chemical indicators
   c) biological indicators
   d) tape indicators

62. A one-of-a-kind instrument has become contaminated during a procedure. The procedure cannot continue without it. In this case, one might employ:
   a) a disinfectant wipe
   b) rapid chemical sterilization
   c) rinse with alcohol
   d) flash sterilization

63. Proper autoclave settings for the average instrument load is:
   a) 20 psi, 150°F, 30 minutes
   b) 10 psi, 300°F, 60 minutes
   c) 15 psi, 250°F, 30 minutes
   d) 30 psi, 120°F, 5 minutes

64. When autoclaving instruments, it is important to:
   a) use only tap water
   b) maintain a logbook of use and maintenance
   c) pack instruments tightly
   d) make sure the instruments are cold

65. Which of the following is *not* usually used to sterilize instruments because it dulls sharp edges and may cause rust?
   a) ultrasound
   b) autoclave
   c) boiling
   d) chemical sterilization

Maintain Surgical Instruments and Equipment

66. You are assisting with a ptosis repair and the surgeon hands you bloody scissors. You should:
     a) wipe them immediately with an instrument wipe
     b) return them to their previous spot on the sterile tray
     c) discard them
     d) open them fully

67. After cleaning, instruments must be rinsed thoroughly to remove all traces of detergent. If detergent residue is left on instruments, this may result in:
     a) pitting
     b) dulling
     c) staining
     d) rust

68. To lubricate moving parts of surgical instruments, one should use:
     a) enzymatic cleaner
     b) ultrasound
     c) instrument oil
     d) instrument milk

69. Which of the following statements regarding instrument milk is *not* true?
     a) Instruments are cleaned prior to dipping in instrument milk.
     b) Instruments are rinsed after dipping.
     c) Instruments are dipped for 30 seconds.
     d) Instrument milk does not sterilize.

70. Using saline solution on instruments may cause:
     a) dulling
     b) pitting
     c) poor sterilization
     d) no problems

71. When cleaning instruments with an ultrasonic unit, contamination from endotoxins can be caused by:
     a) reusing the cleaning fluid
     b) cavitation
     c) leaving the instruments in too long
     d) enzymatic cleaners

72. The phacoemulsification hand piece should be:
     a) flushed with enzymatic cleaner then autoclaved
     b) flushed in and out with distilled water then cold sterilized
     c) placed in an ultrasonic cleaner
     d) flushed with warm distilled water then autoclaved

73. **Which of the following statements about the operating microscope is *false*?**
    a) Check the controls once a week.
    b) Wipe external surfaces with a cloth damp with hot, soapy water.
    c) Insert the foot pedal into a clear plastic bag.
    d) Check the suspension arm before use.

74. **Which of the following regarding the bulbs used in the operating microscope is *true*?**
    a) Storing a bulb on its side will warp the filament.
    b) Only fluorescent lighting may be used.
    c) Bulbs should be replaced weekly.
    d) Allow the bulb to cool before moving the instrument.

75. **Which of the following elements of laser maintenance *cannot* be performed by an ophthalmic tech?**
    a) adjust the power monitors
    b) inspect and clean footswitch
    c) visually inspect cords and hoses
    d) visually inspect for dust and contaminants

Study Notes

Suggested reading in *Principles and Practice in Ophthalmic Assisting: A Comprehensive Textbook:*
    Chapter 37: In-Office Minor Surgery (pp 631-644)
    Chapter 38: Refractive Surgery (pp 645-654)
    Chapter 39: Ophthalmic Laser Surgery (pp 655-663)
    Chapter 40: Surgical Assisting (pp 665-679)
    Correction Note: Please note the following corrections on page 675 left column under *Steam Under Pressure* first paragraph (which is continued from page 674) temperature references should be changed FROM 250°C to 250°F (121°C) and FROM 270°C to 270°F (132°C). The next, full paragraph should be changed FROM 121°C to 250° F (121°C).

Explanatory Answers

1.   b) Instruments for surgery are laid out on the sterile tray in the order in which you expect them to be used. There is no such thing as "more or less" sterile. Either an item is sterile or it's not. The circulator does not handle sterile items.
2.   **Matching:**
    cannula   i)
    clamp   b)
    curette   b)
    dilator   h), i)
    electrolysis unit   e)
    forceps   a), b), c), d), f), g), j), k)
    lacrimal cannula   i)
    needle holder   c), d), g), j)
    phacoemulsification unit   a)
    probe   i)
    scalpel   a), b), c), f), g), j)

scissors	a), b), c), f), g), j)
speculum	a), c)
trephine	c)
vitrector	a)

3. **Matching:**

calipers	d)
cannula	b)
cautery unit	h)
clamp	e)
cryosurgery unit	f)
curette	a)
dilator	e)
electrolysis unit	g)
forceps	c)
needle holder	c)
phacoemulsification unit	i)
probe	e)
scalpel	a)
scissors	a)
speculum	e)
trephine	a)
vitrector	a)

4.   c) A gentian violet skin marker should be used to mark the surgical eye/site. A grease pen or cosmetic eye liner may rub off during prep. A speculum is any instrument used to open an orifice (the eyelids, in ophthalmic practice) so the inside can be inspected.

5.   d) The patient must be alert and oriented when the site is marked so that they are able to verify identification and the procedure. Once sedation has been administered, the patient is no longer considered able to reliably participate. On the table and after being prepped are not appropriate times to mark the site, either.

6.   b) The purpose of the time out is for all present to verify that you have the right patient for the right procedure on the right body part. You must, at some point, also look over the instruments, but that is not part of the official time out.

7.   b) Aseptic technique is not as "strict" as sterile technique and is not suitable for major surgical procedures. *Note:* A few references use the terms *aseptic technique* and *sterile technique* interchangeably.

8.   d) The purpose of asepsis and sterility is to reduce or eliminate infection-causing agents in the area and on objects in that area. Preventing infection is the goal.

9.   c) Touching a sterile item with another sterile item is okay; both are still sterile. However, if something sterile touches or is touched by anything unsterile, then both are contaminated.

10.   a) Only sterile items may be placed in the sterile field. In this question, we are presuming that the suture material itself is sterile, but that the package it's in is not. Sterile gauze is okay as long as the outer packaging does not touch the field.

11.   a) Anything below the level of the waist is contaminated.

12.   a) The circulator is not scrubbed, so you may not touch the edge of the tray (if you do, the tray will have to be considered contaminated). Nudging it with a foot could tip the tray. Instead, grasp the stand, under the drape (this area is nonsterile) and move the stand this way.

13.   d) Prolonged exposure to air renders sterile objects unsterile, but there's no set time limit that I could find in my research. It is clear, however, that the sterile tray with sterile instruments is considered part of the sterile field. As such, it must be under surveillance. Some practices would put a long strip of tape across the room door with a "do not enter" sign. (Foot traffic through the room may increase the chances of contamination.) Others advocate placing a sterile cover over the tray, but I also found a great outcry against this amongst OR nursing sites. The bottom line in sterility is "When in doubt, throw it out," or dismantle the sterile tray and start over.

14.   c) Everyone in the operating room who is a member of the surgical staff should monitor the sterile field and alert the team if sterility has been breached.

15.   b) The sterile part of a surgical gown is the front, between the waist and axillary (armpit) area, as well as the sleeves up to 3 inches beyond the elbow. Everything else is considered nonsterile.

16.   c) A 1-inch edge around the tray is considered nonsterile, so it is not acceptable to have something dangling off the tray edge. Sterile fluid in a sterile container is okay on the tray. Since the outside and edges of sterile packaging are unsterile, it is okay to carefully "dump" the instrument onto the tray, the main point is that the wrapper NOT touch the tray.

17.   b) The margin of safety is 12 inches. This includes anything sterile: scrubbed personnel, the sterile stand, the draped patient, etc.

18.   c) The circulator is not scrubbed, so cannot directly handle any sterile items. The circulator must also not reach across the sterile field. Open the sterile packaging carefully and spread it apart so the assistant can reach between the wrappings and retrieve the sterile item.

19.   b) There have been cases of patient fungal (and other) infections postoperatively where the surgical assistant is wearing artificial fingernails. FYI, if nail polish is worn, it must be free of cracks or flaking, and replaced weekly. Wearing scents in the operating room is discouraged. I hope the thought of dentures causing fungus in the operating room made you laugh!

20.   c) Since the environment used during laser surgery (of any kind) cannot be rendered sterile, laser surgery is considered an aseptic/clean procedure. No one can guarantee success, and it is an elective procedure (ie, not emergent or urgent).

21.   b) SMILE is a relatively new laser refractive procedure where the femtolaser is used to carve a lens-shaped disc of corneal tissue (called a *lenticule*) within the intact cornea. (The shape of the lenticule is predetermined by corneal mapping and other measurements.) The laser then carves a "tunnel" from the top of the lenticule to the corneal surface. This lenticule is then removed under the surgical microscope, thus changing the power of the cornea in order to correct the patient's refractive error. The other "procedures" mentioned are all fabricated.

22.   a) The laser burst of the femtosecond laser is extremely fast (eg, nanoseconds for YAG and smaller femtoseconds for the femtosecond laser). That means that there is more control, and the surgical area is tighter. Collateral tissue damage is the destruction of tissue beyond the desired treatment area; the surgeon is willing to live with it, but it'd be nice to eliminate as much as possible. It is especially used in LASIK and SMILE procedures.

23.   d) Anterior basement membrane dystrophy seems to be the current, popular designation for map-dot-fingerprint dystrophy, Cogan's microcystic dystrophy, and epithelial basement membrane dystrophy. It can cause epithelial sloughing, or corneal erosion. The corneal topography map may be irregular. On slit lamp, you may see the fine parallel lines (like a fingerprint), dots, and/or thicker lines like a geographic map. Patients with anterior basement membrane dystrophy are more likely to have sloughing of the corneal epithelium during or after LASIK.

24. **Matching:**

AK	d)
clear lensectomy/refractive lens exchange	f)
corneal inlay	e)
LASEK	a), b)
LASIK	b), c), g)
phakic IOL/refractive lens implant	f)
PRK	a), b), h), i)
relaxing incisions	d)
RK	d)
SMILE	c)

25. b) The word "laser" is an acronym for light amplification by stimulated emission of radiation. The electrons are provided by a chemical substance (eg, argon gas or YAG crystal). The electrons are "pumped up" by exposing them to a power source such as heat or electricity and are thus excited to such a state that they emit photons of monochromatic (ie, single wavelength) light. The wavelength, direction, and phase of the photons are all the same. This produces a narrow column of light that is extremely intense.

26. c) Of those listed, the carbon dioxide laser has the longest wavelength. From longest to shortest wavelength, commonly used ophthalmic lasers are CO_2, YAG, krypton, argon, and excimer.

27. a) The argon and krypton lasers are absorbed by tissues containing hemoglobin. The absorbed light is transformed into thermal (heat) energy, and coagulation occurs. (To get a mental image of this, it can be compared to welding.) See Table 14-1 for a summary of laser types, actions, and uses.

28. d) Because argon laser light is absorbed by hemoglobin, this laser is wonderfully suited for treating disorders of the blood vessels, such as diabetic retinopathy (both leaking vessels and neovascularization) and vein occlusions. It is also used to treat some retinal detachments (if they are localized and there is no traction) and retinal holes. Its spot size is too large to treat the macula.

29. a) Fluorescein will absorb the 488 nm wavelengths of the argon laser. Thus fluorescein dye should be irrigated from the eye prior to the procedure.

30. a) In order to increase drainage after trabeculectomy, the scleral flap sutures can be lysed by focusing the krypton (or argon) laser right through the conjunctiva.

31. d) The krypton laser is not absorbed by retinal blood vessels (so it passes through hemorrhages), but it is absorbed by melanin (present in the choroid and retinal pigment epithelium). Therefore, it is ideal for the structures listed. (It also passes easily through cataracts.)

32. a) A thin area of corneal stroma can be ablated by the excimer laser to flatten the corneal cap during a refractive procedure known as PRK. The excimer is also used to remove corneal scars.

33. c) Tissues with a high water content are treated with the carbon dioxide laser because water absorbs the laser light.

34. b) Skin cells have a very high water content, ideal for treatment with the carbon dioxide laser. The laser produces an extremely fine line, making it useful in creating incisions during eyelid surgery. The drawback in using it to remove lesions is that there is no specimen left for biopsy, so it is used mainly if the physician is sure that the growth is not malignant. It is also used in performing a sclerectomy, a glaucoma procedure.

35. b) The "tunable" part of a tunable dye laser refers to the ability to select a wavelength (from green to red) that is appropriate to the work being done. (Other lasers have a fixed wavelength which are useful for only specific uses.) The tunable dye laser can be used for iridotomy, iridoplasty, and trabeculoplasty.

36. d) Femtosecond laser–assisted cataract surgery involves using the laser for precise incisions, opening the capsule, breaking up the cataract, and (if desired) relaxing incisions to correct astigmatism.

TABLE 14-1
LASERS IN OPHTHALMOLOGY

Laser	Wavelength	Action	Uses
I. Thermal			
Argon	blue-green (488 to 515 nm) low energy continuous wave	• Photocoagulation • Absorbed by hemoglobin, melanin, and xanthopil	Retinal vascular disease Choroidal neovascularization Trabeculoplasty Iridotomy Suture lysis
Krypton	red (647 nm) continuous wave	• Photocoagulation • Absorbed by melanin, to a lesser degree by hemoglobin (not absorbed by retinal vessels) and xanthopil • Passes more readily through lens opacities and vitreous hemorrhages	Same as Argon but deeper choroid
CO_2	infrared long wavelength low penetration	• Photovaporization (photo-evaporation) • Absorbed by water	Skin lesions Fine, bloodless skin incisions Cautery
Tunable dye	adjustable (green to red)	• Photocoagulation • Variably absorbed by melanin, hemoglobin, and xanthopil	Same as Argon and Krypton
Diode laser	infrared (805 nm)	• Photocoagulation • Sometimes used in conjunction with ICG dye	Retinal vascular disease Choroidal neovascularization
Frequency-doubled YAG	green (532 nm) continuous wave	• Photocoagulation	Same as Krypton
II. Ionizing			
Q-switched YAG	infrared (1064 nm) pulsed laser	• Photodisruption ("cold, cutting") • very tiny spot sizes	Incisions/cutting Synechiotomy Capsulotomy Vitreous adhesions Iridotomy
III. Photochemical			
Excimer	UV light (photo-evaporation)	• Photoablation • Breaks chemical bonds of tissues	Corneal opacities Refractive surgery
Photodynamic therapy	red-infrared (665 to 732 nm)	• Causes chemical changes that result in vascular occlusion and cellular disruption • Used in conjunction with photosensitive agents	Malignant tumors Choroidal neovascularization

Reproduced with permission from Ledford JK. *Certified Ophthalmic Medical Technologist Exam Review Manual.* SLACK Incorporated; 2000.

37.   b) The ionizing (Q-charged) YAG laser results in the ionization of tissue from high heat plus mechanical and acoustic shock waves. This produces a "micro-explosion" (or photodisruption) that destroys the tissue. (It is important to note that the heat itself does not ablate the tissue, but rather the "explosion.")

38.   d) The photodisruptive power of the YAG laser makes it ideal for punching a hole through the iris. Probably the more common use, however, is laser capsulotomy following cataract surgery.

39.   a) The YAG laser might be used in any of the listed procedures except trabeculectomy, which is usually performed with an Argon laser.

40.   a) Jolting can cause the beam to move out of alignment. The instrument should be checked prior to use. Dilithium crystals are used for warp speed in the Star Trek universe. There is no such thing as a "manual density calibration."

41.   d) Any metallic surfaces and mirrors must be removed from a laser room to avoid reflecting of the laser beam. Warning signs/lights are required by OSHA to protect those in the vicinity. There must also be filtering and/or ventilation appropriate to the type of laser being used. Latex is not an issue for laser use.

42.   d) Protective outerwear is not required.

43.   c) The advantages of delivering medication intraocularly is that the medication is placed more or less precisely where it's needed; we are not dependent on a medication having to penetrate numerous tissues before reaching the targeted area. This also decreases the exposure of the entire system (body) to medication.

44.   d) Intravitreal injections are not used in angle closure, where the addition of more volume to the eye could be detrimental. While their most common use is in neovascular macular degeneration, anti–vascular endothelial growth factor injections may also be used to treat diabetic macular edema. Air or oil might be injected to treat retinal detachment, and antibiotic injections may be indicated in infection.

45.   b) Blood thinners make it more likely that the patient will develop a subconjunctival hemorrhage after the injection. Patients should be advised of this since a subconjunctival hemorrhage looks rather scary. However, it is not usually necessary for the patient to discontinue blood thinners prior to the injection.

46.   b) The list is longer, but complications/risks of intravitreal injections include cataract, retinal detachment, and infection/endophthalmitis. Strabismus is not a problem related to intravitreal injections.

47.   c) Even with masks (and shields) on, it is best to limit talking in order to reduce the chances of contamination. Povidone may be used more than once: first for the initial cleansing, then again just prior to injection, and more as directed by the surgeon. Each eye should be prepared individually if both eyes are being treated, including a fresh sterile speculum. Patching is not employed.

48.   c) Items listed in Answer c) would be needed on the tray for intravitreal injections. Saline/BSS would also be provided for rinsing the eye after the procedure. Items in a) might be used for a chalazion, b) for nasolacrimal procedures, and d) for cataract surgery.

49.   **Matching:**

blepharoplasty	e)
corneal scraping	i)
electrolysis	m)
entropion/ectropion repair	g)
excision	c), e), k), p)
extraocular muscle recession/resection	l)
incise and drain	c), d)
intraocular air/gas bubble	j)
iridotomy	h)

lacrimal irrigation and probing	a), f)
phacoemulsification and IOL	b)
ptosis repair	g)
retrobulbar injection	o)
scleral buckle	j)
vitrectomy	j), n)

50. a) Enzymes are added to cleaners to break up organic material (such as proteins, fats, and starches) left on used surgical instruments. They do not impart any degree of sterilization.

51. d) Any instrument with moveable parts, such as scissors and forceps, should be open to the maximum when packaged. This allows the ultrasound or steam access to the maximum amount of surface. Also, once debris is "baked" onto an instrument by autoclaving, it is very difficult to remove.

52. c) Only exposed areas of an instrument gets sterilized. The debris' surface may be sterilized, but the surface under it won't be. And if the debris dislodges while the instrument is in use, the eye is at risk.

53. b) Detergents for cleaning instruments should be pH neutral, that is, have a pH of 7. If the detergent is too basic or too acidic or saline, this can result in stains on the metal.

54. c) Toxic anterior segment syndrome is a noninfective type of sterile endophthalmitis characterized by inflammation inside the eye along with corneal edema. Although rare, it most commonly occurs after cataract surgery. There are various causes, including chemicals released by bacteria as they are destroyed, harmful chemicals in solutions or ointments used during surgery, inadequately flushed instruments, and particulate matter.

55. b) It was found that moist heat could introduce debris (potentially a factor in the occurrence of DLK ["Sands of Sahara Syndrome"]) to subsequent instrument batches if the distillate (residue) from the sterilization process remained in the autoclave. Dry heat eliminates this possibility. Disinfectant spray does not sterilize and would never be used on surgical instruments.

56. c) Incineration means to destroy something by burning. The other answers are viable methods of instrument sterilization. Which method is preferable depends on the nature of the instrument to be sterilized, the speed with which the item is required, and other factors.

57. b) The autoclave (steam under pressure) is the customary and most practical method of sterilizing instruments. Ultrasound is for cleaning only; it does not sterilize.

58. a) A *germicide* is any substance used as a disinfectant, antiseptic, or sterilizing agent. Ethylene oxide is used to sterilize instruments, especially items made of rubber and other materials that would be destroyed by heat or chemicals. It is not commonly used in the average clinic because it is flammable, expensive, and time-consuming. *Note:* Various references use the term germicide differently. Some seem to mean only chemicals. But the property of being germicidal (an adjective) means to kill germs (-*cidal* referring to *kill*), which would include any method of doing so.

59. d) Using chemicals to sterilize instruments is known as cold sterilization. Not all germicides are appropriate for cold sterilization because they do not destroy spores.

60. d) Isopropyl alcohol is not an accepted sterilizing method for surgical instruments because it does not kill spores. An example of glutaraldehyde is Cidex (Johnson & Johnson).

61. c) Biological indicators involve exposing packaged spores to the autoclave process. If the process is working, the spores will not grow (ie, they will have been rendered unviable). Mechanical indicators involve monitoring the gauges and settings on the autoclave itself to be sure that desired pressure, temperature, steam, and time are reached and properly maintained; they do not guarantee sterility. Chemical indicators (of which tape indicators are a type) turn color when exposed to the proper pressure, temperature, steam, and time. They cannot guarantee sterility, either, although they should be used.

62. d) Flash sterilization (also called *immediate use*) is used when instruments must be processed quickly, and is done (at proper pressure, temperature, and time) using an autoclave that is equipped for such a cycle. While many resource materials will suggest a pressure, temperature, and time, the best method is to proceed according to your autoclave's user's manual. Otherwise, you will see variations from 3 minutes up to 15 minutes. Not all autoclaves can accomplish flash sterilization.

63. c) The correct setting for the autoclave when sterilizing an average load of instruments is 15 psi, 250°F, for 30 minutes.

64. b) A logbook of use, testing, maintenance, and repairs will help ensure that the unit is working properly. Distilled, deionized water must be used, as tap water contains minerals that may build up in the unit. Instruments should not be packed but loaded so that the steam will reach every part of every packet. Instruments should be room temperature, as cold ones may cause condensation and staining.

65. c) Boiling instruments is not generally recommended for several reasons, chief of which is that it may not be sufficient to kill bacterial spores. In addition, boiling tends to dull sharp edges (so critical in eye surgery) and may cause rusting.

66. a) An instrument that may be required again but is handed to you dirty should not be returned to the sterile, unused part of the tray or thrown out. Wipe them immediately with an instrument wipe and place on a different part of the tray.

67. c) The usual cause of stained instruments is detergent left on cleaned instruments. It will generally wipe off easily and does not affect the sterility of the instrument, but does need to be addressed by more thorough rinsing. It can also be caused if the steam contains certain minerals (notably calcium and magnesium). Rust does not wipe off. Pits affect the integrity of the instrument's surface.

68. d) Instrument milk (or surgical milk) is used to lubricate the moving parts of instruments. It also protects stainless steel and inhibits corrosion, helping to prevent staining and rusting. There are many brands and formulas. Follow the directions for the particular liquid you are using. Oil is not used as a lubricant because it interferes with the autoclaving process.

69. b) Commonly, the instruments are first cleaned, then dipped into the solution for 30 seconds, removed, and allowed to air dry prior (not rinsed) to packaging for the autoclave. Instrument milk does not sterilize.

70. b) Pitting is surface damage caused by exposure to saline solutions. The only remedy is to have the instrument refinished or replaced.

71. a) After use, the solution used in an ultrasound may be contaminated by bacteria. When the bacteria are destroyed (by cavitation), their toxic contents are released into the solution. Fresh solution should be used, and the unit (and basket) properly cleaned between uses.

72. d) The phaco hand piece should be flushed with warm distilled water, not with any type of chemical agent. It should be flushed out only, not drawn back into the hand piece. It is not placed into an ultrasonic cleaning unit. It may be sterilized using autoclave, flash sterilization, or high vacuum.

73. a) The controls (foot pedal, etc) should be checked prior to use. External surfaces are cleaned as indicated in b). The optics should be cleaned weekly as per manufacturer's instructions. Putting the foot pedal into a bag protects the pedal from any spilled fluids (cleaning or otherwise). The suspension arm should be checked prior to use. It is the one part that, if it malfunctions and releases, could potentially harm the patient.

74. d) Moving the microscope when the bulb is hot may damage the filament. In addition, allow the bulb to cook before removal, and do not handle a new bulb with bare fingers.

75. a) Only specially trained factory reps or service personnel should adjust the power monitors.

Bibliography

Cordero I. Understanding and caring for an operating microscope. *Comm Eye Health J.* 2014;27(85):17. Accessed March 17, 2023. www.ncbi.nlm.nih.gov/pmc/articles/PMC4069782/

Chapter 15

Ophthalmic Patient Services and Education

Ledford JK.
*Certified Ophthalmic Technician Exam
Review Manual, Third Edition* (pp 275-308).
© 2023 Taylor & Francis Group.

ABBREVIATIONS USED IN THIS CHAPTER

- ADA   Americans with Disabilities Act
- AED   automated external defibrillator
- CPR   cardiopulmonary resuscitation
- EMS   emergency medical services
- F   Fahrenheit (temperature)

Note: See also Question 13.

Part I*

Effective Communication

1. **In addition to language differences, barriers to communication with patients can include:**
    a) cognitive disabilities
    b) hearing impairments
    c) education level
    d) all of the above

2. **Nonverbal communication includes all of the following *except*:**
    a) vocabulary
    b) body language, facial expressions, and gestures
    c) voice volume and tone
    d) clothing

Care for Diverse Populations

3. **Diversity includes not only people groups of varied appearance, language, and ability, but also respecting different:**
    a) customs
    b) beliefs
    c) gender orientations
    d) all of the above

4. **Your patient has advancing dementia. Communicating effectively with them includes:**
    a) speaking more loudly
    b) using simple sentences
    c) using expansive gestures
    d) avoiding direct communication

---

* Sections have been inserted into this lengthy chapter for ease of study, to allow for a logical "break" point.

5.   Your patient is a 4-year-old you have seen before, whom you know to be fearful. To make the exam easier, you might consider:
     a) speaking to the guardian only, not the patient
     b) offering the child a soft drink
     c) removing your lab coat before entering the exam room
     d) sending the guardian out of the room

Interpersonal Relationship Skills

6.   Your colleague is extremely knowledgeable about all things "eye." However, she has difficulty connecting to patients in a positive way. The subject of "bedside/chair-side manner" is known as:
     a) transactional analysis
     b) sales pitch
     c) service recovery
     d) interpersonal relationship skills

7.   Connecting with patients in an appropriate emotional way is important because:
     a) patients will then buy glasses from the practice
     b) they will give more honest answers to objective testing
     c) there is a relationship between healing and human interaction
     d) it's nice to be nice

8.   Considering the patient as a whole being in need of health and healing vs as "an eye" is a function of:
     a) whole-unit treatment
     b) the Zen of eye care
     c) holistic medicine
     d) wholesome medical care

9.   Possibly one of the greatest barriers to effective communication with patients in the exam room is:
     a) lack of eye contact
     b) automated equipment
     c) electronic medical records
     d) lack of physical touch

10. You walk by an open door and notice that a coworker is having difficulty getting a patient to fixate for a Tono-Pen pressure check. You ask, "Can I help?" and your coworker shuts the door in your face. You approach the coworker later, in private. Which of the following statements is an example of good interpersonal skills?
     a) "You were really rude to me in front of that patient."
     b) "I feel confused about what happened, and I'd like to talk about it."
     c) "Don't ever shut the door in my face again."
     d) "I won't ever try to help you again."

The Dissatisfied Patient

11.   **The process taken when reaching out to a dissatisfied patient in order to rectify the situation and regain patient loyalty is known as:**
    a) complaint handling
    b) performance managing
    c) service recovery
    d) customer service

12.   **Which of the following would be an example of reflective listening on your part, in the case where a patient is unhappy about having to hold a book too close when reading with their new glasses?**
    a) "I have confirmed the prescription of the new glasses, and it is correct."
    b) "When we measured you for the glasses, you said you *wanted* to hold a book at 11 inches."
    c) "You don't like having to hold a book so close for reading with your new glasses."
    d) "I'm sorry you're unhappy. We'll just have the optician make you a new pair."

Patient Education*

13.   **Match the test to the description you would give the patient about the test.**
    <u>Test</u>
    Amsler grid
    anomaloscope
    autorefractor
    break up time
    brightness acuity test
    color vision arrangement test
    color vision plates
    contrast sensitivity
    corneal sensitivity test (anesthesiometer)
    corneal topography
    dark adaptation test
    electrooculogram
    electroretinogram
    exophthalmometer
    fluorescein angiography
    fluorescein dye
    gonioscopy
    Heidelberg retina tomography
    Humphrey visual fields
    keratometer
    laser interference biometry
    macular photostress test
    optical coherence tomography
    pachymeter
    potential acuity meter

* See also Chapter 16: General Medical Knowledge, section *Eye Diseases and Conditions*, for more questions regarding this material. While the knowledge base itself is being tested in Chapter 16, it is expected that the tech will describe these things to a patient using terms the patient can understand.

pupillometer
retinoscopy
Schirmer test
slit lamp
specular microscope
tear osmolarity
tonometry
ultrasound
visual evoked potential/visual evoked response

Description to Patient
I look at the way this light reflects from your eye. This gives me an idea of what lenses may help you see better.
The grids on this test evaluate your ability to detect varying degrees of light and dark.
The patterns on these pages will help us detect color vision problems.
The pattern of how you arrange these little caps will help us know if there are any color vision problems.
This instrument detects color vision problems.
This instrument is used to measure for any protrusion of the eye.
This instrument makes a map of the curvature of the cornea, the clear covering over the front of your eye.
This instrument measures how long it takes your eyes to adapt from bright light to darkness.
This instrument measures the curvature of the cornea, the clear covering over the front of your eye.
This instrument measures the distance between your pupils in order to line your glasses up correctly.
This instrument measures the thickness of the cornea, the clear covering over the front of your eye.
This instrument measures/images your eye using sound waves.
This instrument scans your eye and comes up with a possible glasses prescription.
This instrument takes several measurements needed to select the proper intraocular lens for cataract surgery.
This instrument uses light to scan and create a cross-section of the tissues of the eye.
This is a microscope that helps me see the front of your eye in detail.
This is a scanning laser that creates a 3-dimensional image of the optic nerve and surrounding tissue.
This is a special camera that images the inner cell layer of your cornea, which will give us an idea of the health of the cornea.
This is to test your tear production.
This liquid glows in the microscope's blue light.
This little lens is used to be able to see the part of your eye where the aqueous fluid drains out.
This test evaluates and records the response of a specific cell layer of the retina.
This test evaluates the composition of your tears.
This test evaluates the overall health of the retina.
This test evaluates the pathway that light takes as it travels from your eye to the brain.
This test gives us an idea of how long your tears stay on your eye.
This test gives us an idea of what your vision is like when glare hits you.
This test gives us an idea of what your vision might be if your cataract was removed.
This test helps us evaluate the sensitivity of the nerves in your cornea.
This test helps us evaluate your central vision, checking for distortion.
This test makes images the doctor will use to study the blood flow in your retina.
This test maps out your vision, especially in the periphery/edges.
This test measures how quickly your vision recovers after seeing a really bright light.
This test measures the pressure inside your eye.

14. **Match the procedure to the description you would give the patient about the procedure.**

Procedure

biopsy
blepharoplasty
cataract surgery
cautery
centesis
corneal transplant
cryo
ectropion repair
electrolysis
entropion repair
incise and drain
intraocular injection
laser capsulotomy
laser iridotomy
laser trabeculectomy
panretinal photocoagulation
probe and irrigation
punctal plugs
refractive surgery
scleral buckle
strabismus surgery

Description to Patient

any procedure that changes your glasses prescription, usually to eliminate the need for glasses
inserting tiny plastic stoppers into the openings of the tear drainage system (usually the lower lids)
opening a fluid or pus-filled lesion to empty it
opening the nasolacrimal duct and flushing the tear drainage system
sending tissue to a pathologist to find out what it is (usually looking for cancer)
surgery that removes scarred cornea and uses clear donor tissue to replace it
surgery that removes the cloudy lens from inside the eye; a clear plastic lens implant is put in its place to allow clearer vision
surgery that uses a silicone band to repair a retinal detachment
surgery to "loosen" the lids (usually the lower) so they lie against the eyeball instead of flipping in and rubbing the cornea
surgery to "tighten" the lids (usually the lower) so they lie against the eyeball instead of turning out
surgery to remove excess skin (and sometimes fat) from the eyelids (usually the upper)
surgery to straighten "crossed" eyes
using a cold probe to freeze tissue
using a laser to "seal" tiny areas all over the retina to prevent diabetic damage
using a laser to open the cloudy membrane behind an intraocular lens implant
using a syringe to deliver medication inside the eye
using a syringe to remove fluid, usually from the front of the eye
using a tiny electric charge to kill a hair follicle
using heat to burn tissue, such as sealing off a bleeding blood vessel
using laser to make an opening in the iris so that fluid inside the eye can drain
using laser to make openings in the drainage system inside the eye so fluid doesn't build up

Prevention

15. **Using sunglasses and lenses with ultraviolet filtering is advisable for patients with:**
    a) angle-closure glaucoma
    b) keratoconus
    c) retinal detachment
    d) macular degeneration

16. **Smoking can exacerbate each of the following conditions *except*:**
    a) lid ptosis
    b) cataracts
    c) glaucoma
    d) macular degeneration

17. **The single most important feature for prevention of eye injuries in industry and sports is:**
    a) ocular vitamins
    b) minimize contact
    c) proper eye protection
    d) proper refractive correction

18. **Your patient is monocular and has no refractive error. Best advice for this patient is to:**
    a) wear glasses with safety lenses at all times
    b) use artificial tears 4 times per day
    c) have an eye exam every 6 months
    d) wear sunglasses at all times

19. **Your 63-year-old patient's mother and grandmother have a history of dry macular degeneration. Best advice to this patient is:**
    a) use artificial tears
    b) avoid using a hot tub
    c) get 8 hours of sleep every night
    d) take a good multivitamin

20. **A patient wearing contact lenses who is experiencing pain and redness should be advised to:**
    a) rewet the lens on the eye
    b) see if it goes away after 1 hour
    c) splash water in the eye
    d) remove the lens

21. **The best way for a patient with dry eye to prevent tearing is to:**
    a) instill artificial tears as directed
    b) instill artificial tears as needed
    c) rub the eyes periodically
    d) irrigate with homemade saline

Compliance

22. A patient who is postop after cataract surgery stopped using the topical steroid drops after 3 days. This patient runs the risk of:
     a) elevated intraocular pressure
     b) rebound inflammation
     c) rebound infection
     d) poor refractive result

23. To which of the following ocular medications might instructions to the patient include "Don't let yourself run out of drops. If you go out of town, take them with you."
     a) tear drops
     b) allergy drops
     c) macular degeneration drops
     d) glaucoma drops

24. Your patient has been given oral antibiotics for cellulitis. You tell them:
     a) take them until you feel better
     b) take them all until they're gone
     c) take half and save the other half in case of recurrence
     d) apply directly to the affected area

25. Your patient with glaucoma admits to not using latanoprost and dorzolamide/timolol as directed. You should:
     a) scold them
     b) ask why they don't use them as directed
     c) try to scare them with stories of blindness
     d) dismiss them from the practice

26. An important part of counseling patients regarding treatment compliance is to:
     a) avoid mentioning side effects
     b) go over the package insert with them
     c) help the patient identify barriers
     d) insist on a schedule that you supply

27. The parent of an active 4-year-old being patched for amblyopia states matter-of-factly that she doesn't "force" him to wear the patch because he doesn't like it. You should:
     a) help her identify positive reinforcement tactics
     b) suggest parenting classes
     c) provide written instructions
     d) suggest she discipline the child

Acceptance

28. **Your patient has macular degeneration and recently had to give up her driver's license. Today her demeanor is angry, and she expresses frustration with the situation. The most helpful thing for you to say might be:**
     a) "No one ever said this would be easy."
     b) "It'll be nice to have someone chauffeur you everywhere!"
     c) "I'd be angry, too, if it happened to me."
     d) "You didn't do anything to cause this."

29. **In order to reach a point of acceptance to new, debilitating vision loss, one must:**
     a) allow various emotions to run their course
     b) be regimented with treatments
     c) begin at once to learn adaptive techniques
     d) keep a positive attitude

Side Effects of Drops Being Administered

30. **You are about to dilate a 5-year-old with cyclogyl. Which of the following is *not* appropriate to tell the parent?**
     a) "Your child might still be a little dilated tomorrow."
     b) "Your child might be a bit light sensitive for several hours."
     c) "Your child won't be able to see for several hours."
     d) all of the above

31. **Which of the following statements to your patient regarding routine dilation is *false*?**
     a) Most people can see to drive.
     b) It may blur your reading vision.
     c) Your pupils will look larger.
     d) Lights might seem dimmer.

32. **Your patient wears a soft contact lens and also has glaucoma. She removed the lens and had an intraocular pressure check with Goldmann applanation. You have irrigated the fluorescein out of her eye the best you can. You advise her:**
     a) to insert a fresh, new lens
     b) to leave the lens out the rest of the day
     c) to wait 1 hour before reinserting the lens
     d) she may reinsert the lens immediately

Patient Empathy

33. **Your patient is a teary 5-year-old who is still sniffling after getting dilating drops. You drop to one knee to his eye-level and say, "I'm sorry I had to do something you didn't like." This is an example of:**
     a) pity
     b) sympathy
     c) compassion
     d) "I messages"

34. **Which of the following does *not* involve showing empathy for a patient?**
    a) Jotting a note in the patient's chart telling the physician how to pronounce the patient's name.
    b) Leaving the exam room door slightly ajar for your patient who is claustrophobic.
    c) Allowing a child patient to sit on a guardian's lap in the exam chair.
    d) Sending the patient a card reminding them of an upcoming appointment.

Greeting

35. **When greeting a patient in person or on the phone, you should state your name and then:**
    a) take the patient history
    b) verify patient identity
    c) explain what you'll be doing for the patient
    d) obtain contact information

36. **Which of the following is *not* part of a successful patient greeting?**
    a) eye contact
    b) smiling
    c) using the patient's name
    d) shaking hands

Assist Patients With Disabilities

37. **The key in transferring any patient from a wheelchair to an exam chair is to always:**
    a) use a transfer board
    b) get assistance
    c) lock the wheelchair
    d) use a mechanical lift

38. **When assisting a patient using a cane or walker, the patient should be encouraged to:**
    a) use a wheelchair while in your office
    b) walk on their own as much as possible
    c) lean on you as necessary
    d) use the device all the way to the exam chair

39. **The clinic clerk asks for your advice in scheduling a child patient with autism. You suggest asking the patient's guardian:**
    a) if the patient is ever violent
    b) what time of day is the patient most alert and calm
    c) is the patient in a wheelchair
    d) if the patient can recognize letters

40. **For which situation in an adult patient might you need to speak in simple, short sentences?**
    a) post-traumatic stress disorder
    b) fellow eye techs
    c) dementia
    d) anxiety/depression

41. The patient with post-traumatic stress disorder may require any of the following except:
     a) warning if there is going to be a loud noise
     b) speak loudly and clearly
     c) door left partially opened
     d) emotional support dog

42. The parent of a child with intellectual disabilities has called to inquire about an eye exam. The father says that the child's ability to communicate is limited and wants to know if an eye exam is even possible. This parent can be told:
     a) A lot of our tests, even for glasses, can usually be done without input from the patient.
     b) What we can do is limited, but we'll be glad to see your child.
     c) We can do pretty much everything for your child except prescribe glasses.
     d) The exam will be no different than that for any other child.

43. Your patient has epilepsy. It is important to inquire:
     a) Is a dark environment likely to trigger a seizure?
     b) Will the dilating drops counteract your medication?
     c) Will covering one eye trigger a seizure?
     d) Are flashing lights likely to trigger a seizure?

44. Which of the following is *least* likely indication that your patient is very anxious?
     a) heavy breathing, sweating
     b) complaints of being dizzy or light-headed
     c) patient trying hard to give the "right" answer
     d) patient refuses all eye drops

45. The civil rights law that requires a medical practice to provide adequate communication for persons with disabilities is:
     a) the Americans with Disabilities Act (ADA)
     b) the Equal Communications Act (ECA)
     c) the Medical Explanations Act of Equality (MEAE)
     d) the Prevention of Misunderstanding Act (PMA)

46. Using pen and paper to communicate with a deaf patient:
     a) is as adequate as providing an interpreter
     b) may not meet the requirements of civil rights laws
     c) is as effective as the patient reading lips
     d) is a violation of the Equal Communications Act

Patient Referrals

47.   **Match the condition to the specialty ophthalmic clinic the patient might be referred to. Answers may be used more than once.**
Specialty Clinic
a) cornea
b) glaucoma
c) neuro-ophthalmology
d) ocular genetics
e) ocular immunology
f) oculoplastics
g) oncology
h) vitreous/retina

Condition
___ albinism
___ basal cell carcinoma of lid
___ coloboma of eyelid
___ cranial nerve palsy
___ diabetes
___ Fuchs' dystrophy
___ infant with large, "cloudy" eyes
___ keratoconus
___ lung cancer patient with new iris lesion
___ multiple sclerosis
___ nystagmus
___ patient who is not responding to latanoprost, brimonidine, and timolol
___ patient with scarring from herpes simplex infection
___ premature infant with questionable vision
___ presumed ocular histoplasmosis syndrome
___ pseudotumor cerebri
___ ptosis over the pupil in a 2-year-old
___ reconstruction of eyelid
___ retinal detachment
___ retinitis pigmentosa
___ retinoblastoma
___ sarcoidosis
___ unexplained diplopia
___ unexplained visual field loss

Apply/Remove Eye Dressings and Shields

48.   **Which of the following is most likely to require the application of an eye dressing?**
a) loss of vision
b) bacterial keratitis
c) corneal abrasion
d) keratitis sicca

49. **An eye dressing ("pressure patch") is properly applied by:**
     a) directly taping the eye shut
     b) strips of tape angled from upper nasal forehead down to cheek
     c) weaving strips of tape in and out over the patch and onto the skin
     d) strips of tape horizontally across the patch and onto the forehead/temple

50. **Which of the following is commonly applied after cataract surgery?**
     a) very tight pressure patch
     b) butterfly closures
     c) patch and shield
     d) bandage contact lens

Counsel and Assist With Medication Reimbursement Programs

51. **Your patient with glaucoma admits that she uses her twice-a-day glaucoma drops only once daily "to make them last longer." You learn that the cost of the drops is prohibitive for her. How can you help?**
     a) Find out if the drug company can help.
     b) Reassure her that once is enough.
     c) Remind her that the drug will not work well unless used as directed.
     d) Suggest a different, less expensive medication.

Phone Calls: Respond and Document*

52. **The receptionist hands you the following note:** *Joe Smith, feels like there's something in eye, call back at 123-456-7890.* **You follow up by calling the patient. Proper documentation of your call should include:**
     a) details of the problem
     b) patient education given
     c) follow-up plans
     d) all of the above

53. **In addition to medical details, your properly documented phone call must include some notation regarding:**
     a) the patient's satisfaction with the information given
     b) the patient's comprehension of information and/or directions
     c) the patient's consent to discuss the situation with the physician
     d) the patient's "no show" history

* See also *Triage and Appoint* in this chapter.

Forms

54. **Which of the following is *not* true?**
    a) A filled-out form is part of the patient's record.
    b) An improperly filled-out form could be used as evidence in court.
    c) A properly filled-out form will ensure that the patient obtains their license.
    d) A filled-out form falls under privacy rules while it is in possession of the clinic.

Adjust/Repair Spectacles

55. **The patient's glasses sit too low on their face. This can be adjusted by:**
    a) bending the nose pads closer together
    b) tightening the temples
    c) loosening the temples
    d) spreading the nose pads apart

56. **Before adjusting a plastic frame, it is important to:**
    a) warm the frames
    b) cool the frames
    c) clean the frames
    d) remove the lenses

57. **In most cases, frames should be adjusted so that there is a:**
    a) retroscopic tilt
    b) maximum pupillary distance
    c) pantoscopic tilt
    d) minimum vertex distance

58. **Which of the following is *not* modifiable by adjusting the frames?**
    a) segment position
    b) physical comfort
    c) effective power of the lens
    d) base curve

59. **In general, the top of a bifocal segment is positioned so that it:**
    a) aligns with the upper lid margin
    b) aligns with the lower lid margin
    c) bisects the pupil
    d) aligns with the bottom of the pupil

60. **In general, the top edge of a trifocal segment is positioned so that it:**
    a) aligns with the top edge of the pupil
    b) aligns with the upper lid margin
    c) aligns with the bottom edge of the pupil
    d) aligns with the lower lid margin

61. **A child patient is wearing a segment bifocal to help correct for an accommodative esotropia. The usual alignment in this case is that the upper segment edge:**
    a) aligns with the lower lid margin
    b) falls 2 mm below the lower lid margin
    c) falls 4 mm below the lower pupil margin
    d) splits the pupil

Care and Handling*

62. **Which of the following is *not* a step in cleaning a prosthetic eye?**
    a) always wash hands first
    b) line sink/counter with soft towel
    c) wipe gently with disinfectant wipe
    d) dry before reinserting

63. **Which of the following is an accepted method of cleaning a prosthetic eye?**
    a) soft toothbrush
    b) mild soap and water
    c) soak in alcohol
    d) scrub with detergent

64. **What can happen if soap residue remains on the prosthesis after cleaning?**
    a) surface scratches
    b) dulling of finish
    c) socket irritation
    d) crazing of the acrylic

65. **Which of the following is *not* true?**
    a) After enucleation, the patient should remove the implant at night.
    b) A cosmetic shell should be removed before sleep.
    c) A prosthesis is usually replaced every 3 to 5 years.
    d) Artificial tears may be used with a prosthesis.

66. **Your patient complains that their artificial eye feels scratchy. Proper cleaning and artificial tears don't help much. Which of the following is likely to be most helpful?**
    a) increase cleaning schedule
    b) have eye professionally polished
    c) use artificial tear ointment
    d) irrigate socket daily with contact lens solution

67. **The average replacement schedule for an ocular prosthesis is:**
    a) annually
    b) every 3 to 5 years
    c) every 8 to 10 years
    d) they do not need replacing

* Care and handling of contact lenses is covered in Chapter 18.

68. **Cleaning of spectacles and lenses is best accomplished by using:**
     a) rubbing alcohol
     b) fingernail polish remover (acetone)
     c) a dry tissue
     d) warm water and soap

69. **One of the most common causes for a temple breaking is:**
     a) removing the glasses with one hand
     b) using improper cleaning techniques
     c) poor frame design
     d) intentional abuse

Part II

Triage and Appoint

70. **Match the terms with the definitions.**
     Term
     emergent
     priority
     routine
     urgent

     Definition
     _____ needs to be seen within days
     _____ needs to be seen immediately
     _____ needs to be seen next available
     _____ needs to be seen same day

71. **Which of the following would *not* be categorized as emergent or urgent?**
     a) painful, red eye
     b) sudden, painless loss of vision
     c) tearing and blurred vision after reading for 1 hour
     d) foreign body sensation after grinding metal

72. **Which of the following phone messages requires your *most* immediate attention?**
     a) hit in eye with tennis ball
     b) glaucoma medication refill where patient has one dose left
     c) red eyes matted shut in the mornings
     d) watery, gritty eyes

73. **Sudden, painless loss of vision might be caused by any of the following *except*:**
     a) retinal artery occlusion
     b) retinal vein occlusion
     c) open angle glaucoma
     d) transient ischemic attack

74. A mother calls in to make an appointment for her 12-month-old because a recent photograph of the child showed a red reflex in one eye and a white reflex in the other. This may be caused by:
    a) retinoblastoma
    b) anisocoria
    c) anisometropia
    d) infantile glaucoma

Ocular First Aid

75. Every chemical splash is considered emergent. But which of the following substances would cause the *most* concern for ocular damage?
    a) bleach
    b) beer
    c) battery acid
    d) vinegar

76. Your patient got some furniture cleaning solution in one eye and has brought the bottle to the office with them. How can you find out more about the solution?
    a) look it up in the *Physician's Desk Reference*
    b) read the ingredients label
    c) look it up in *Principles and Practice in Ophthalmic Assisting*
    d) look up the Safety Data Sheet

77. Which of the following is *most* problematic if not evaluated as soon as possible after the injury?
    a) laceration of upper lid
    b) laceration of brow
    c) laceration of lower lid
    d) laceration of lateral canthus

78. Your patient reports a foreign body sensation after grinding metal. This happened about 1 hour ago. Vision is 20/20, there is slight injection, and the pupil is peaked at 8:30. What is your next step?
    a) lightly cover the eye and summon the physician
    b) instill topical anesthetic
    c) perform applanation tonometry
    d) measure interpupillary distance

79. Your patient was in a car accident and the air bag deployed. They present with a black eye and subconjunctival hemorrhage in OD, double vision, and some facial numbness on the right. Which of the following is the most probable situation?
    a) hyphema
    b) blow-out fracture
    c) subluxed lens
    d) retinal detachment

80.   **You are cleaning house and splash some ammonia in your left eye. You immediately:**
a) report to the emergency room
b) phone your boss to meet you at the clinic
c) instill artificial tear drops
d) rinse your eye with water for 20 minutes

81.   **Which of the following would *not* be considered a side effect of a topical eye drop?**
a) stinging
b) tearing
c) dizziness
d) redness

82.   **The most severe adverse drug reaction is:**
a) anaphylaxis
b) dizziness
c) fainting
d) irregular heartbeat

83.   **Symptoms of anaphylaxis may include any of the following *except*:**
a) swelling or itching of lips, tongue, throat
b) tingling of extremities, yellow mucosa, swelling of joints
c) coughing, wheezing, shortness of breath
d) confusion, weakness, paleness

84.   **Which of the following is likely at *most* risk for experiencing anaphylaxis?**
a) patient having dilated exam
b) patient having applanation tonometry
c) patient being fit with contact lenses
d) patient having a fluorescein angiography

85.   **Which of the following injectables is most important to have in your crash cart to deal with anaphylactic reactions?**
a) fluorescein
b) epinephrine
c) antivenin
d) botulinum

86.   **Your patient says they feel faint. You should:**
a) administer epinephrine
b) have them put their head down between their knees
c) have them stand and tilt their head back
d) reassure them that they'll be fine in a moment

Rx to Pharmacy

87.   **The proper steps when faxing a patient prescription include all of the following *except*:**
a) inclusion of patient release form
b) verify the number before calling
c) use of a cover sheet
d) verifying receipt of the prescription

88. **You are handed a written Rx for medication to call in for a patient. You notice some abbreviations on your clinic's "do not use" list. The purpose of the list is to avoid mistakes caused when different medications or orders fall into any of the following categories *except*:**
    a) sound alike
    b) look alike
    c) are banned by the FDA
    d) are easily miswritten

Patient Flow

89. **The progression of a patient's visit, from coming in the front door to walking back out into your parking lot, is known as:**
    a) patient flow
    b) traffic pattern
    c) streaming
    d) surge

90. **Places or times where patient flow is repeatedly "bogged down" is known as a:**
    a) dead space
    b) spike
    c) trough
    d) bottleneck

91. **Your clinic is running at least 45 minutes behind schedule. You should:**
    a) say nothing and hope no one notices
    b) inform patients and offer to reschedule them
    c) inform patients and let them decide to wait or not
    d) Answers b) and c)

Patient Charts

92. **To whom does the information in the chart belong?**
    a) the patient
    b) the practice
    c) the American Academy of Ophthalmology
    d) the patient's insurance company

93. **Your patient has requested a copy of today's visit. Which of the following is *true*?**
    a) A release must be signed by the patient.
    b) This practice is prohibited.
    c) A disclaimer must be signed by the physician.
    d) The practice may withhold the records if the patient owes money.

Schedule Nonophthalmic Tests

94. **You are scheduling blood work for a patient, and the scheduler tells you to remind the patient that these are fasting tests. You tell the patient:**
   a) The test is quick and you won't be there long at all.
   b) Don't eat or drink anything for 12 hours before the test.
   c) Don't take any medications for 12 hours before the test.
   d) The test will involve running on a tread mill.

95. **You are scheduling an MRI for a patient and notice on his history that he is a Vietnam veteran. Which of the following questions is *most* important?**
   a) Have you ever been shot?
   b) Do you have any retained shrapnel in your body?
   c) Do you have post-traumatic stress disorder?
   d) Are you claustrophobic?

Vital Signs

96. **Vital signs include each of the following *except*:**
   a) respiration
   b) blood pressure and pulse rate
   c) blood sugar level
   d) body temperature

97. **Normal resting pulse rate for an adult is:**
   a) 30 to 40
   b) 40 to 55
   c) 60 to 100
   d) 100 to 120

98. **In an adult, the appropriate pulse to take is usually the:**
   a) radial pulse
   b) brachial pulse
   c) carotid pulse
   d) temporal pulse

99. **Normal resting respiration rate per minute for an adult is:**
   a) 8 to 10
   b) 12 to 20
   c) 20 to 25
   d) 25 to 30

100. **Which of the following is an indication for checking the patient's blood pressure?**
   a) use of topical prednisolone
   b) use of oral erythromycin
   c) use of topical polyvinyl alcohol
   d) use of topical timolol

101. **Above what body temperature is a person considered to have a fever?**
    a) 97.0°F
    b) 98.6°F
    c) 99.0°F
    d) 100.4°F

CPR*

102. **The most common airway obstruction in an unconscious adult is:**
    a) food
    b) the tongue
    c) displaced dentures
    d) ice

103. **Which group is at most risk for developing cardiopulmonary arrest?**
    a) those with cardiovascular problems
    b) those with diabetes
    c) those with emphysema
    d) those with cancer

104. **If breathing and pulse are not present, brain death will usually occur:**
    a) in 2 to 4 minutes
    b) in 4 to 6 minutes
    c) in 6 to 10 minutes
    d) in 10 to 14 minutes

105. **How many people survive cardiac arrest outside a hospital if no one performs chest compressions or CPR?**
    a) 1 in 5
    b) 1 in 10
    c) 1 in 20
    d) 1 in 25

106. **"Hands-only" CPR has been introduced to the public because:**
    a) few people take CPR training
    b) previously only health care workers could perform CPR
    c) bystanders are reluctant to administer mouth-to-mouth breathing
    d) many areas are remote, and EMS is more than 15 minutes away

107. **The rate of compressions in hands-only CPR is:**
    a) 30 per minute
    b) 1 per second
    c) 100 per minute
    d) 140 per minute

108. **The correct rescuer position for performing chest compressions on an adult is:**
    a) straddling the victim, hands interlaced, elbows straight
    b) at the victim's side, both hands on chest, elbows bent
    c) at the victim's head, heel of one hand on chest, elbow straight
    d) at the victim's side, hands interlaced, elbows straight

* Proof of CPR training is no longer required by IJCAHPO® to sit for certification exams, but does list it as a test criteria.

109. **The correct depth for chest compressions in an adult is:**
    a) 1 to 1.5 inches
    b) at least 2 inches
    c) 4 inches
    d) until the rib cage crackles

Note: Questions 110 to 112 refer to the following scenario: You are walking alone on a local hiking trail and come upon an adult man lying on the ground by the pond.

110. **What is the *first* thing you need to do?**
    a) check for responsiveness
    b) make sure the scene is safe
    c) call 911
    d) go look for an AED

111. **The victim is nonresponsive, gasping, and has a pulse. What is your next step?**
    a) start CPR
    b) observe carefully until EMS arrives
    c) attach AED and administer shock
    d) open the airway and give rescue breaths

112. **The victim is now nonresponsive, has no pulse, and is not breathing. You should:**
    a) punch on his chest to re-start the heart
    b) observe until EMS arrives
    c) initiate CPR
    d) begin rescue breathing

113. **Which of the following regarding CPR is *not* true?**
    a) Two rescuers should switch places every 5 minutes.
    b) Adult compressions are 100 per minute.
    c) The ratio of 2-rescuer CPR is 30 compressions and 2 breaths.
    d) It is OK to stop if no help has arrived and you're too worn out to continue.

114. **All of the following are *true* regarding AEDs *except*:**
    a) They can be used by any bystander.
    b) They are appropriate to use on adults and children.
    c) They provide a shock to restart the heart.
    d) They are used until EMS arrives.

115. **Number in order the steps for using an AED. You have already determined that the scene is safe, and that the victim is unconscious with no pulse. EMS has been activated but is some minutes away.**
    ＿＿ attach AED pads and plug them in
    ＿＿ designate someone specific to get AED
    ＿＿ if shock is recommended, order all to stand clear
    ＿＿ open victim's shirt
    ＿＿ press shock button if ordered to do so
    ＿＿ push analyze button
    ＿＿ resume CPR as directed
    ＿＿ turn on the unit
    ＿＿ wipe victim's chest dry

Study Notes

Suggested reading in *Principles and Practice in Ophthalmic Assisting: A Comprehensive Textbook:*
> Chapter 7: History Taking (*Communication Skills* pp 78-80, *AIDET Model of Patient Satisfaction* p 81, *Patient Services/Escorting Patients With Special Needs* p 89)
> Chapter 41: Around the Office (pp 683-688)
> Chapter 42: Record Keeping and Electronic Medical Records (pp 689-694)
> Chapter 44: Health Care Compliance and Regulatory Issues (pp 705-714)

Note: Many chapters in the book have a section entitled Patient Services, usually toward the end of the chapter; you might consult these as well.

Explanatory Answers

Part I

1. d) Every item listed can create difficulty when communicating. Cognitive disabilities involve the reasoning, learning, and memory parts of the brain. Poor hearing may mean that the patient smiles and acts like they understand what you've said, but really doesn't. A person's level of education may be a hindrance as well if you're using words outside their experience and knowledge.

2. a) Nonverbal communication is when you DON'T "use your words," literally. So even the volume and tone of your voice is considered nonverbal communication. The words you use would, necessarily, be verbal communication. The cue from facial expressions has been greatly curtailed by the necessity of wearing face masks, so you need to pay more attention to your patients' body language and other cues (as well as your own). Maybe you've never considered clothing as a form of nonverbal communication, but it is. For example, if all the techs in the office wear scrubs, it says "I am a member of the medical team." Or a clean, crisp lab coat over street clothes suggests that you are a professional.

3. d) When caring for diverse populations, you must take into account much more than the obvious. Other people groups may have customs and belief systems that are different from your own. For example, in some cultures making prolonged eye contact might be considered disrespectful or aggressive.

4. b) To be more effective when communicating with a person who has dementia, use short, simple sentences. Avoid asking rapid-fire questions. Be aware that the last thing you say (if you're giving them a list, for example, "sore throat, fever, shortness of breath, or tiredness") is probably going to be the only thing they catch from said list and they will often just repeat that word. Speaking more loudly (unless there is also a hearing impairment) may actually come off as being aggressive, as may exaggerated gestures. But *do* talk directly to the patient.

5. c) Visits to a doctor's office can be stressful. Some people (not just kids!) have a negative reaction to anyone in a lab jacket (dubbed "white coat syndrome"). Ditch the lab coat and see if the exam goes more smoothly. Speak directly to the child and use the guardian as a back-up for information. If for some reason you must send the guardian out of the exam room (not a good idea in most cases), make sure someone else is with you to act as chaperone.

6. d) Connecting to patients at chair-side is an element of interpersonal relationship skills.

7. c) Doubtless you have heard the saying, "They may forget what you said, but they will never forget how you made them feel." (This is often misattributed to the gifted poet laureate Maya Angelou. My research indicates that it's actually a quote from Carl W. Buehner. No matter who said it first, it is pretty much true.) And healing is enhanced in an environment of positive human interaction. Objective testing, remember, does not require a response from the patient.

8.   c) *Holistic* refers to treating something as the sum of its parts, a realization that recognizes the interconnectedness of the parts. Thus, holistic medicine takes into account the entire person: physical, intellectual, mental, emotional, spiritual (ie, mind and body).

9.   a) In general, lack of eye contact is a barrier to effective communication and therefore to care of the patient. If your clinic uses electronic medical records, this can be a real problem. It is easy to get into the habit of facing the computer screen instead of the patient and ask your history questions without your eyes leaving the screen. This leaves the patient feeling ignored or worse, unimportant.

10.   b) This answer is what is known as an *I message*. The intent of using an *I message* is to avoid sounding accusatory and avoid putting the other person on the defensive. (The word *you* should rarely be used in an *I message*, as it assigns blame). It is a method of owning your emotions and identifying the triggering event as 2 separate entities, and without escalating the conflict. It is beyond the scope of this book to go into detail, but the point is to use your words to defuse adverse situations.

11.   c) Service recovery involves the steps taken to resolve problems perceived by a patient. The theory of service recovery is that when contacted immediately and effectively, the dissatisfied patient is "recovered" to the practice, and actually becomes more loyal than before.

12.   c) Reflective listening requires that first you listen, without judgment, without interruption, without interpretation. Then you repeat back to the patient (or whomever) the gist of what you heard them say. You don't have to parrot them word for word, but make sure you state back to them what they said to you. This lets the patient know you are listening. If you have not understood what they said, this is their cue to set you straight. Keep reflecting back to the patient until both of you are sure you got it right.

13.   **Matching:**
      Amsler grid: this test helps us evaluate your central vision, checking for distortion
      anomaloscope: this instrument detects color vision problems
      autorefractor: this instrument scans your eye and comes up with a possible glasses prescription
      break up time: this test gives us an idea of how long your tears stay on your eye
      brightness acuity test: this test gives us an idea of what your vision is like when glare hits you
      color vision arrangement test: the pattern of how you arrange these little caps will help us know if there are any color vision problems
      color vision plates: the patterns on these pages will help us detect color vision problems
      contrast sensitivity: the grids on this test evaluate your ability to detect varying degrees of light and dark
      corneal sensitivity test (anesthesiometer): this test helps us evaluate the sensitivity of the nerves in your cornea
      corneal topography: this instrument makes a map of the curvature of the cornea, the clear covering over the front of your eye
      dark adaptation test: this instrument measures how long it takes your eyes to adapt from bright light to darkness
      electrooculogram: this test evaluates the overall health of the retina
      electroretinogram: this test evaluates and records the response of a specific cell layer of the retina
      exophthalmometer: this instrument is used to measure for any protrusion of the eye
      fluorescein angiography: this test makes images the doctor will use to study the blood flow in your retina
      fluorescein dye: this liquid glows in the microscope's blue light
      gonioscopy: this little lens is used to be able to see the part of your eye where the aqueous fluid drains out
      Heidelberg retina tomograph: this is a scanning laser that creates a 3-dimensional image of the

optic nerve and surrounding tissue

Humphrey visual fields: this test maps out your vision, especially in the periphery/edges

keratometer: this instrument measures the curvature of the cornea, the clear covering over the front of your eye

laser interference biometry: this instrument takes several measurements needed to select the proper intraocular lens for cataract surgery

macular photostress test: this test measures how quickly your vision recovers after seeing a really bright light

optical coherence tomography: this instrument uses light to scan and create a cross-section of the tissues of the eye

pachymeter: this instrument measures the thickness of the cornea, the clear covering over the front of your eye

potential acuity meter: this test gives us an idea of what your vision might be if your cataract was removed (*Note:* May also be called the super pinhole)

pupillometer: this instrument measures the distance between your pupils in order to line your glasses up correctly

retinoscopy: I look at the way this light reflects from your eye. This gives me an idea of what lenses may help you see better.

Schirmer test: this is to test your tear production

slit lamp: this is a microscope that helps me see the front of your eye in detail

specular microscope: this is a special camera that images the inner cell layer of your cornea, which will give us an idea of the health of the cornea.

tear osmolarity: this test evaluates the composition of your tears

tonometry: this test measures the pressure inside your eye

ultrasound: this instrument measures/images your eye using sound waves

visual evoked potential/visual evoked response: this test evaluates the pathway that light takes as it travels from your eye to the brain

14. **Matching:**

biopsy: sending tissue to a pathologist to find out what it is (usually looking for cancer)

blepharoplasty: surgery to remove excess skin (and sometimes fat) from the eyelids (usually the upper)

cataract surgery: surgery that removes the cloudy lens from inside the eye; a clear plastic lens implant is put in its place to allow clearer vision

cautery: using heat to burn tissue, such as sealing off a bleeding blood vessel

centesis: using a syringe to remove fluid, usually from the front of the eye

corneal transplant: surgery that removes scarred cornea and uses clear donor tissue to replace it

cryo: using a cold probe to freeze tissue

ectropion repair: surgery to "tighten" the lids (usually the lower) so they lie against the eyeball instead of turning out

electrolysis: using a tiny electric charge to kill a hair follicle

entropion repair: surgery to "loosen" the lids (usually the lower) so they lie against the eyeball instead of flipping in and rubbing the cornea

incise and drain: opening a fluid or pus-filled lesion to empty it

intraocular injection: using a syringe to deliver medication inside the eye

laser capsulotomy: using a laser to open the cloudy membrane behind an intraocular lens implant

laser iridotomy: using laser to make an opening in the iris so that fluid inside the eye can drain

laser trabeculectomy: using laser to make openings in the drainage system inside the eye so fluid doesn't build up

> **panretinal photocoagulation**: using a laser to "seal" tiny areas all over the retina to prevent diabetic damage
>
> **probe and irrigation**: opening the nasolacrimal duct and flushing the tear drainage system
>
> **punctal plugs**: inserting tiny plastic stoppers into the openings of the tear drainage system (usually the lower lids)
>
> **refractive surgery**: any procedure that changes your glasses prescription, usually to eliminate the need for glasses
>
> **scleral buckle**: surgery that uses a silicone band to repair a retinal detachment
>
> **strabismus surgery**: surgery to straighten "crossed" eyes

15. d) Macular degeneration has been associated with ultraviolet exposure. The other disorders are not at risk from ultraviolet light.

16. a) Smoking can adversely affect many eye conditions. I was once told, "Of the 3 major causes of blindness [ie, cataracts, glaucoma, and macular degeneration], smoking makes them all worse" (source unknown). Smoking also notoriously affects dry eye. Ptosis is a drooping eyelid, basically unaffected by smoking.

17. c) While it's important to correct any refractive error (and indeed, this may play a role in safety!), proper eye protection is the number one feature in eye safety at work and play. Minimizing contact is great, too, but in many sports that's not going to happen. Vitamins are great, but do not lower the risk for eye injury.

18. a) When a patient has useful vision in only one eye, it is recommended that they wear glasses with safety lenses full time, even if optical correction is not needed, and even if they are not performing at-risk activities. The frequency of eye exams will be determined by the practitioner according to the problems the patient is having. Full time wear of sunglasses is not needed.

19. d) Since the patient's family history for macular degeneration is so strong, it could be preventative to begin taking a good multivitamin. The practitioner may even recommend an "eye vitamin" (not listed as an option).

20. d) Immediately removing the lens is always the right answer if there is pain or redness. Better yet, if the eye is red and painful, don't even put the lens in! Rewetting the lens isn't a bad idea, but removal is best. Splashing tap water in an eye with a contact is not advised. The lens may become dislodged, or the water may be contaminated.

21. a) This always sounds backward to patients. "My eyes don't need tear drops; they're already watering!" However, using the tear drops as directed (whether the patient thinks they need them or not) can actually prevent excessive tearing. Rubbing the eyes now has a very bad reputation and has been implicated in keratoconus. [1] Homemade saline is contraindicated for use in the eye under any circumstances, as it may harbor Acanthamoeba.

22. b) Suddenly stopping the steroid (anti-inflammatory) drop after surgery may cause a resurgence (rebound) of inflammation. The patient may call with a red, painful eye, and blurry vision. This can also happen if the patient is taking the drop as directed but fails to shake it. Elevated intraocular pressure may be associated with steroid use, not its discontinuance. Steroids are not antibiotics that treat infection. If inflammation is controlled, there should not be any effects on the postop refraction.

23. d) While tear drops and allergy drops (both of which can probably be bought over the counter if necessary) may be important to the patient's comfort, the most vital of those listed is the glaucoma drops. Without them, the patient's intraocular pressure may run high. There is no such thing as drops for macular degeneration.

24. b) Antibiotics should be taken until they are gone. Otherwise, there is a risk of the infection rebounding. Unfortunately, many people stop when they begin to feel better, and the infection doesn't get knocked out. You would not apply an oral medication to the eye.

25. b) The best thing you can do is try to help the patient discover why they are having a problem with compliance. Once you know that, you can work with the patient to find a solution.

26. c) Work with the patient to identify the reasons that compliance is a challenge. Then encourage the patient to come up with practical ways that they can overcome the problems. For example, if remembering to take medication is the difficulty, then perhaps use of a timer or reminder would be useful, but only if the patient has and can use the timer. Be creative. Remember that it's best if the patient can come up with their own solutions instead of being told what to do.

27. a) Help the parent identify rewards for the child's compliance. Even better if you can enlist the child's help. ("What are some things you really like to do?")

28. c) By acknowledging her feelings, you are giving her permission to be angry. Anger is an important step along the road to acceptance. Statements a) and b) are not helpful at all. While reassuring the patient that she did not do anything to blame herself for, she is not at that point yet. (Of course, if she asks if she brought it on herself, you can reassure her.)

29. a) Feeling angry, sad, and depressed are just a few of the emotions one goes through when experiencing loss or change of any kind. Other feelings might include guilt, denial, shame, and grief. It is of great help to know that these feelings and thoughts are normal, and even a part of healing. Let your patients know that these emotions will likely ebb and flow, maybe for a long time. Being overly regimented with treatment, and diving right into rehab, are probably ways a person might cope with the emotions. But emotions need to be *felt*. "Keep your chin up" is a useless maxim offered by people who have no idea what a person is going through. Sometimes "chin down" is necessary for a while, as one moves toward acceptance.

30. c) I usually tell the parent, "If it was you being dilated, you'd still be able to see to drive." That way when Junior says, "I CAN'T SEE!" the parent knows that he's not been "blinded" by the drops.

31. d) Because the pupils are larger, many patients are sensitive after being dilated because lights seem brighter. The other statements are true.

32. c) Even though you have irrigated the fluorescein out of the eye, some will remain; this can potentially stain the lens. Best case scenario, wait 1 hour. If she doesn't mind the stain, she could put the lens back in after the exam, if the physician permits. There's no need to go without a lens for the rest of the day.

33. b) Sympathy acknowledges another person's pain along with a desire for their well-being. It is different from empathy, where you are able to put yourself in the position of the other and feel what they are feeling. (So in this situation, you might be sympathetic or empathetic, depending on how much you feel the child's distress.) Pity is an acknowledgment of the pain of another, but you may be devoid of feelings yourself. Compassion involves empathy to the point where you "do something" to relieve the other's stress. For info on "I messages," see Answer 10.

34. d) Of the activities listed, the recall card is the most impersonal. Not that that makes it bad, per se. The idea here is to identify what having empathy might look like.

35. c) The patient needs to know who you are, but also what your role is in the clinic and in today's exam/call. An example is, "Good morning! I'm Jan, and I'll be working with you before you see Dr. Davis today." More information can follow as you go through the exam.

36. d) The 3 parts of greeting someone are: (1) eye contact, (2) the smile, and (3) using the patient's name. Eye contact acknowledges that you know the patient is present. The smile conveys friendliness. Using the patient's name affirms the uniqueness of them as an individual. Patients don't really expect to shake hands, which has definitely fallen out of vogue since COVID-19.

37. c) Always, always, always lock the wheelchair. The other items may be necessary with some patients, but not all. Always lock the wheelchair.

38. d) I don't know why, but patients tend to set aside a cane or walker once they get inside the exam room door, and try to walk on their own to the exam chair. The patient should be told and encouraged to use the device until seated; then you can move it to some out-of-the way spot.

39. b) Schedule the appointment for a time when the patient will be most alert and calm. In autism, aggression can occur, but violence is rare. Ask the guardian (or the patient, if appropriate) what can be done to make the patient more comfortable. Some persons with autism do not want to be touched, for example. Select optotypes for this patient as you would anyone else: based on their ability.

40. c) The patient with dementia may have difficulty with comprehension, so keep it short and sweet. See also Answer 4. Hope I made you laugh on the "fellow eye techs" answer! Some days this is me!

41. b) Hearing problems aside, the patient with post-traumatic stress disorder does not require special communication techniques. Depending on the nature of the trauma, there may be a high startle reflex, claustrophobia, and other challenges. These may be better controlled if the patient who has an emotional support dog is permitted to bring the animal with them.

42. a) Many tests are objective (not requiring a response from the patient) or have objective modalities (eg, retinoscopy vs refraction). The parent should be encouraged to bring the child so that their ocular health can be evaluated. Present a positive, can-do attitude that reflects the philosophy of your practice.

43. d) Flashing lights, repeating patterns, and contrasting patterns can all precipitate an epileptic seizure in certain individuals with the disorder. This response to visual stimuli is called photosensitive epilepsy. If your patient has seizures, it is important to know if lights affect them prior to the exam. You may have to forgo certain tests.

44. d) A patient who refuses all eye drops may have many reasons for doing so other than anxiety. (Granted, the thought of the eye drops may be what is making the patient feel anxious!) The anxious patient may tremble, feel faint or weak, have trouble concentrating, breath heavily or rapidly, sweat, and other symptoms. They may also respond to testing in a way that leaves you feeling that they're trying to please you with their answers or are overly eager to give you the "right" answer.

45. a) The ADA is a piece of civil rights law that was enacted in 1990. Among other things, it requires that state and federal agencies, and "places of public accommodation" provide information in a format that is accessible to those with disabilities (including deafness).[2] The other "acts" are fabricated.

46. b) The ADA requires communication with persons of disability to be "adequate." Not all deaf persons are adept with pen and paper. Of interest, the syntax of American Sign Language is not the same as the written word. This means that things might get lost in translation. "Adequate" usually means using the manner in which the person best communicates. Not what's easiest or most convenient for the practice.[2] There is no "Equal Communications Act."

47. **Matching**:

albinism	d)
basal cell carcinoma of lid	g), also f)
coloboma of eyelid	f)
cranial nerve palsy	c)
diabetes	h), also c) if nerves become involved
Fuchs' dystrophy	a)
infant with large, "cloudy" eyes	b)
keratoconus	a)
lung cancer patient with new iris lesion	g)
multiple sclerosis	e), also c)
nystagmus	c)
patient who is not responding to latanoprost, brimonidine, and timolol	b)
patient with scarring from herpes simplex infection	a)
premature infant with questionable vision	h)
presumed ocular histoplasmosis syndrome	h), also e)
pseudotumor cerebri	c)
ptosis over the pupil in a 2-year-old	f)
reconstruction of eyelid	f)
retinal detachment	h)
retinitis pigmentosa	d), h)
retinoblastoma	g), h), also d)

sarcoidosis	e), also c)
unexplained diplopia	c)
unexplained visual field loss	c)

48. c) Were looking for "none of the above? If that had been listed as a possible answer, it would have been the correct one. Of the situations listed, the only one that *might* require patching is the corneal abrasion; however, this practice has fallen into disuse. except, perhaps, for deep abrasions.

49. b) The tape is angled over the patch, from the upper nasal side of the forehead down to the temporal side of the cheek, avoiding the mouth. (You have no idea how much I wanted to use *duct tape* as a possible answer!)

50. c) A patch (but not a tight pressure patch) and a shield are applied to the eye after cataract surgery. (Another case where I wanted to put *duct tape* as a wrong answer!)

51. a) Many drug companies offer assistance to patients who qualify for this help. The patient will need to submit an application, which will include the doctor's verification of the patient's need. You can be most helpful by being aware of these programs, finding them online, and then filling out as much of the application as possible for the patient. While it is true that the medication should be used as directed, the patient already knows this. Knowledge is not the problem. Money is. Only the physician can make the decision to change to a different medication.

52. d) Your documentation in the chart must include date and time you spoke to the patient, a brief history (much like you'd note in the chart if the patient were in the office), what you told the patient, and the next step that needs to be taken (including informing the physician).

53. b) In addition to a summary of the patient's problem and your instructions/education of the patient, it is important to make a note whether or not the patient understood what you told them. "Patient voiced understanding" and "patient agreed to this plan" are common wording for this. You don't need consent to discuss the patient's issues with the physician. Patient satisfaction isn't usually documented per se, and the patient's "no show" history is not pertinent to the call.

54. c) Some patients mistakenly believe that if they get a form filled out and signed by the physician, they will obtain their objective. But I always tell patient to remember that we are just filling out the paperwork with the results of our tests. The licensing board (or whomever) is the one that decides if they get their license. The other statements are true. Once a filled-out form is in the patient's hand, it's their duty to safeguard the information.

55. a) Moving the nose pads closer together will make the frames sit higher on the frame. (Moving them farther apart would lower them.) Adjusting the bend of the temples (not tightening or loosening) may help as well.

56. a) Plastic frames should be gently warmed before bending. This is usually done with a frame warmer, but you can use a hairdryer or warm water. Heat gently, taking take care not to melt the frame. Bend carefully; even heated plastic can snap.

57. c) Most patients' glasses will be adjusted to provide a pantoscopic tilt. That is, the bottom of the frame is closer to the cheek and the top tilts away from the face slightly. A retroscopic tilt would be the opposite, where the frame top is closer to the brow and tilts away from the face as you approach the cheek. Pupillary distance is measured initially so that the lenses are properly positioned when placed into the frame. The vertex distance is an optical measurement used to help determine the lens power needed (mainly for strong lenses) according to how far the lenses will sit from the eyes.

58. d) The base curve is a set feature of the lens and is not modifiable by adjusting frames or any other method available in the average eye clinic. The position of the bifocal or trifocal segment(s) can be raised or lowered, at least to some degree, by adjusting the frame to change its vertical alignment. Adjustment can also make the frames more comfortable. The effective power of a lens is changed when the lens is tilted or moved closer to/farther from the eye. (The actual power doesn't change, of course.)

59.   b) There are exceptions, but the most common practice is to align the top of a bifocal segment with the edge of the patient's lower lid.

60.   c) In the case of a trifocal, the top edge is usually placed at the bottom edge of the pupil.

61.   d) A child is more likely to avoid using a bifocal segment because they can use the top segment and see well up close by accommodating. In order for this treatment to be successful, the patient must use the bifocal segment for near. So for children, the segment is raised so that the line bisects ("splits") the pupil, to increase the chances that they will use the bifocal.

62.   c) Disinfectants are not used on a prosthetic eye. In addition, the "fabric" of a wipe may be too harsh. Teach your patient to wash hands first, put down a soft towel in case the eye is dropped, and (after cleaning and rinsing, see Answers 63 and 64) dry with a soft cloth before reinserting.

63.   b) Only mild soap (no perfumes or additives) and water should be used to gently clean the prosthesis. No brush should be used, just the fingers.

64.   c) After cleaning with mild soap, the prosthesis should be thoroughly rinsed. Tap water or saline can be used. Soap residue won't damage the prosthesis, but it can cause irritation to the socket tissues.

65.   a) The comment about removing the implant is incorrect. The implant is the "marble" placed in the socket to keep the orbit formed and is sewn in under the conjunctiva. It is thus inaccessible to the patient. The other statements are true. A cosmetic shell goes over a disfigured eye (ie, the globe is still in place) and should be removed before sleeping. Regarding replacement, see Answer 67. It's fine to use artificial tears with a prosthesis.

66.   b) The current trend is to remove the prosthesis as little as possible, so increasing the cleaning schedule isn't a great idea. Tear ointment would smear on the prosthesis' surface. Irrigating the socket daily would necessitate removing the prosthesis daily, and contact lens solution is not meant to be used on socket tissues. The prosthesis should be professionally cleaned and polished, on the average, once every year. More often, if the patient is prone to developing deposits.

67.   b) On average, most people will need to replace an artificial eye every 3 to 5 years. There may be more frequent replacements if the socket changes (ie, due to growth or shifting), or the prosthesis gets chipped.

68.   d) Items in Answers a) to c) will damage coatings and/or mar the lenses. A dry tissue should never be used; wood particles in a paper towel, tissue, etc, can scratch the lens. Stick to the warm water and soap, drying with a soft cloth.

69.   a) Taking glasses off with one hand involves a "tearing" motion that weakens the temple, stresses the hinge, and wreaks havoc on the adjustment. Patients should be encouraged to use 2 hands, where pressure is applied evenly on both sides of the frame.

Part II

70.   **Matching**:

emergent	needs to be seen immediately
priority	needs to be seen within days
routine	needs to be seen next available
urgent	needs to be seen same day

71.   c) Tearing and blurred vision after reading for a while can be annoying and bothersome and is probably caused by dry eye. It is not emergent or urgent and can be seen within several days. A painful, red eye has a multitude of possibilities, including angle-closure glaucoma, which is emergent. Sudden, painless loss of vision is also emergent, as it can signal an occlusion in the ocular circulation. A foreign body sensation in a patient who gives a history of using a metal grinder is at least urgent and perhaps emergent. Differential diagnoses for many emergent and urgent cases can only be narrowed down accurately by seeing the patient.

72. a) Blunt, concussive trauma to the eye can cause rupture (to lids, globe or its contents), bleeding, hyphema, blow-out fracture, retrobulbar hematoma, retinal detachment, detachment/dislocation of the lens, bruising, swelling, nerve damage, extraocular muscle damage, and other problems. Glaucoma patients should be counseled not to run out of their medications, and this is not an urgent inquiry. Red, matted eyes are likely some sort of infection, and watery, gritty eyes are probably related to dryness. In these 2 scenarios the patient is uncomfortable, but they are not urgent cases.

73. c) Sudden, painless loss of vision is an ocular emergency. Of those entities listed, open angle glaucoma does not cause these symptoms. I was originally going to list angle-closure glaucoma as the answer, then discovered that on occasion it can be painless. Retinal artery and vein occlusion is also known as an "eye stroke". Transient ischemic attack (TIA) is also related to an occlusion of blood flow, but the body's own defenses are able to clear the clot relatively quickly. A TIA can have any of the symptoms of a stroke. If there is temporary vision loss with a TIA, it is specifically known as *amaurosis fugax*.

74. a) Retinoblastoma is a cancer of the retina, usually found in children. Left untreated, the cancer can invade the brain and cause death. Early detection is key; it is generally treated by enucleating the eye. Anisocoria is unequal pupils; anisometropia is unequal refractive error (ie, between the 2 eyes); infantile glaucoma is not associated with a white reflex. Of interest is the term *pseudoleukocoria*, a white pupil seen in a picture that is simply a photographic artifact and not ocular at all.

75. a) Answers b), c), and d) are all acidic and may cause painful surface burns. Bleach, however, is alkaline (or basic). In addition to a surface burn, a base can penetrate the tissues. This makes it the more concerning of those listed. Other basic/alkaline baddies: cement, mortar, lime, ammonia, and lye.

76. d) Safety Data Sheets contain all kinds of information on most any type of compound, cleaner, solution, etc, that is in use. The data include flammability, freezing temperature, and adverse reactions to bodily contact. The sheets are available online.

77. c) Of those listed, the lacerated lower lid can be potentially problematic if the nasolacrimal system is involved (punctum, canaliculus, etc). If the structures are not properly realigned, the patient may suffer permanent watering.

78. a) The peaked pupil is a clue that there may be an intraocular foreign body. Do not instill any drops or put any pressure on the globe. Cover it lightly and notify the doctor. Measuring pupillary distance will not provide any useful information.

79. b) Blunt trauma to the face could cause any of the mentioned problems. The fact that there is double vision and some facial numbness points to a blow-out fracture where extraocular muscles and nerves have herniated through the fractured bones.

80. d) You should do for yourself what you would tell a patient to do: irrigate with water for at least 20 minutes. *Then* you can call your boss, go to the ER, or whatever.

81. c) Dizziness is considered an *adverse reaction*. The other 3 answers are possible *side effects*, which generally subside on their own. Information on every drug will have a list of these. Adverse reactions, however, are unpredictable and may be quite severe to the point of life-threatening. Intervention is thus required.

82. a) Anaphylaxis is a severe allergic reaction. The most common causes are food and drugs. If the victim lapses into shock, the situation is then known as *anaphylactic shock*, which can be life-threatening. Anaphylaxis requires quick intervention, so health care workers must be able to recognize the symptoms (see Answer 83). The clinic should have a plan and materials in place beforehand, in case this emergency occurs.

83. b) In addition to those listed, other symptoms/signs can include rash, dizziness, sneezing, rapid heartbeat, weak pulse, vomiting, diarrhea, and cramps, among others. The 2 hallmarks, however, are respiratory difficulty and dropping blood pressure. These 2 things are basically responsible for the symptoms seen in anaphylaxis and can lead to shock and death.

84.   d) Of those listed, the patient who is going to have a fluorescein angiography is at highest risk for an anaphylactic reaction. Eye drops of any kind could potentially cause anaphylaxis, but the risk is much higher when an injected medication is involved. The contact lens fit is least likely to have any kind of allergic reaction, although it is vaguely possible if the patient was allergic to something in the lens material.

85.   b) Epinephrine (also called adrenalin) counteracts the over-blown allergic response of the body. It dilates airways and constricts blood vessels. This results in increased air flow and increased blood pressure. Injectable fluorescein is probably the most likely substance in the eye clinic to cause anaphylaxis. Antivenin is administered to counteract certain toxic bites and stings. Botulinum is used in cosmetic procedures (and unlikely to cause such a severe reaction, although it is possible); it would not be used to treat anaphylaxis.

86.   b) When a patient feels dizzy or faint, your response should be to get the patient's head lower than the heart. The easiest way to do this is have the seated patient bend over with the head between the knees. Reassurance can be offered at this point. Epinephrine is used in anaphylaxis (and administered by the physician). Having a dizzy patient stand is going to almost guarantee they will actually faint.

87.   a) It is not necessary to fax a patient release form when sending a prescription using this method. Ideally, you should call the company/office and verify their fax number, use a cover sheet over the prescription (for privacy), and then call to verify that the company received the fax.

88.   c) Abbreviations and acronyms get placed on your clinic's "do not use" list because they look alike (eg, timolol and timolol/dorzolamide), sound alike (eg, Tobrex and TobraDex, or my favorite Zantac and Xanax); physically resemble each other (such as tryphan blue and methylene blue), or are easily miswritten (eg, qid instead of qd). The FDA does not "ban" abbreviations.

89.   a) Patient flow begins when the patient walks in your door and continues through registration, waiting time, preliminary examination and special testing, dilation (and waiting some more), seeing the physician, treatment, patient education, arranging follow-up visits, and check out.

90.   d) Bottlenecks are places (such as a narrow hallway where people are going both ways), times (perhaps your clinic schedule regularly backs up at 3 o'clock), or procedures (waiting for special testing, maybe?) where patient flow bogs down or actually grinds to a near-halt. If you want to improve patient flow, you must identify and rectify bottlenecks.

91.   d) Although patients obviously know when you're running behind, it's good form to let them know that you're aware. By giving them options, you restore some level of control to them. Another option is to inform patients and let them leave and come back in 30 minutes or so.

92.   a) The physical chart (on paper or electronic device) belongs to the practice. The information therein belongs to the patient.

93.   a) A release of information must be signed any time the patient receives a hard copy of their records. The practitioner doesn't have to sign anything. The practice cannot refuse to furnish the patient's records just because the patient has an outstanding bill.

94.   b) Fasting means that the patient should not eat or drink anything, usually for 12 hours prior to the test. Ask the scheduler to elaborate, if necessary. Usually water or black coffee (no sweetener!) are OK. Patients usually take their normal medication with a sip of water, but check on this too, especially if the patient is diabetic.

95.   b) Since the MRI uses strong magnetism, it is vital to know whether the patient has any metal in his body. Normally you might think of plates and screws, but some veterans (and others) have retained shrapnel in their bodies. Asking "have you ever been shot?" is not a very "gentle" inquiry and still may not elicit the desired information. Answers b) and c) are pertinent, but sedation may help these patients relax. The most vital question is about retained metal.

96.   c) The patient's blood sugar level may be important in some cases, but it is not considered a part of vital signs. *Note:* some references have added oxygen saturation to vital signs.

97. c) According to the American Heart Association, normal pulse rate for an adult is between 60 and 100.

98. a) The radial pulse (in the wrist) is usually taken in the adult. Brachial pulse is in the upper arm and is usually used for checking infants and young children. The carotid pulse is in the neck, and the temporal in the temple; these are not commonly used for evaluating pulse in the clinic.

99. b) References differ. Some say 12 to 16, others 12 to 18, yet others 12 to 20.

100. d) Timolol is a beta-blocker, which can affect blood pressure.

101. d) The old standard of normal body temperature being 98.6°F has gone by the wayside. Now, normal is considered variable among individuals, ranging from 97°F to 99°F.[3] Above 100.4°F is now considered "having a fever."

102. b) The victim's own tongue is the most common obstruction to the airway. This occurs after the victim loses consciousness.

103. a) People with heart problems are most at risk for cardiopulmonary arrest, with over 17.9 million deaths worldwide attributable to cardiovascular disorders.[4]

104. b) Brain death occurs approximately 4 to 6 minutes after pulse and breathing cease.

105. b) Only 1 in 10 victims (approximately) will survive outside-of-hospital cardiac arrest if chest compressions or CPR is not performed.[5] If CPR is started immediately, survival rates can double or triple.[5]

106. c) In 2010, a report was released that found hands-only (or compression-only) CPR to be about as effective as CPR that includes emergency breathing on adults.[6] This is good news because bystanders are increasingly reluctant to perform mouth-to-mouth breathing on a person whose medical background (especially COVID and HIV status) is unknown.
     Note: The American Heart Association and the International Liaison Committee on Resuscitation periodically update and change the CPR guidelines. As of publication, laymen are taught that if they *witness* an adult or teen collapse, they are to immediately call 911, then begin compressions.[7] The rationale behind this recommendation is that a victim in cardiac arrest will lose their pulse within 10 seconds of the attack.

107. c) The compression rate in hands-only CPR is the same as in CPR that includes rescue breathing: 100 per minute. (If you press to the tune of the Bee Gees' song *Stayin' Alive*, you will be delivering about 100 compressions per minute.)

108. d) When performing compressions on an adult, the rescuer is kneeling at the victim's side, hands interlaced and placed on the victim's chest (2 finger-widths above the xiphoid process), elbows straight. The rescuer's shoulders, elbows, and hands should be in line. Compressions originate from the shoulders and arms, not by bending the elbows or rocking the body.

109. b) In order for the compressions in an adult to be effective, they must be at least 2 inches deep.

110. b) Make sure the scene is safe. You can't be of any help if you get into trouble, too. Granted, this scenario looks pretty benign. But you never know. Just take a quick look around.

111. d) Gasping is not breathing, so you cannot wait. Open the airway and attempt to give rescue breaths. Since the patient has a pulse, administering CPR or giving a shock with the AED is not appropriate.

112. c) This victim has no pulse and is not breathing. You must initiate CPR, with effective compressions and breaths. Thumping on the chest (termed a *precordial thump*) can cause injury to the patient if not properly placed, and can actually backfire. It is not recommended that laymen attempt this maneuver. Since there is no pulse, rescue breathing alone is not enough.

113. a) In 2-rescuer CPR, the rescuers should switch places every 2 minutes (5 cycles). This helps to prevent fatigue. Adult compressions are 100 (so are child and infant compressions). And as much as you'd hate to, it is okay to stop if no help has arrived and you're too worn out to keep going. You did your best.

114. a) While many AEDs actually tell you what to do step-by-step, they are to be used only by trained personnel. There are now pediatric-sized pads, and some AEDs have a switch to deliver a pediatric-appropriate shock.

115. **Numbering**:

5 attach AED pads and plug them in

1 designate someone specific to get AED

7 if shock is recommended, order all to stand clear

3 open victim's shirt

8 press shock button if ordered to do so

6 push analyze button

9 resume CPR as directed

2 turn on the unit

4 wipe victim's chest dry

References

1. Eye rubbing MRI1 [video]. Posted November 9, 2019. Accessed March 7, 2021. www.youtube.com/watch?v=piy1C8PG4aI

2. Hay M, Duncan K. What ODs need to know about the Americans with Disabilities Act (ADA) and effective communication. CovalentCareers Website. Published April 10, 2018. Accessed December 17, 2020. Covalentcareers.com/resources/ada-and-optometrists/

3. Fischer K. Forget 98.6°F. Humans are cooling off—here's why. Healthline. Posted January 12, 2020. Accessed April 2, 2021. www.healthline.com/health-news/forget-98-6-humans-now-have-lower-body-temperature-on-average-heres-why

4. Cardiovascular diseases. World Health Organization Website. Accessed March 18, 2023. www.who.int/health-topics/cardiovascular-diseases/#tab=tab_1

5. CPR facts & stats. American Heart Association Website. Accessed March 18, 2023. https://cpr.heart.org/en/resources/cpr-facts-and-stats

6. Svensson L, Bohm K, Castren M, et al. Compression-only CPR or standard CPR in out-of-hospital cardiac arrest. *N Engl J Med*. 2010;363:434-442. Accessed March 18, 2023. www.nejm.org/doi/full/10.1056/NEJMoa0908991

7. American Heart Association. Hands-only CPR: 2 steps to save a life [video]. Posted May 20, 2020. Accessed March 18, 2023. www.youtube.com/watch?v=M4ACYp75mjU (*Note*: Methods change. Search for Hand-only-CPR for the current year.)

Bibliography

Allergies and anaphylaxis. June 14, 2020. Accessed November 21, 2020. www.webmd.com/allergies/anaphylaxis

American Heart Association. CPR & first aid emergency cardiovascular care. Accessed March 18, 2023. https://cpr.heart.org/en/resuscitation-science/cpr-and-ecc-guidelines/algorithms#adult (*Note*: Methods change. Search for CPR for the current year)

Resnick R. 10 strategies to improve patient compliance with medication. Cureatr Website. January 22, 2020. Accessed December 10, 2020. blog.cureatr.com/10-strategies-improve-patient-compliance-with-medication

Tips for documenting calls. Risk Management, Webpage of National Chiropractic Mutual Insurance Company (NCMIC). Posted June 21, 2018. Accessed November 22, 2020. www.ncmic.com/insurance/malpractice/risk-management/tips-for-documenting-calls/

Turner A, Rabiu M. Patching for corneal abrasion. Cochrane Database Syst. Updated July 26, 2016. doi:10.14651959.CD004764.pub3

Chapter 16

General Medical Knowledge

Ledford JK.
*Certified Ophthalmic Technician Exam
Review Manual, Third Edition* (pp 309-390).
© 2023 Taylor & Francis Group.

ABBREVIATIONS USED IN THIS CHAPTER

- ACG   angle-closure glaucoma
- AMD   age-related macular degeneration
- CN   cranial nerve
- D   diopter
- mm   millimeters
- μ   "mu" (denotes 10^{-6} power)
- NLD   nasolacrimal duct
- RNFL   retinal nerve fiber layer
- RP   retinitis pigmentosa
- RPE   retinal pigment epithelium
- TIA   transient ischemic attack
- UV   ultraviolet
- VEGF   vascular endothelial growth factor

Note: See also Question 320.

Part I*

Body Systems (Function/Processes)

1. **Match each entity to the appropriate body system. Answers may be used more than once.**
   <u>Body System</u>
   a) cardiovascular/circulatory
   b) endocrine
   c) gastrointestinal/digestive
   d) musculoskeletal
   e) nervous
   f) respiratory

   <u>Entity</u>
   __ adrenal glands
   __ afibrillation
   __ aorta
   __ arteriosclerosis
   __ arthritis
   __ atria
   __ biceps
   __ brain
   __ bronchi
   __ carotid
   __ CN VII
   __ colon
   __ diabetes

---

* Sections have been inserted into this lengthy chapter for ease of study, to allow for a logical "break" point.

__ diaphragm
__ duodenum
__ esophagus
__ femur
__ fight or flight response
__ gall bladder
__ gonads
__ Graves' disease
__ hormones
__ human growth hormone
__ insulin
__ islets of Langerhans
__ larynx
__ lateral rectus
__ liver
__ lymph nodes
__ mitral valve
__ optic nerve
__ orbicularis oculi
__ orbit
__ pancreas
__ parathyroid
__ pharynx
__ pituitary
__ plasma
__ platelets
__ pulse
__ spinal cord
__ stomach
__ thyroid
__ trachea
__ ulna
__ vena cava
__ ventricle
__ vertebrae
__ xiphoid

2.   **Which of the following is involved in delivering hormones to various parts of the body?**
     a) respiratory system
     b) endocrine system
     c) cardiovascular system
     d) digestive system

3.   **Which of the following is involved in transferring nutrients and removal of waste?**
     a) cardiovascular system
     b) digestive system
     c) respiratory system
     d) all of the above

4.   Which of the following is/are involved in movement of the eye?
      a) musculoskeletal system
      b) nervous system
      c) endocrine system
      d) just a) and b)

Ocular Anatomy, Structure, and Function

5.   The primary goal of the eye's components is to:
      a) interpret what is seen
      b) focus incoming light onto the lens
      c) focus incoming light onto the retina
      d) maintain proper intraocular pressure

6.   The ocular media consist of:
      a) the lens correction for ametropia
      b) contact lenses and intraocular lenses
      c) the eyelid, sclera, uvea, and optic nerve
      d) the tear film, cornea, humors, and lens

7.   Which of the following ocular structures has the *highest* refractive power?
      a) tear film
      b) cornea
      c) lens
      d) aqueous and vitreous (combined)

8.   Which of the following occupies the space between the back of the iris and the front of the crystalline lens?
      a) anterior chamber
      b) vitreous chamber
      c) posterior chamber
      d) posterior segment

9.   You have applied for a job with a retina practice. This is known as:
      a) posterior chamber
      b) uveal segment
      c) vitreous chamber
      d) posterior segment

10.   Collectively, the orbit, extraocular muscles, lacrimal apparatus, lids, and optic nerve are referred to as the:
      a) uvea
      b) ocular adnexa
      c) exterior segment
      d) ophthalmonexa

Cranial Nerves

11. **CNs are usually designated by:**
    a) Arabic numerals
    b) metric numerals
    d) letters
    d) Roman numerals

12. **Which of the following CNs is *not* directly associated with ophthalmology?**
    a) I
    b) II
    c) IV
    d) VI

13. **Which of the following CNs are associated with the extraocular muscles?**
    a) I, X, XII
    b) II, V, VII
    c) III, IV, VI
    d) I, VI, VII

Orbit

14. **How many bones make up the orbit?**
    a) 5
    b) 7
    c) 8
    d) 12

15. **Which of the following is the more delicate bone in the orbit?**
    a) frontal
    b) zygomatic
    c) ethmoid
    d) maxillary

16. **Through what opening does the optic nerve enter the orbit?**
    a) optic foramen
    b) supraorbital foramen
    c) suborbital foramen
    d) lacrimal foramen

17. **A sinus infection can sometimes feel like pressure behind the eyes. This is because:**
    a) there is a rise in intraocular pressure
    b) there are sinus cavities behind some of the orbital bones
    c) steroids are used to treat it
    d) exophthalmos occurs

18. **Which of the following is the bone at the very back of the orbit?**
    a) maxillary
    b) sphenoid
    c) lacrimal
    d) frontal

Extraocular Muscles*

19.   **The 4 rectus muscles originate from the:**
      a) optic foramen
      b) Tenon's membrane
      c) Annulus of Zinn
      d) palpebral conjunctiva

20.   **The trochlea serves to:**
      a) anchor the superior oblique
      b) anchor the inferior oblique
      c) act as a sling for the superior oblique
      d) innervate the superior rectus

21.   **Which of the following is *not* true regarding the extraocular muscles?**
      a) They are part of the voluntary nervous system.
      b) They are innervated by 1 of 3 CNs.
      c) They attach to the globe behind the limbus.
      d) They are smooth muscle.

Globe

22.   **The outermost layer of the globe is the:**
      a) sclera
      b) choroid
      c) Dua's layer
      d) episclera

23.   **Blood is supplied directly to the globe via the:**
      a) internal carotid artery
      b) ophthalmic artery
      c) external carotid artery
      d) aorta

24.   **Which of the following is *not* a role of orbital fat?**
      a) cushions the globe
      b) allows extraocular muscles to glide smoothly
      c) provides volume in the socket
      d) stimulates growth of the infant orbit

25.   **Which of the following is a sheath-like layer that surrounds the globe, separating it from the orbital fat?**
      a) Annulus of Zinn
      b) sclera
      c) Tenon's capsule
      d) conjunctiva

* For questions on the actions of the extraocular muscles, see Chapter 7, Questions 16 to 27.

Lids

26. Which of the following is *not* true?
a) The skin of the eye lids is among the thinnest in the body.
b) There is almost no fat directly under the skin of the eye lids.
c) The lids serve to protect against noxious light.
d) It is rare for the skin of the lids to swell.

27. Which of the following is *not* found in the eyelid?
a) goblet cells
b) glands of Moll
c) glands of Zeis
d) meibomian glands

28. Which muscle is involved with closing the eye?
a) orbicularis oculi
b) superior rectus
c) superior tarsal
d) blinkus superiorus

29. Which of the following is *not* part of the mechanism to open the eye?
a) CN VI
b) levator muscle
c) superior tarsal muscle
d) tarsus

30. Which of the following is a layer of connective tissue within the eyelid?
a) sclera
b) bulbar conjunctiva
c) tarsus
d) limbus

31. Which nerves supply motor impulses to the upper lid?
a) CNs III and VII
b) CNs III and IV
c) CNs IV and VI
d) CNs VI and VII

32. The extra fold of skin in the nasal canthi that can sometimes cause the appearance of esotropia is:
a) dermatochalasis
b) ptosis
c) epicanthal fold
d) blepharoptosis

33. How many puncti are in each set of lids?
a) 1
b) 2
c) 4
d) 8

34.   **The proper term for the "corner" of the eye is:**
    a) canthus
    b) fornix
    c) fissure
    d) angle

35.   **The area between the upper and lower lid margins where the globe is exposed is the:**
    a) superior lid fold
    b) inferior lid crease
    c) visual margin
    d) fissure

Conjunctiva

36.   **The conjunctiva is a:**
    a) connection point for muscles in the lids
    b) mucous membrane
    c) conduction point for nerve endings
    d) muscle tendon

37.   **Which of the following is *not* a part of the conjunctiva?**
    a) cilia
    b) bulbar
    c) palpebral
    d) fornix

38.   **A patient calls and says they've lost a soft contact lens behind their eye. You tell them:**
    a) insert another contact
    b) go to the emergency room
    c) use a plunger to try to find it
    d) it can't actually get behind the eye

39.   **Which of the following statements about the conjunctiva is *false*?**
    a) It helps lubricate the eye.
    b) It lines the eyelids.
    c) It generates the arcus senilis.
    d) It stops at the corneal limbus.

40.   **Which of the following are *not* found in the conjunctiva?**
    a) trabecular glands
    b) glands of Wolfring
    c) glands of Krause
    d) goblet cells

41.   **Into what area of the lower lid are eye medications usually instilled?**
    a) nasal canthus
    b) medial canthus
    c) cul-de-sac
    d) punctum

42. **The small fold of bulbar conjunctiva situated just in front of the caruncle is the:**
    a) punctum
    b) plica
    c) cul-de-sac
    d) nasal canthus

Lacrimal System and Tears

43. **Which of the following is *not* a function of the tear film?**
    a) supply oxygen to the cornea
    b) drainage of aqueous
    c) moisten the external eyeball
    d) provide clear vision

44. **The layers of the tear film are:**
    a) epithelium, stroma, and endothelium
    b) capsule, cortex, and nucleus
    c) mucin, water (aqueous), and oil
    d) vitreous, aqueous, and lipid

45. **The main lacrimal gland is involved in what part of lacrimation?**
    a) mucin production
    b) sweat production
    c) oil production
    d) reflex tearing

46. **Which of the following contributes mucin to the tear film?**
    a) goblet cells
    b) glands of Moll
    c) glands of Zeis
    d) meibomian glands

47. **Which of the following helps to "fill in" tiny surface irregularities on the corneal surface?**
    a) oily layer of the tear film
    b) watery layer of the tear film
    c) mucin layer of the tear film
    d) epithelial cells

48. **On average, how often does the human adult blink?**
    a) every 2 seconds
    b) 5 to 10 times per minute
    c) 15 to 20 times per minute
    d) over 25 times per minute

49. **The collection of tears that pool at the nasal canthus is known as the:**
    a) lacrimal lake
    b) reflex tears
    c) caruncle
    d) plica

50. **Which CN provides sensory innervation to the lacrimal gland?**
     a) CN III
     b) CN IV
     c) CN V
     d) CN VI

51. **The action of the lids in moving the tear film into the lacrimal drainage system is known as:**
     a) the blink reflex
     b) the lacrimal pump
     c) the lacrimal reflex
     d) nasolacrimal duct stimulation

52. **The flow of tears off the eye occurs in the following order:**
     a) nasolacrimal duct, canaliculus, nasolacrimal sac, punctum, nasal cavity
     b) canaliculus, punctum, nasolacrimal duct, nasolacrimal sac, nasal cavity
     c) punctum, canaliculus, nasolacrimal sac, nasolacrimal duct, nasal cavity
     d) punctum, nasolacrimal duct, canaliculus, nasolacrimal sac, nasal cavity

Sclera/Episclera

53. **The episclera provides:**
     a) a portion of the tear film
     b) blood supply for the sclera
     c) drainage for aqueous humor
     d) blood supply for the retina

54. **Which of the following statements about the sclera is *not* true?**
     a) It is formed of the same type of fibers as the cornea.
     b) The color may vary somewhat.
     c) It can affect intraocular pressure readings.
     d) It maintains a state of dehydration.

55. **The point where the sclera meets the cornea is the:**
     a) lamina cribrosa
     b) trabeculum
     c) scleral spur
     d) limbus

56. **The portion of the sclera that is in the angle of the eye is the:**
     a) scleral spur
     b) ora serrata
     c) trabecular meshwork
     d) ciliary body

57. **The portion of the sclera that is in the optic nerve cup is the:**
     a) disc
     b) sieve of Orbiculum
     c) lamina cribrosa
     d) ora serrata

Cornea*

58. **What is the average central thickness of the cornea?**
a) 480 to 510 μm
b) 535 to 545 mm
c) 551 to 565 μm
d) 590 to 600 μm

59. **The average refractive power of the cornea is:**
a) 30 to 34 D
b) 35 to 39 D
c) 40 to 44 D
d) 45 to 50 D

60. **The corneal tissue is largely composed of:**
a) collagen fibers
b) tendons
c) crystallins
d) neurons

61. **The cornea receives sensory innervation by which of the following?**
a) optic nerve
b) ophthalmic nerve
c) maxillary nerve
d) frontal nerve

62. **Which of the following is a normal blood supply for the cornea?**
a) neovascularization at the limbus
b) ophthalmic artery
c) lymphatic system
d) none of the above

63. **Which of the following represents the meeting of the cornea with the trabecular meshwork?**
a) Schlemm's canal
b) Schwalbe's line
c) limbus
d) scleral spur

64. **Which of the following is *not* a layer of the cornea?**
a) Bowman's membrane
b) pigment epithelial cells
c) Descemet's membrane
d) stroma

65. **Which of the following is the thickest corneal layer(s)?**
a) epithelium
b) endothelium
c) stroma
d) Bowman's and Descemet's membranes

*For more on the role of the cornea in refractive errors/astigmatism, see Chapter 6, Questions 1 to 3.

66. Which of the following about the corneal epithelium is *not* true?
    a) Its cells cannot regenerate.
    b) It protects against external fluids.
    c) It is 5 to 7 layers thick.
    d) It provides a smooth refractive surface.

67. The corneal epithelium overlies:
    a) the stroma
    b) Descemet's membrane
    c) Bowman's layer
    d) the anterior lens capsule

68. Which of the following corneal layers can regenerate?
    a) epithelium
    b) endothelium
    c) Bowman's membrane
    d) none of the above

69. Which of the following could be described as the cornea's "dehydration pump"?
    a) stroma
    b) canaliculus
    c) nasolacrimal sac
    d) endothelial layer

70. The endothelial cells have what shape?
    a) round
    b) hexagonal
    c) cuboid
    d) rod-shaped

71. The density of the corneal endothelial layer is:
    a) 2 cell layers thick
    b) 1 mm thick
    c) 50 μm thick
    d) a single cell thick

72. On what do the endothelial cells rest?
    a) stroma
    b) Bowman's membrane
    c) nucleus
    d) Descemet's membrane

73. Your physician is planning cataract surgery for a patient and has requested an endothelial cell count. The reason for this is:
    a) to estimate the patient's potential vision if the cataract was removed
    b) to evaluate the curvature of the inner cornea
    c) to determine what type of lens implant to use
    d) to determine the risk to the endothelial layer

Part II

Anterior Chamber/Angle/Aqueous Humor*

74.   **The aqueous humor is produced by the:**
a) corneal endothelium
b) ciliary processes
c) iris
d) trabecular meshwork

75.   **The physical nature of the aqueous is most like:**
a) blood plasma
b) cerumen
c) whole blood
d) mucin

76.   **From its generation to drainage, aqueous flows in which order?**
a) angle, posterior chamber, pupil, anterior chamber
b) angle, anterior chamber, pupil, posterior chamber
c) pupil, posterior chamber, anterior chamber, angle
d) posterior chamber, pupil, anterior chamber, angle

77.   **Which of the following are part of the angle's aqueous drainage system?**
a) trabecular meshwork
b) Schlemm's canal
c) Answers a) and b)
d) none of the above

78.   **Intraocular pressure is a result of:**
a) systolic and diastolic blood pressure
b) rate of aqueous production and resistance to outflow
c) pressure in the ophthalmic artery and vein
d) cranial pressure transferred to the eye through the optic nerve

79.   **The "diurnal curve" of intraocular pressure refers to:**
a) the fluctuation of intraocular pressure levels in a 24-hour period
b) the fluctuation of intraocular pressure levels over a 6-month period
c) the relation of intraocular pressure to the shelf-life of glaucoma medications
d) the level of uric acid in the aqueous

80.   **The purpose of the inflowing aqueous humor is to:**
a) keep the surface of the eye moist
b) provide nutrients to the retina
c) provide nutrients to the cornea and lens
d) provide major refractive power to the ocular media

* Aqueous humor dynamics and IOP are discussed in Chapter 5, Questions 1-5 and this chapter, Questions 232-242.

81. **The aqueous also functions to:**
    a) transport cells and chemicals into the anterior chamber
    b) prevent medications from penetrating the anterior chamber
    c) detoxify waste products of the tissues
    d) provide a primary refracting surface

82. **The purpose of the outflowing aqueous humor is to:**
    a) increase the intraocular pressure
    b) bathe the retina with nutrients
    c) bathe the back of the lens with nutrients
    d) remove waste products

Iris/Pupil*

83. **The muscles of the iris are:**
    a) medial and lateral irides
    b) sphincter, dilator
    c) superior and inferior irides
    d) interior and lateral sphincters

84. **Which of the following is stimulated by the parasympathetic system to cause miosis?**
    a) iris sphincter muscle
    b) iris dilator muscle
    c) ciliary muscle
    d) orbicularis oculi

85. **If the sympathetic system is stimulated, it causes what ocular response?**
    a) blurred vision
    b) reflex tearing
    c) dilation
    d) convergence

86. **Which of the following supply motor impulses to the iris?**
    a) CN II
    b) CNs III and V
    c) CNs V and VII
    d) CN VII

87. **The junction between the dilator and sphincter muscles of the iris is called the:**
    a) fundus
    b) ora serrata
    c) collarette
    d) frill

88. **Which pigment is found in the backside of the iris?**
    a) visual purple
    b) melanin
    c) cyanin
    d) chlorophyll

* See also Chapter 4, Questions 2, 3, 8, 12 to 16, and 40 to 42.

Crystalline Lens*

89. **Which of the following regarding the crystalline lens is *not* true?**
     a) The anterior surface is flatter than the posterior surface.
     b) It gets thinner over the years, liquefying the center.
     c) The interior is putty-like at birth.
     d) It is made up of a capsule, cortex, and nucleus.

90. **What supplies the lens with nutrients and waste removal?**
     a) lenticular blood vessels
     b) ciliary body
     c) aqueous
     d) anterior capsule

91. **The crystalline lens is held in place by means of:**
     a) ciliary muscle
     b) ciliary body
     c) vitreous
     d) zonules

92. **The shape of the crystalline lens is controlled by the:**
     a) extraocular muscles
     b) ciliary muscle
     c) orbicularis lenticuli
     d) CN II

93. **What is the main cause of presbyopia?**
     a) loss of muscle tone in the ciliary muscle
     b) increased flexion of the capsule
     c) sustained accommodation
     d) increased rigidity of the lens nucleus

94. **With age, the crystalline lens becomes more compact and forms more layers. This is called:**
     a) syneresis
     b) matriculation
     c) lamination
     d) liquefaction

95. **When presented with a near object:**
     a) the ciliary body contracts
     b) the orbicularis lenticuli relaxes
     c) the ciliary muscle contracts
     d) the pupils dilate

96. **The phenomenon described in Question 95 is known as:**
     a) accommodation
     b) convergence
     c) near vision
     d) divergence

* See also Chapter 9, Questions 4 to 6.

97. The phenomenon where the lens accommodates, the pupil gets smaller, and the eyes converge in response to a near object, is known as the:
    a) focusing triad
    b) accommodative reflex
    c) presbyopic reflex
    d) divergence insufficiency

Uvea/Choroid

98. Which of the following is *not* a part of the uveal tract?
    a) choroid
    b) ciliary muscle
    c) iris
    d) ciliary body

99. Which of the following statements is *not* true regarding the uvea?
    a) it is pigmented
    b) it is avascular
    c) in Latin, the term means "grape"
    d) it is referred to as the "middle" layer of the eye

100. The choroid is situated:
    a) between the sclera and retina
    b) between the retina and the vitreous
    c) in the center of the retina
    d) behind the optic nerve

101. Which of the following does *not* depend on the choroidal blood supply?
    a) macula
    b) outer layer of the retina
    c) inner layer of the retina
    d) middle layer of the retina

Vitreous

102. Which of the following is *not* true regarding the vitreous humor?
    a) The anterior face may be visible with the slit lamp.
    b) It adheres to the anterior capsule of the crystalline lens.
    c) It is avascular.
    d) It is about 98% water.

103. Which of the following statements about the vitreous humor is *true*?
    a) It is regenerated by the ciliary body.
    b) It helps provide nourishment to the retina.
    c) It is nourished by the sclera and ciliary muscle.
    d) It plays a role in maintaining the shape of the globe.

104. **In the case of a concussive injury, the vitreous acts as a(n):**
    a) intraocular pressure stabilizer
    b) stabilizer for the iris
    c) shock absorber
    d) cushion for the cornea

105. **With age, the vitreous begins to liquefy and lose some of its gel-like quality. This is called:**
    a) cyclitis
    b) syneresis
    c) presbyopia
    d) floaters

106. **In cases of treating macular degeneration, the vitreous may function as a(n):**
    a) drug reservoir
    b) barrier to antioxidants
    c) retinal blood barrier
    d) anti-inflammatory agent

Retina

107. **The portion of the eye's interior that is visible with an ophthalmoscope is commonly called the:**
    a) posterior chamber
    b) fundus
    c) optic nerve
    d) macula

108. **Your physician has requested posterior pole photos. Which of the following is meant?**
    a) center the optic nerve in the photo
    b) center the macula in the photo
    c) position the optic nerve in the superior part of the frame
    d) include the nerve and the macula in the photo

109. **This structure lies between the vitreous and the choroid.**
    a) sclera
    b) episcleral
    c) crystalline lens
    d) retina

110. **The retina of the eye is sometimes compared to:**
    a) film in a camera
    b) a movie screen
    c) a pixel
    d) a satellite dish

111. **The function of the retina is to:**
    a) reflect light onto the optic nerve
    b) provide stereo acuity
    c) receive light and convert it into electrical impulses
    d) provide blood supply to the choroid

112. **Each eye is situated in the head so that incoming images fall on the:**
    a) optic nerve
    b) macula
    c) posterior pole
    d) fundus

113. **Which of the following is *false*? (Consider the retinal anatomy in the direction from the vitreous to the choroid.)**
    a) Incoming light first strikes the inner limiting membrane.
    b) The nerve fiber layer lies under the inner limiting membrane.
    c) The RPE lies under the photoreceptor cells.
    d) The external limiting membrane abuts the choroid.

114. **Which is the area of absolute finest, best vision?**
    a) macula
    b) foveola
    c) fovea
    d) optic nerve

115. **This part of the retina is avascular and has the largest concentration of cone cells:**
    a) periphery
    b) choroid
    c) macula
    d) vitreous

116. **The main blood supply for the retina is the:**
    a) choroidal vessels
    b) central retinal vein
    c) central retinal artery
    d) vitreous vessels

117. **The main nerve involved with the retina is:**
    a) CN II
    b) CN II
    c) CN VI
    d) CN VII

118. **Through which does light first pass?**
    a) choroid
    b) rods and cones
    c) nerve fiber layer
    d) pigment epithelium

119. **The retinal nerve fiber layer is made up of:**
    a) connective tissue
    b) blood vessels
    c) rod and cone cells
    d) axons of ganglion cells

120. **The orderly arrangement of the ganglion fibers makes it possible to identify:**
    a) distortions in visual acuity
    b) the area of the visual pathway involved in a visual field defect
    c) diabetic and hypertensive retinopathy
    d) the amount of vision lost to degeneration

121. **Nerve fibers from the portion of the optic nerve that is farthest from the macula course around the macula to converge at the:**
    a) horizontal raphe
    b) equator
    c) angle
    d) vertical raphe

122. **Which of the following statements is *false*?**
    a) Vision in low light is referred to as scotopic.
    b) The rod cells provide no color vision.
    c) The cone cells do not function well in dim light.
    d) The rod and cone cells attach directly to the nerve fiber layer.

123. **Rod cells are:**
    a) evenly scattered throughout the retina
    b) are concentrated in the fovea
    c) are concentrated around the optic nerve
    d) mainly concentrated about 4 to 5 mm from the macula

124. **Which of the following about rod cells is *false*?**
    a) They are outnumbered by cone cells.
    b) They are adapted for vision in dim light.
    c) They contain the pigment rhodopsin.
    d) Light causes a biochemical reaction which the rods convert to an electric signal.

125. **Bright light causes the breakdown of rhodopsin in a process known as:**
    a) regeneration
    b) bleaching
    c) dilution
    d) mitigation

126. **The process of the rods coming to full functionality in the absence of light is called:**
    a) dark adaptation
    b) twilight vision
    c) contrast sensitivity
    d) photomacular stress

127. **Which of the following statements regarding cone cells is *false*?**
    a) There are 3 types of cone cells.
    b) There is some overlap in the color range of the cones.
    c) All cones have exactly the same photosensitive pigment.
    d) If all cones are stimulated equally, we see white.

128. **You have walked out of a dark movie theater into the bright sun. Approximately how long will it take your healthy eyes to light adapt?**
    a) 30 seconds
    b) 1 minute
    c) 2 minutes
    d) 20 minutes

129. **Which of the following is *not* a function of the RPE?**
    a) absorbs harmful light rays
    b) recycles photoreceptor pigments
    c) provides energy for the rods and cones
    d) permits full access of toxic material to the rods and cones

130. **The RPE overlies which of the following?**
    a) rod and cone cells
    b) Bruch's membrane
    c) the choroid
    d) ganglion fibers

Optic Nerve

131. **Which of the following regarding the optic nerve is *true*?**
    a) It is the area of sharpest vision.
    b) The eye is situated in the skull so that incoming light focuses here.
    c) There is an equal distribution of rods and cones here.
    d) It is known as the physiologic blind spot.

132. **The portion of the optic nerve that is visible in a fundus exam is the:**
    a) lamina cribrosa
    b) fovea
    c) optic disc
    d) chiasm

133. **The average dimensions of the adult optic disc is approximately:**
    a) 1 x 1 mm
    b) 2 x 1.5 mm
    c) 2 x 2 mm
    d) 2 x 2.5 mm

134. **Roughly in the center of the optic disc is a depression called the:**
    a) physiologic cup
    b) rim
    c) macula
    d) fossa

135. **An evaluation of the fundus generally includes an estimation of:**
    a) axial length
    b) cup-to-disc ratio
    c) disc-to-macula distance
    d) fundus curvature

136. **The nerve fibers that meet at the optic nerve are the:**
    a) rods and cones
    b) ganglion cell axons
    c) optic radiations
    d) brain stem

137. **At the optic nerve cup, the sclera forms which of the following?**
    a) trabecular meshwork
    b) ora serrata
    c) lamina cribrosa
    c) limbus

Visual Pathway*

138. **Images pass through the optic nerve and thence to the:**
    a) lateral geniculate body, chiasm, occipital cortex, and brain stem
    b) optic tract, lateral geniculate body, and cerebral cortex
    c) chiasm, optic tract, lateral geniculate body, and occipital cortex
    d) chiasm, optic tract, lateral geniculate body, and cerebellum

Physiology of Color Vision**

139. **Color vision is a product of:**
    a) the wavelength of light
    b) retinal photoreceptor cells and proteins
    c) the brain's interpretation
    d) all of the above

140. **Retinal cone cells are differentiated from each other by:**
    a) their color
    b) their position in the retinal periphery
    c) the wavelength they are "tuned" to
    d) their shape

141. **How many different types of cone cells are normally found in the human retina?**
    a) 2
    b) 3
    c) 4
    d) 5

142. **The presence of different types of cone cells that are sensitive to various wave lengths of light is the basis of the:**
    a) island of color vision theory
    b) the bi-color theory
    c) the full-hue theory
    d) trichromatic theory of color vision

* For questions about the visual pathway, see Chapter 3, Questions 1 to 20.
** See Questions 115 and 127, this chapter, concerning the cone photoreceptor cells.

143. If all 3 of the cone types are equally stimulated, which of the following is perceived?
    a) gray
    b) black
    c) full spectrum
    d) white

Part III

Inflammation Versus Infection

144. Which of the following might cause an infection?
    a) trauma
    b) virus
    c) allergens
    d) paralysis

145. Which of the following would likely be associated with inflammation?
    a) allergic conjunctivitis
    b) chalazion
    c) iritis
    d) all of the above

146. Hallmarks of inflammation include all of the following *except*:
    a) swelling/pain
    b) redness
    c) bleeding
    d) heat/fever

147. Which of the following is an inflammation?
    a) papillomacular bundling
    b) papilloma
    c) papillitis
    d) papilla

Eye Diseases and Conditions*

148. Match each disorder to the ocular part affected. Some disorders may have more than one answer.
    Ocular Part
    a) cranial nerves
    b) orbit
    c) extraocular muscles
    d) globe
    e) lids
    f) lacrimal

* For question on surgical treatments of certain disorders, see Chapter 14, Question 49.

Disorder
__ afferent or efferent pupillary defect
__ anophthalmos
__ Bell's palsy
__ blepharitis
__ blepharospasm
__ blow-out fracture
__ Brown syndrome
__ buphthalmos
__ canaliculitis
__ cellulitis
__ chalazion
__ coloboma
__ corneal or facial numbness
__ dacryocystitis
__ dermatochalasis
__ Duane's syndrome
__ duct obstruction
__ entropion/ectropion
__ epiphora
__ exophthalmos
__ lagophthalmos
__ meibomian gland deficiency/disease
__ microphthalmia
__ *molluscum contagiosum*
__ myasthenia gravis
__ prolapsed lacrimal gland
__ ptosis
__ strabismus
__ sty
__ sympathetic ophthalmia
__ tonic pupil
__ trichiasis
__ xanthelasma

149. **Match each disorder to the ocular part affected. Some disorders may have more than one answer.**
     Ocular Part
     a) conjunctiva
     b) sclera/episclera
     c) cornea
     d) anterior chamber/angle/aqueous
     e) iris and ciliary body
     f) pupil
     g) lens

Ocular Disorder
__ albinism
__ angle closure
__ aniridia
__ anisocoria
__ arcus senilis
__ buphthalmos
__ cataract
__ cells/flare
__ coloboma
__ cyclitis
__ dry eye syndrome
__ episcleritis
__ erosion
__ exfoliation
__ Fuchs' dystrophy
__ heterochromia
__ hyphema
__ hypopyon
__ iritis
__ keratitis
__ Krukenberg's spindle
__ Marcus Gunn
__ Mittendorf's dot
__ narrow angle
__ *ophthalmia neonatorum*
__ pannus
__ pinguecula
__ prolapse
__ prolapsed lacrimal gland
__ pterygium
__ scleritis
__ subconjunctival hemorrhage
__ subluxation
__ synechea (anterior/posterior)
__ trachoma
__ ulcer

150. **Match each disorder to the ocular part affected. Some disorders may have more than one answer.**
    Ocular Part
    a) uvea
    b) vitreous
    c) retina (*not* including macular or optic nerve)
    d) macula
    e) optic nerve (CN II)
    f) visual pathway (*not* including retina or optic nerve)

Disorder
__ age-related degeneration
__ albinism
__ asteroid hyalosis
__ central serous chorioretinopathy
__ coloboma
__ color vision deficiencies
__ cotton wool spots
__ cupping
__ degenerations
__ detachment
__ diabetic retinopathy
__ drusen
__ epiretinal membrane
__ floaters/scoots
__ glaucoma
__ hemorrhage
__ hypertensive retinopathy
__ macular hole
__ papilledema
__ papillitis (inflammation of disc)
__ pituitary tumor
__ presumed ocular histoplasmosis syndrome
__ prolapse
__ quadrantanopsia visual field defect
__ RP
__ retinoblastoma
__ retinopathy of prematurity
__ tears/holes
__ toxoplasmosis
__ traumatic brain injury
__ uveitis (anterior/posterior)
__ vascular occlusion

Cranial Nerves/Neurology

151. Which of the following is a rhythmic jerking of the eyes that the patient can't control?
    a) saccades
    b) strabismus
    c) nystagmus
    d) CN II palsy

152. A nerve palsy in which of the following CNs would *not* result in a problem with the extraocular muscles?
    a) CN II
    b) CN III
    c) CN IV
    d) CN VI

Extraocular Muscles*

Orbit/Globe

153. Which of the following is a potentially life-threatening condition?
     a) preorbital cellulitis
     b) molluscum contagiosum
     c) corneal abrasion
     d) orbital cellulitis

154. You are performing a range of motion test on your patient. When you move the pen light from straight up, downward into primary position, you notice that the eyelids' movement lags behind the movement of the eyes themselves. This can be a sign of:
     a) Sarah's palsy
     b) diabetes
     c) malnutrition
     d) Graves disease

155. What is the difference between proptosis and exophthalmos?
     a) Proptosis refers specifically to the eye.
     b) The terms are largely interchangeable.
     c) Proptosis means only one eye is pushed forward; exophthalmos means both eyes.
     d) Exophthalmos means that there is a tumor behind the globe.

Lids and Skin

156. Matching, one answer:
     Entity
     blepharitis
     blepharospasm
     cellulitis
     chalazion
     dermatochalasis
     ectropion
     entropion
     hordeolum
     lagophthalmos
     ptosis
     trichiasis
     xanthelasma

     Description
     _____ blocked meibomian gland
     _____ drooped eyelid
     _____ inward-growing eyelash
     _____ incomplete lid closure

* For questions about extraocular muscle disorders, see Chapter 7, Questions 11, 13, 28 to 40, and 104 to 110.

_____ infected hair follicle
_____ infected, inflamed tissues of lid/orbit
_____ in-turned eyelid
_____ lid infection
_____ lid twitch
_____ out-turned eyelid
_____ sagging skin of upper lid
_____ yellow lipid skin deposit

Lacrimal

157. Obstructed NLD is most often seen:
a) in persons with autoimmune disease
b) in teens
c) in children
d) after injury

158. Symptoms of NLD obstruction include all of the following *except*:
a) mattering
b) tearing
c) redness/swelling
d) limited eye movement

159. Initial treatment of NLD obstruction in an infant may include:
a) hospitalization
b) surgery
c) massages and antibiotic drops
d) placement of a stent

160. Inflammation/infection of the nasolacrimal sac is called:
a) canaliculus
b) chalazion
c) dacryocystitis
d) blepharitis

161. Your patient says, "How can I have dry eye when my eyes are watering all the time?" The phenomenon described is called:
a) epiphora
b) trichiasis
c) contralacrimation
d) entropion

162. Which of the following is *not* typically associated with dry eye?
a) burning
b) tearing
c) blurred vision
d) halos around lights

163. When a patient complains of dry eye symptoms, pertinent questions might include any of the following *except*:
    a) Do you use oxygen at night for sleep apnea?
    b) Are you exposed to smoke?
    c) Do you sleep with a fan blowing on you?
    d) Do you sleep with a humidifier running?

164. Treatment for dry eye often includes warm compresses and gentle lid massages. The purpose of this is to:
    a) increase tear production
    b) decrease tear drainage off the eye
    c) increase patient comfort
    d) open and stimulate the meibomian glands

165. The scenario described in Question 164 is indicated in the case of:
    a) chalazia formation
    b) sty formation
    c) meibomian gland dysfunction
    d) lacrimal sac obstruction

166. The purpose of punctal plugs or punctal ablation is to:
    a) decrease tear production
    b) open the canaliculi
    c) keep tears on the eye
    d) increase tear formation

167. In the evaluation of dry eye, a test that can indicate the salt content of tears is:
    a) meibography
    b) tear osmolarity
    c) Schirmer's test I
    d) Schirmer's test II

168. Meibomian gland dysfunction is the most frequent cause of:
    a) systemic dryness
    b) nasolacrimal obstruction
    c) evaporative dry eye
    d) conjunctivitis

Conjunctiva

169. On slit lamp exam, your patient has a small, clear-looking nodule on the temporal conjunctiva. Most likely this is a:
    a) pinguecula
    b) pterygium
    c) nevus
    d) melanoma

170. **Which of the following would be initially treated with a topical antibiotic drop?**
   a) fungal conjunctivitis
   b) viral conjunctivitis
   c) bacterial conjunctivitis
   d) allergic conjunctivitis

171. **A patient with "pink eye" has now developed corneal involvement. This is known as:**
   a) epidemic conjunctivitis
   b) episcleritis
   c) keratoconus
   d) keratoconjunctivitis

172. **You are examining the conjunctiva of a contact lens wearing patient. When you flip the upper lid, you see tiny, red, raised lesions that make the surface look like cobblestones. Most likely this is:**
   a) Acanthamoeba infection
   b) giant papillary conjunctivitis
   c) viral infection
   d) fungal infection

173. **A patient calls in, stating "My eye is bleeding!" As you go through triage with them, they state that there is no discharge, no pain, no change in vision. The redness is a large spot on the white of their eye. They take aspirin daily. Most likely this is a:**
   a) retinal hemorrhage
   b) lid laceration
   c) pterygium
   d) subconjunctival hemorrhage

174. **Other factors causing the previous scenario could include any of the following *except*:**
   a) infection
   b) taking blood thinners
   c) hard coughing or sneezing
   d) heavy lifting

Sclera/Episclera

175. **What condition might result in yellow-looking sclera?**
   a) sun exposure
   b) chronic exposure to dust
   c) jaundice
   d) drinking too much lemonade

176. **Thin sclera might appear bluish. This is because of:**
   a) excessive crying
   b) elevated intraocular pressure
   c) elevated blood pressure
   d) the underlying choroid

177. **Your patient has complaints of a moderately red, uncomfortable eye. The other eye is clear; vision is good in both eyes. You are using the slit lamp and see a raised, red nodule just under the bulbar conjunctiva. The palpebral conjunctiva looks normal, and there is no discharge. This scenario may be due to:**
    a) episcleritis
    b) conjunctivitis
    c) angle closure
    d) iritis

178. **Which of the following statements about scleritis is *not* true?**
    a) Pain can be severe.
    b) It is often associated with autoimmune disease.
    c) Men are more likely to have it.
    d) It can result in death of scleral tissue.

Cornea*

179. **Your patient has iritis. What corneal signs might you see with the slit lamp?**
    a) punctate keratopathy
    b) corneal edema
    c) corneal ulcer
    d) precipitates

180. **At the slit lamp you notice cornea neovascularization in the upper limbal area. What would you ask the patient next?**
    a) Do you use any kind of eye drops?
    b) Do you see halos around lights?
    c) Do you sleep in contact lenses?
    d) Have you had any floaters recently?

181. **At the slit lamp, you notice fine lines and dots just under the epithelium. This can be a sign of:**
    a) keratitis
    b) anterior basement membrane dystrophy
    c) Fuchs' dystrophy
    d) corneal abrasion

182. **At the slit lamp, you notice a vertical "bar" of fine, dark dots on the corneal endothelium. Most likely, this is:**
    a) corneal dystrophy
    b) intraocular foreign body
    c) Krukenberg's spindle
    d) corneal scar

---

* For more questions on cornea, see Questions 58 to 73 in this chapter. For corneal problems related to contact lenses see Chapter 18, Questions 114 to 124, 126, 127, and 132.

183. **In the scenario in Question 182, the patient is at higher risk for developing which of the following?**
     a) keratoconus
     b) macular degeneration
     c) retinal detachment
     d) glaucoma

184. **Which of the following statements regarding Fuchs' corneal dystrophy is *false*?**
     a) It can cause corneal edema.
     b) It is a risk factor in cataract extraction surgery.
     c) One of the first symptoms may be blurred vision in the evening.
     d) Descemet's membrane thickens and the endothelial cells are damaged.

185. **You are examining a patient at the slit lamp. When they look down, you notice that the cornea pushes the lower lid forward. This could be:**
     a) exophthalmos
     b) proptosis
     c) keratoconus
     d) ectropion

186. **Which of the following is *not* used in treatment of keratoconus?**
     a) corneal transplant
     b) topical steroids
     c) intracorneal rings
     d) corneal cross-linking

187. **Your patient has a left Bell's palsy. Of concern in a case like this is:**
     a) corneal exposure keratitis
     b) conjunctivitis
     c) ectropion
     d) eyelid tic

188. **A contact lens patient has called complaining of fairly sudden onset of pain, light sensitivity, and redness. What is the most logical question to ask?**
     a) Are these daily disposable lenses?
     b) How long are you wearing the contacts?
     c) What type of lenses are you wearing?
     d) Have you gotten anything under the contact?

189. **Your 75-year-old patient presents with a complaint of a "white ring" around the eyes. You look at them with the slit lamp and see a creamy-white/gray circle just inside the corneal limbus all the way around the eye. Most likely this is:**
     a) a cataract
     b) a pterygium
     c) limbal cancer
     d) a benign arcus senilis

190. **Which of the following statements regarding a pterygium is *false*?**
     a) It can be associated with chronic exposure to ultraviolet light.
     b) It can be associated with chronic exposure to dust and wind.
     c) It may require surgical removal if it encroaches on the optic zone.
     d) Infants are frequently born with it.

191. Your patient had LASIK several months ago. Today at the slit lamp you see some whitish-gray-looking areas, some with feathered edges, under the flap. This could be:
    a) a viral dendrite
    b) stromal rejection
    c) epithelial ingrowth
    d) pingueculum

Anterior Chamber/Aqueous/Angle*

192. Your patient has been dealing with a rather severe bout of uveitis. On slit lamp exam, you see a collection of whitish material at the bottom of the angle. This is probably a(n):
    a) hyphema
    b) arcus senilis
    c) hypopyon
    d) pigment dispersion

193. In the scenario in Question 192, if you use a pinpoint beam to visualize the anterior chamber, you will probably find:
    a) floaters
    b) cells and flare
    c) lashes
    d) flashes

194. In the scenario in Question 193, you are looking at the cells in the anterior chamber with a pinpoint beam and see them moving. This is caused by:
    a) amoeba-like movement of the cells
    b) an optical illusion
    c) light reflecting off of floaters
    d) circulation of the aqueous

Iris/Ciliary Body

195. Your practitioner has diagnosed a patient with iritis and has prescribed homatropine drops. This is done in order to:
    a) immobilize the iris
    b) prevent photophobia
    c) sharpen the patient's vision
    d) cure the infection

196. Which of the following is another term for iritis?
    a) anterior uveitis
    b) posterior uveitis
    c) shipyard eye
    d) panuveitis

* Regarding the angle, see Questions 77 (anatomy) and 247, 251, 261, 263, and 264 (glaucoma) in this chapter.

197. **A concerned foster parent has brought in a 6-month-old for examination because "his pupils look funny." With your pen light, you can see that the pupil is open at the bottom. This is most likely a(n):**
    a) sign of child abuse
    b) iris coloboma
    c) result of Cesarean birth
    d) result of oxygen given just after birth

198. **Which of the following may have an unusually pale iris and photophobia?**
    a) infant born prematurely
    b) person with Down syndrome
    c) older adult
    d) person with albinism

199. **Which of the following structures plays a role in glaucoma?**
    a) ciliary body
    b) ciliary muscle
    c) choroid
    d) crystalline lens

200. **Which of the following structures may play a role in obstruction of the angle?**
    a) cornea
    b) ciliary body
    c) iris
    d) pupil

Pupil*

Lens

201. **Matching, one answer:**
    Term
    congenital
    cortical
    hypermature
    incipient
    nuclear sclerotic
    posterior subcapsular

    Definition
    _____ early; just beginning
    _____ lens opacity present at birth
    _____ opacity between the epithelium and nucleus
    _____ opacity in the hardened center of the crystalline lens
    _____ opacity in the membrane behind the crystalline lens
    _____ whitish cataract with breakdown of the cortex

* For questions about pupillary defects, see Chapter 4, Questions 1, 9 to 11, and 17 to 39.

Uvea

202. **Symptoms of uveitis include:**
   a) sudden, painless loss of vision
   b) lid swelling and redness
   c) pain, redness, light sensitivity
   d) discharge and redness

203. **Another name for iritis is:**
   a) posterior uveitis
   b) cyclitis
   c) anterior uveitis
   d) choroiditis

204. **Your employer has diagnosed a patient as having panuveitis. This means that:**
   a) the iris and ciliary body are involved
   b) the entire uvea is involved
   c) a record number of people have uveitis at the same time
   d) the entire cornea is involved

205. **Which of the following is the most common type of intraocular malignancy in adults?**
   a) choroidal nevus
   b) choroidal melanoma
   c) neurofibroma
   d) retinoblastoma

206. **Which of the following patients must be especially monitored for the appearance of choroidal cancer?**
   a) leukemia
   b) fibromyalgia
   c) cutaneous melanoma
   d) lung and breast cancer

Vitreous

207. **The finding of multiple opacities in the vitreous is known as:**
   a) amaurosis fugax
   b) aura
   c) TIA
   d) asteroid hyalosis

208. **Which of the following is associated with posterior vitreous detachment?**
   a) visual aura
   b) loss of part of the visual field
   c) painless loss of vision in one eye
   d) floaters and flashes

209. **Symptoms of a posterior vitreous detachment are considered an urgent case to be seen in within 24 hours because:**
    a) retinal detachment can have the same symptoms
    b) they are a sign of elevated intraocular pressure
    c) after 24 hours the lids swell shut
    d) after 24 hours the double vision will be permanent

Retina*

210. **A new patient says that their last doctor gave them a paper "checkerboard" to take home and look at. Of the following, what is the most likely reason?**
    a) cataracts
    b) glaucoma
    c) macular degeneration
    d) corneal dystrophy

211. **Which of the following regarding AMD is *false*?**
    a) It is the most common cause of blindness in persons over 65 in the United States.
    b) There is no treatment for the wet form.
    c) Risk factors include high blood pressure and high cholesterol.
    d) Prevention includes avoiding ultraviolet exposure and stop smoking.

212. **Symptoms of AMD include:**
    a) floaters
    b) distorted central vision
    c) tunnel vision
    d) gritty sensation

213. **Which of the following retinal findings is *not* generally associated with dry AMD?**
    a) cherry red spot
    b) drusen
    c) geographic atrophy
    d) pigment changes

214. **Retinal changes in wet AMD might include any of the following *except*:**
    a) new, abnormal blood vessels
    b) swelling of macula
    c) macular hole
    d) subretinal fluid

215. **Which of the following statements regarding epiretinal membranes is *not* true?**
    a) It is also referred to as cellophane maculopathy.
    b) It can cause distorted central vision.
    c) It is caused by vitreomacular traction.
    d) It is most commonly seen in middle age.

* Diabetic retinopathy is covered in Questions 295 and 296 in this chapter. Hypertensive retinopathy is in Question 300.

216. **Which of the following is a disorder where there is progressive night blindness and loss of peripheral vision?**
    a) glaucoma
    b) RP
    c) macular degeneration
    d) epiretinal membrane

217. **Which of the following statements regarding RP is *false*?**
    a) It is a genetic/hereditary disorder.
    b) Ocular signs of the disorder are usually present at birth.
    c) It generally affects the rod cells first.
    d) Blindness usually occurs by age 40 years.

218. **Which of the following might be of help to a patient with RP?**
    a) anti-VEGF injections
    b) low vision aids
    c) long-term oral steroids
    d) topical steroids

219. **Which of the following is *not* associated with retinopathy in a newborn?**
    a) cardiac arrest
    b) prematurity
    c) respiratory distress
    d) low birth weight

220. **Retinopathy of prematurity is primarily a problem of:**
    a) hyperpigmentation
    b) lack of cone cells
    c) neovascularization
    d) drusen

221. **There has been an increase in the cases of retinopathy of prematurity. This is due to:**
    a) increase in birth rate
    b) increase in induced births
    c) increase in Cesarean deliveries
    d) premature infants surviving earlier and earlier births

222. **In retinal detachment, the retina no longer functions properly because:**
    a) the optic nerve is detached
    b) the vitreous is destroyed
    c) the macula is still attached
    d) it has been separated from its blood supply

223. **A retinal detachment that forms when there is a retinal tear and fluid has accumulated between the retina and choroid is called a:**
    a) traction detachment
    b) horseshoe detachment
    c) rhegmatogenous detachment
    d) recurrent detachment

224. Which of the following is *not* considered a risk factor for retinal detachment?
a) macular degeneration
b) high myopia
c) previous ocular injury or surgery
d) mature cataracts

225. Your patient with diabetic retinopathy has called in today with a sudden, painless shower of floaters and flashing lights. This may indicate a(n):
a) macular degeneration
b) macular pucker
c) tractional retinal detachment
d) iritis

226. In a scenario where vitreous is tugging on the macula, which of the following might develop?
a) hypertensive changes
b) macular hole
c) glaucoma
d) retinal ulcer

227. Your new, adult patient gives a history of having had a "stroke" in the right eye. This layperson's term probably is referring to some type of:
a) fungal infection
b) vascular occlusion
c) wet macular degeneration
d) amblyopia

228. Which of the following might cause a sudden, painless loss of peripheral vision?
a) central artery/vein occlusion
b) acute angle closure
c) cortical cataracts
d) branch artery/vein occlusion

229. Which of the following represents the greatest emergency?
a) central retinal vein occlusion
b) branch retinal vein occlusion
c) branch retinal artery occlusion
d) central retinal artery occlusion

230. You suspect that your patient is presenting with a central retinal artery occlusion. What might you expect the practitioner to see on fundus examination?
a) cherry-red spot of the optic disc
b) vitreous hemorrhage
c) cherry-red spot of the macula
d) retinal detachment

231. Which of the following statements is *false*?
a) Branch occlusions affect a specific part of the retina.
b) Risk factors for retinal vascular occlusions include diabetes and hypertension.
c) Vein occlusions affect blood supply to the entire retina.
d) Smoking increases the risk of having a retinal vascular occlusive event.

Optic Nerve (CN II)/Glaucoma*

232. **Intraocular pressure is determined by:**
    a) systolic and diastolic blood pressure
    b) rate of aqueous production and resistance to outflow
    c) pressure in the ophthalmic artery and vein
    d) cranial pressure transferred to the eye through the optic nerve

233. **Which of the following regarding aqueous and intraocular pressure is *not* true?**
    a) Intraocular pressure is generally higher in the morning than in the evening.
    b) Intraocular pressure is slightly higher in the posterior chamber than in the anterior chamber.
    c) Aqueous has no effect on the optical system of the eye.
    d) Aqueous provides nutrition and waste removal for internal ocular structures.

234. **The physiologic cup of the optic nerve:**
    a) is an abnormal finding in glaucoma
    b) represents the normal opening in the sclera
    c) is the area of finest central vision
    d) is a normal depression in the macular area

235. **In glaucoma, the term "cupping" refers to:**
    a) a pale optic disc
    b) a decrease and "pinching" in the size of the physiologic cup
    c) an enlargement and "caving in" of the physiologic cup
    d) dips in the retinal veins and arteries

236. **A comparison of the proportion of damaged disc to visually functioning disc is termed:**
    a) abnormal retinal correspondence
    b) the cup-to-disc ratio
    c) the AC/A ratio
    d) the glaucoma ratio

237. **A large cup would be represented by:**
    a) 0.2
    b) 0.9
    c) 20/400
    d) 30 mm Hg

238. **The first area of the optic nerve to be damaged by elevated intraocular pressure is often:**
    a) the center of the disc
    b) the interior of the disc
    c) the nasal side of the disc
    d) the upper and lower portions of the rim

239. **In glaucoma, areas of optic nerve damage directly relate to:**
    a) the visual field pattern
    b) the diurnal curve of intraocular pressure
    c) laser treatment
    d) areas of neovascularization

* For questions about glaucoma as related to visual fields, see Chapter 3, Questions 183 to 189. For questions regarding tonometry, see Chapter 5. Regarding central corneal thickness, see Chapter 11, Questions 44 and 45.

240. **Reduction and control of elevated intraocular pressure is based on:**
    a) lowering the diastolic and systolic blood pressure
    b) lowering cranial pressure
    c) increasing aqueous production and/or decreasing outflow
    d) decreasing aqueous production and/or increasing outflow

241. **Glaucoma is classically characterized by the triad of increased intraocular pressure, visual field damage, and:**
    a) pigment in the trabecular meshwork
    b) decreased facility outflow
    c) fluctuating visual acuity
    d) optic nerve head damage

242. **Physicians do not rely on intraocular pressure measurements alone when evaluating a patient for glaucoma because:**
    a) some eyes cannot tolerate even "normal" pressure
    b) tonometers are difficult to calibrate
    c) only Goldmann tonometry is reliable
    d) inaccuracies are common

243. **In addition to tonometry, the diagnosis of glaucoma may be based on all of the following tests *except*:**
    a) corneal pachymetry
    b) gonioscopy
    c) retinoscopy
    d) perimetry

244. **Gonioscopy is used to evaluate:**
    a) the angle structures
    b) the optic nerve
    c) peripheral vision
    d) corneal edema

245. **Vision lost by glaucoma damage:**
    a) can be recovered if the intraocular pressure is brought under control
    b) can be recovered if laser treatment is used
    c) can be recovered with certain topical or oral medications
    d) generally cannot be recovered

246. **The diurnal curve of intraocular pressure in a glaucoma patient:**
    a) may vary by 4 mm
    b) may vary up to 10 mm
    c) is less than in an eye without glaucoma
    d) produces intraocular pressure that is lower in the morning

247. **The most common type of glaucoma is:**
    a) congenital
    b) secondary
    c) open-angle
    d) angle-closure

248. **Risk factors for open-angle glaucoma include all of the following** *except*:
    a) being under age 40 years
    b) positive family history
    c) Black heritage
    d) history of ocular trauma

249. **Which of the following regarding open-angle glaucoma is** *false*?
    a) It is more prevalent in the Black population.
    b) It can be cured.
    c) Optic nerve damage cannot be reversed.
    d) It might be controlled with a single medication.

250. **The dangerous element of open-angle glaucoma is:**
    a) pain
    b) rapid, irreversible visual loss
    c) lack of symptoms
    d) lack of signs

251. **In open-angle glaucoma:**
    a) the iris blocks off the angle structures
    b) the pressure damages the ciliary body
    c) the angle allows too much aqueous to drain out
    d) the angle looks normal

252. **A patient known to have open-angle glaucoma:**
    a) should not be dilated
    b) should have their pressures checked with an air-puff tonometer
    c) should be checked annually with confrontation fields
    d) needs annual dilation, gonioscopy, and formal visual fields

253. **A patient in the end stages of open-angle glaucoma:**
    a) may have a small island of vision temporally
    b) may have a small island of vision centrally
    c) may have a small island of vision nasally
    d) still has enough peripheral vision to get around

254. **A patient with open-angle glaucoma has missed an appointment for a pressure check. The practice should:**
    a) wait for the patient to call and reschedule, then emphasize the importance of intraocular pressure checks
    b) inform the patient's relatives, and stress the importance of having intraocular pressure checks
    c) have the pharmacist ask the patient to call the office when medication needs to be refilled
    d) contact the patient immediately to reschedule, emphasizing the importance of intraocular pressure checks

255. **If a patient experiences an increase in intraocular pressure while using corticosteroids, this is known as:**
    a) ocular hypertension
    b) glaucoma suspect
    c) steroid regulator
    d) steroid responder

256. **Symptoms of congenital glaucoma may include:**
    a) redness and decreased vision
    b) swelling, photophobia, and diplopia
    c) epiphora, redness, and mattering
    d) photophobia, blepharospasm, and epiphora

257. **Ocular hypertension is a situation in which there is elevated intraocular pressure:**
    a) but the cup-to-disc ratio is less than 0.4
    b) but no damage has occurred to the optic nerve or visual field
    c) and nerve damage has remained stable over a period of years
    d) and the patient also has a visual field defect

258. **A patient who is a "glaucoma suspect" is:**
    a) at risk for developing glaucoma
    b) a candidate for immediate laser treatment
    c) a candidate for preventative laser iridotomies
    d) 100% sure of eventually developing glaucoma

259. **Symptoms and signs for acute ACG may include all of the following *except*:**
    a) severe pain
    b) decreased vision
    c) vomiting/nausea
    d) miotic pupil

260. **A patient phones in with a painful red eye. In addition to an ACG attack, you must ask questions to discern whether the patient might, instead, have any of the following *except*:**
    a) iritis
    b) conjunctivitis
    c) subconjunctival hemorrhage
    d) keratoconjunctivitis

261. **In ACG:**
    a) the iris closes off the anterior chamber angle
    b) there is a sudden surge of aqueous production
    c) a miotic pupil prevents aqueous passage
    d) corneal edema closes off the anterior chamber angle

262. **Emergency treatment during an ACG attack includes pressure lowering medications and:**
    a) miotics
    b) mydriatics
    c) antibiotics
    d) corticosteroids

263. **All of the following may trigger an ACG attack *except*:**
    a) being dilated in the office
    b) being in a dark room
    c) sudden exposure to bright light
    d) sitting in a movie theater

264. **Which of the following conditions gives a higher risk for developing an ACG attack?**
   a) high hyperopia
   b) high myopia
   c) aphakia
   d) keratoconus

265. **The appearance of halos around lights during an attack of ACG is due to:**
   a) lens edema
   b) corneal edema
   c) vitreous hemorrhage
   d) optic nerve damage

Optic Nerve, Other

266. **Which of the following statements about optic nerve pallor (paleness) is *false*?**
   a) It extends along the visual pathway to the visual cortex.
   b) It is not a disease in and of itself.
   c) It can be a sign of inflammation.
   d) It can be associated with elevated intracranial pressure.

267. **Optic nerve pallor is usually associated with:**
   a) decreased vision and afferent pupillary defect
   b) systemic hypertension
   c) diabetic retinopathy
   d) retinal detachment

268. **Swelling of the optic nerve due to increased intracranial pressure is called:**
   a) papilloma
   b) papilledema
   c) ocular hypertension
   d) glaucoma suspect

269. **Which of the following are *not* symptoms of the disorder mentioned in the previous scenario?**
   a) headache, vomiting
   b) flickering vision, double vision
   c) severe eye pain and redness
   d) blurred vision, transient loss of vision

270. **Sometimes the cup-to-disc ratio is high, but there are no other hallmarks of glaucoma. This is called:**
   a) glaucoma suspect
   b) physiologic cupping
   c) normal tension glaucoma
   d) tilted nerves

271. **Which of the following is a disorder that damages the nerve axons as well as the myelin sheath of the optic nerve?**
a) uveitis
b) Graves' disease
c) Jacob's retinopathy
d) optic neuritis

272. **With what disorder is the scenario in Question 271 usually associated?**
a) multiple sclerosis
b) fibromyalgia
c) cystic fibrosis
d) muscular dystrophy

273. **Which of the following are *not* symptoms of optic neuritis?**
a) pain in eye, pain on moving eye
b) sudden or advancing vision loss
c) scintillating aura
d) distorted vision, gray vision

Part IV

Color Vision Defects*

274. **Which of the following terms represents a color deficiency in the "red" cones?**
a) protanopia
b) tritanopia
c) monochromatism
d) protanomaly

275. **What is the most common type of inherited color vision deficiency?**
a) deuteranomoly
b) protanopia
c) rod monochromatism
d) blue cone monochromatism

276. **Which of the following statements is *false*?**
a) Most people with color vision deficiency can see colors.
b) The term "color blindness" is actually inaccurate.
c) Acquired color vision deficiency is the most common type.
d) Red-green color deficiency is an X-linked genetic trait.

277. **Which patient with a color vision defect might experience improvement?**
a) patient with X-linked color deficiency
b) patient born with 2 functioning cone types
c) patient who is no longer taking Plaquenil (hydrochloroquine)
d) none of the above

* For additional questions on color vision defects, see Chapter 11, Questions 36 to 39.

Infectious Diseases*

Trauma**

278. The patient has a severely injured eye with no hope of recovery. The physician has recommended an enucleation. This recommendation is based on the concern that:
    a) a prosthesis will be more cosmetically appealing than the injured globe
    b) endophthalmitis may develop
    c) sympathetic ophthalmia may develop
    d) secondary glaucoma may develop

279. Which of the following is an example of radiation injury?
    a) contact lens over-wear
    b) battery acid splash
    c) snow blindness
    d) bleach splash

280. Which scenario carries the highest risk of globe rupture?
    a) penetrating trauma
    b) blunt trauma
    c) thermal trauma
    d) chemical trauma

281. "Pepper spray" works to incapacitate an attacker because it:
    a) is abrasive
    b) precipitates a retinal detachment
    c) fogs glasses
    d) is a lachrymatory agent

282. Your patient burned their upper lid with their curling iron. The area is red and blistered. This is an example of a:
    a) first-degree burn
    b) second-degree burn
    c) third-degree burn
    d) fourth-degree burn

283. Your patient was driving when an accident caused the air bag to deploy. Now they have double vision. What may have happened?
    a) retinal detachment
    b) subconjunctival hemorrhage
    c) corneal abrasion
    d) blow-out fracture

* See Chapter 12: Microbiology.
** For more questions on trauma, see also Chapter 15, Questions 75 to 80.

284. **Your patient complains of awakening in the middle of the night with a foreign body sensation in the right eye. That's the same eye that got scratched by a tree limb last year. The most likely cause is:**
     a) lacrimal obstruction
     b) trichiasis
     c) recurrent erosion syndrome
     d) entropion

285. **Your patient was hit in the eye with a tennis ball at speed. When you look at the eye with the slit lamp, you cannot see the pupil or the iris. Everything behind the cornea just looks black. This is probably a(n):**
     a) hyphema
     b) hypopyon
     c) subconjunctival hemorrhage
     d) ulcer

286. **A metallic corneal foreign body should be removed as soon as possible to avoid:**
     a) elevated intraocular pressure
     b) bruising
     c) development of a rust ring
     d) impairment of color vision

287. **Your patient was grinding metal and felt something go in their eye. While they have no pain now, they wanted to get the eye checked out. On slit lamp exam, you notice a small, dark lesion on the sclera. Your next action for this patient should be:**
     a) Pressure patch and let the patient wait their turn.
     b) Apply a shield and get the doctor at once.
     c) Irrigate the eye and get the doctor at once.
     d) Instill numbing drops and let the patient wait their turn.

288. **Which sport probably has the highest risk of injury if no eye protection is worn?**
     a) golf
     b) paintball
     c) swimming
     d) fencing

289. **A social worker has brought in a 4-month-old child for evaluation. Your exam has found unequal pupils, tiny red blotches on the sclera, and failure to fix and follow. The most important part of this child's exam will be:**
     a) electrophysical testing to better determine vision
     b) dilated fundus exam
     c) tonometry
     d) full strabismus workup

290. **In the scenario in Question 289, permanent vision loss is usually the result of:**
     a) external damage to the eye
     b) retinal hemorrhage
     c) damage to the cerebral cortex
     d) retinal detachment

Ocular Manifestations of Systemic Disease

291. **Match each finding to the appropriate disorder group. Answers may be used more than once, with some disorder groups having more than one answer.**
    Finding
    a) autoimmune/inflammatory disease
    b) cancer (primary and metastatic)
    c) cardiovascular disease
    d) diabetes
    e) infectious disease (including AIDS and TB)
    f) neurologic disorder
    g) nutritional
    h) thyroid

    Disorder Group
    __ A-V crossing
    __ cataracts
    __ dry eye
    __ emboli
    __ exophthalmos
    __ herpes zoster
    __ Kaposi's sarcoma
    __ keratitis sicca
    __ melanoma
    __ "night blindness"
    __ nystagmus
    __ ptosis
    __ retinoblastoma
    __ retinopathy
    __ Sjögren's syndrome
    __ squamous cell of the lid
    __ strabismus
    __ uveitis/ocular inflammation

292. **The most serious ocular effects of malnutrition are due to the lack of:**
    a) Vitamin A
    b) Vitamin C
    c) zinc
    d) Vitamin E

293. **The ocular disorder most commonly supplemented with "eye vitamins" is:**
    a) macular degeneration
    b) cataracts
    c) glaucoma
    d) optic neuritis

294. **The *most* common ocular problem associated with smoking is:**
    a) increased risk of nuclear sclerotic cataract
    b) increased risk of macular degeneration
    c) more severe optic nerve damage in glaucoma patients
    d) chronic conjunctival irritation

295. **The occurrence of diabetic retinopathy is mainly related to:**
    a) visual acuity
    b) whether or not the patient is obese
    c) the duration of the diabetes
    d) the presence or absence of other eye disease

296. **Other ocular problems seen in diabetics include:**
    a) recurrent infections
    b) early onset of presbyopia
    c) cataracts, refractive fluctuations, and muscle palsies
    d) optic neuropathy, nystagmus, and diplopia

297. **The main cause of unilateral or bilateral exophthalmos in adults is:**
    a) pseudotumor
    b) neuroblastoma
    c) Graves' disease
    d) orbital cellulitis

298. **Rheumatic arthritis is an auto-immune disease often associated with:**
    a) extreme dry eye
    b) corneal dystrophy
    c) subconjunctival hemorrhages
    d) hypopyon

299. **The most common ocular findings in patients with human immunodeficiency virus are:**
    a) retinal scarring
    b) keratoconjunctivitis
    c) changes in retinal and conjunctival blood vessels
    d) H. zoster infection

300. **Serious visual impairment in the patient with hypertension most often occurs as the result of:**
    a) associated cataracts
    b) associated retinal scarring
    c) blood vessel damage
    d) retinal detachment

301. **The most common effect of atherosclerosis on the eye is:**
    a) artery obstruction
    b) hemorrhage
    c) traction retinal detachment
    d) formation of microaneurysms

302. **Which of the following is *not* generally associated with neurological disorders?**
    a) double vision
    b) pupil abnormality
    c) visual field defect
    d) cataract

303. **The symptoms caused by brain tumors are often related to:**
    a) increased pressure inside the head
    b) cancer spreading to the orbit
    c) cancer spreading to the uvea
    d) interruptions to ocular blood flow

304. **Symptoms of brain tumor can include:**
    a) floaters, flashes, curtain over vision
    b) decreased vision, shortness of breath, halos around lights
    c) optic nerve cupping, retinal hemorrhage, elevated intraocular pressure
    d) headache, double vision, decreased vision, nausea and vomiting

305. **Which of the following is *not* a malignant eyelid tumor?**
    a) basal cell carcinoma
    b) squamous cell carcinoma
    c) melanoma
    d) papilloma

306. **Which of the following is a congenital tumor that is generally diagnosed by age 3 years?**
    a) RP
    b) leukocoria
    c) retinoblastoma
    d) intraocular dermoid

307. **A patient presents with unilateral keratoconjunctivitis, a painful rash on one side of the face, and a history of chicken pox infection as a child. It is very likely that this patient has:**
    a) herpes simplex
    b) herpes zoster
    c) rubella
    d) contact dermatitis

Part V

Medical Terminology

308. **Match the prefix to its meaning. Some meanings have more than one answer:**
    Prefix
    a/an-
    ab-
    abo-
    aniso-
    auto-
    bio-
    blepharo-
    bruno-
    chloro-
    cyano-
    e/ex-
    en-

endo-
entero-
eso-
exo-
hyper-
hypo-
infero-
infra-
kerato-
leuko-
mal-
myo-
osteo-
pan-
para-
pseudo-
pulmo-
retro-
rubeo-
supra-
xanth-

Meaning
all
around
bad
behind
blue
bones
brown
cornea
different
eye lids
false
green
in
life
muscles
out
over
red
respiration
self
under
up
white
without
yellow

309. **Match the suffix to its meaning:**
    Suffix
    -algia
    -duct
    -itis
    -ology
    -oma
    -ometry
    -opsia/-opia
    -osis
    -tropia

    Meaning
    condition of
    deficient vision
    inflammation
    measurement
    move
    pain
    study of
    tumor
    turn

    Terms

310. **Which term refers to movement/motion?**
    a) transient
    b) stationary
    c) kinetic
    d) static

311. **Which term refers to something that is hidden, or seen only when specifically revealed?**
    a) latent
    b) patent
    c) idiopathic
    d) external

312. **What term refers to an entity that is obvious without testing?**
    a) occult
    b) clandestine
    c) obscured
    d) manifest

313. **Which term refers to a possible medical concern that a patient notices about themself?**
    a) autocratic
    b) hypochondria
    c) symptom
    d) paranoia

314. **Which term refers to a test you perform that requires no response from the patient (such as retinoscopy)?**
    a) self-limiting
    b) objective
    c) subjective
    d) catch trial

315. **Which term refers to an eye that has an intraocular lens implant?**
    a) pseudophakic
    b) aphakic
    c) pseudophoric
    d) phakic

316. **Which term refers to the hormonal system?**
    a) lymphatic
    b) sympathetic
    c) parasympathetic
    d) endocrine

317. **In order to be deemed acceptable, an abbreviation used in a patient's chart must:**
    a) be documented in your clinic's policies manual
    b) appear in a valid medical dictionary
    c) be viewed as valid by professional peers
    d) be published in a professional journal

318. **In addition to a clinic list of approved abbreviations, there should also be a:**
    a) list of banned abbreviations
    b) list of banned terms
    c) list of approved terms
    d) protocol for office memos

319. **In which of the following would it be allowable to use office-approved abbreviations?**
    a) informed consent paperwork
    b) patient discharge instructions
    c) note to a co-worker
    d) clinic privacy notice

320. **Matching, one answer:**
    <u>Abbreviation</u>
    AMD
    AT
    c̄
    COAG
    DME
    EOM
    gtt
    IOP
    NLP
    NSAID
    NTG
    OWS
    PD

PH
PI
prn
PRP
PVD
s̄
SCH
SPK
ung
W4D
YLC

Meaning
__ drops
__ ointment
__ laser procedure for diabetic retinopathy
__ method of checking eye pressure
__ with glasses on
__ without glasses on
__ disk with tiny hole(s) in it
__ anti-inflammatory drug that doesn't have steroids in it
__ patient has no vision; can't even see light
__ most common form of glaucoma
__ glaucoma that is present in a patient with normal pressures
__ pressure inside the eye
__ as needed
__ fine dots of corneal staining
__ muscle(s) responsible for eye movement
__ laser treatment to remove cloudiness of posterior capsule
__ laser treatment to help prevent angle closure
__ the distance between one pupil and another
__ thickening/swelling of the macula associated with diabetes
__ deterioration of the macula associated with aging
__ painful condition resulting from wearing contact lenses longer than recommended
__ test for binocular vision or suppression
__ bloody-looking area on the white of the eye
__ jelly inside the eye has pulled away from the retina

Safety

321. **Which of the following is *not* considered biohazardous waste?**
     a) tissue removed from xanthelasma excision
     b) used batteries
     c) used scalpel blades
     d) blood-soaked gauze from surgery

322. **Disposal of which of the following is subject to specific rules and regulations?**
    a) sterile cotton swab used to obtain material for culturing
    b) all medical waste
    c) gloves worn when instilling eye drops
    d) paper gown worn during lacrimal irrigation

323. **Contaminated sharps may be disposed of:**
    a) in puncture-proof containers
    b) with any medical waste
    c) by double-bagging in red bags
    d) by wrapping in surgical linen

324. **Someone in the clinic has accidentally dropped some test tubes that contained cultures from a patient with a possible infectious corneal ulcer. Two of the tubes broke. How should the broken glass be disposed of?**
    a) sprayed with disinfectant and placed in the trash
    b) placed in a sharps container
    c) placed in doubled biohazard bags
    d) infection control should be contacted

325. **Which of the following is pathological biohazardous waste that must be disposed of by incineration or other approved means?**
    a) freshly removed biopsy specimen
    b) enucleated eye
    c) used needles from intravitreal injections
    d) blood-dotted gauze

326. **Which of the following is considered to be "other potentially infectious material"?**
    a) vomitus
    b) extracted aqueous
    c) bloody tears
    d) blood

327. **Which of the following should be disposed of in a red biohazard bag?**
    a) used #10 blade
    b) blood-soaked gauze
    c) tissue a patient sneezed into
    d) gloves used during a routine eye exam

Study Notes

Suggested reading in *Principles and Practice in Ophthalmic Assisting: A Comprehensive Textbook*:
    Chapter 2: Ocular Anatomy (pp 11-26)
    Chapter 3: Ocular Physiology (pp 27-37)
    Chapter 10: Ocular Motility, Strabismus, and Amblyopia (*Basic Sciences*, pp 137-138)
    Chapter 23: Microbiology (pp 439-457)
    Chapter 24: Genetics (pp 459-472)
    Chapter 25: Neuro-Ophthalmology (pp 473-484)
    Chapter 26: Ocular Disorders and Conditions: External and Anterior Segment (pp 485-498)

Explanatory Answers

Part I

1. **Matching:**

adrenal glands	b)
afibrillation	a)
aorta	a)
arteriosclerosis	a)
arthritis	d)
atria	a)
biceps	d)
brain	e)
bronchi	f)
carotid	a)
CN VII	e)
colon	c)
diabetes	b)
diaphragm	f)
duodenum	c)
esophagus	c)
femur	d)
fight or flight response	e)
gall bladder	c) (also has secondary endocrine functions)
gonads (testes/ovaries)	b)
Graves' disease	b)
hormones	b)
human growth hormone	b)
insulin	b)
islets of Langerhans	b)
larynx	f)
lateral rectus	d)
liver	c) (also has secondary endocrine functions)
lymph nodes	a) (the lymph system is considered a subset of the circulatory system)
mitral valve	a)
optic nerve	e)
orbicularis oculi	d)
orbit	d)
pancreas	b)
parathyroid	b)
pharynx	f)

pituitary	b)
plasma	a)
platelets	a)
pulse	a)
spinal cord	e)
stomach	c)
thyroid	b)
trachea	f)
ulna	d)
vena cava	a)
ventricle	a)
vertebrae	d)
xiphoid	d)

2.   b) The endocrine system involves formation of hormones and releasing them to have their effects on the target organ/system.

3.   d) Certainly the digestive system involves breaking down materials so that nutrients enter the blood stream and waste material is eliminated from the body. The respiratory system sends oxygen through the blood stream and removes carbon dioxide from it. The cardiovascular system is the highway by which nutrients are made available to the body's cells.

4.   d) Eye movements originate in the nervous system (CN VI, IV, and VII). The muscles (which are anchored to the skeletal system) are stimulated by the nerves. Voilá! Motion!

5.   c) Incoming light is focused on the retina in the healthy eye. (Interpretation occurs in the occipital cortex of the brain.)

6.   d) The ocular media are the transparent structures of the eye through which light passes. Some references might not include the tear film. The term "the humors" refers to the aqueous humor and vitreous humor.

7.   b) The cornea has more refractive power than even the lens. The average crystalline lens has 15 diopters of plus power. The cornea has 40 to 44 (references vary).

8.   c) The posterior chamber is between the backside (interior) side of the iris and the front of the lens. The anterior chamber is between the interior side of the cornea and the front of the iris. The vitreous chamber is from the back of the lens to the retina. The posterior segment includes the vitreous, retina, optic nerve, and choroid.

9.   d) See Answer 8.

10.   b) *Ocular adnexa* is a term referring to the "accessories" of the eye: things that aren't a part of the eyeball itself but attach to it. The uvea is the vascular coat of the eye, including the iris, ciliary body, and choroid. Exterior segment is not a term that is in use, and ophthalmonexa is a term I made up.

11.   d) CNs are usually designated by Roman numerals or name (Table 16-1).

12.   a) The CNs that do *not* have an effect on the eye or its structures are I (olfactory), VIII (vestibulo-cochlear), IX (glossopharyngeal), X (vagus), XI (accessory), and XII (hypoglossal). One might argue for CN X, as instilling eyedrops in certain patients can cause a "vasovagal response" that includes fainting, but the reaction is stimulated by *triggers* (such as seeing blood, getting an injection, having your eyes "messed with"). CN X has lots of little fingers throughout the body, but none that go directly to the eye.

13.   c) The CNs that are responsible for the motor function of the extraocular muscles are III, IV, and VI. Remember the mnemonic "LR6 SO4 all others 3." The lateral rectus is innervated by CN VI, the superior oblique by CN IV, and the superior/medial/inferior recti and the inferior oblique are served by CN III.

14.   b) Seven bones make up the orbit: frontal, sphenoid, zygomatic, maxillary, palatine, ethmoid, and lacrimal.

TABLE 16-1

CRANIAL NERVES AFFECTING THE EYES

Name	Designation	Ocular/Vision Affect*	Action**
Optic nerve	CN II	Visual acuity, color vision, peripheral vision	Sensory
Oculomotor	CN III	Ocular alignment (MR, SR, IO, IR), opens the eye, constricts pupil, accommodation	Motor and Parasympathetic
Trochlear	CN IV	Ocular alignment (SO)	Motor
Trigeminal	CN V	Lacrimal gland, upper lid, conj (sensory)	Both (mixed)
Ophthalmic	V_1	Upper lid and palpebral conj, lacrimal gland, cornea, ciliary body, iris, forehead and scalp, sinuses *Also* pupil dilation	Sensory Motor
Maxillary	V_2	Lower lid and palpebral conj, cheek, sinuses	Sensory
Abducens	CN VI	Ocular alignment (LR)	Motor
Facial	CN VII	Closes the eye, facial expression (motor) Lacrimal gland stimulation	Both (mixed) and Sympathetic

15. c) The ethmoid bone, in the orbital floor, is porous. This makes it very fragile and prone to fracture in concussive injury to the socket. The frontal, zygomatic, and maxillary bones make up part of the orbital rim, which is thick in order to protect the globe. Some references will name the lacrimal bone as the most fragile, but that was not given as an option here.

16. a) The optic foramen (a foramen is an opening or passage through bone) of the sphenoid bone admits the optic nerve, as well as the ophthalmic artery, into the orbit. The supraorbital foramen is in the frontal bone under the brow; the supraorbital nerve (a branch of the orbital nerve [which is a branch of the trigeminal nerve]), artery, and vein enter here. The suborbital foramen is below the orbit, in the maxillary bone; the infraorbital nerve (a branch of the maxillary), artery, and vein pass through it. The lacrimal foramen is an opening in the lacrimal bone through which the lacrimal duct passes.

17. b) There are 4 groups of sinuses: frontal, maxillary, sphenoid, and ethmoid. Because of the proximity of the eye to these sinuses, pressure in the sinuses can sometimes give the sensation of pressure in the eyes.

18. b) The sphenoid bone is at the very back of the orbit. Portions of the maxillary and frontal bones make up the orbital rim. The lacrimal bone is within the orbit on the nasal side.

19. c) The Annulus of Zinn is a ring-like tendon that surrounds the optic nerve. The 4 rectus muscles all originate here.

20. c) The trochlea is a little "ring" of fibrous cartilage material that is attached to the frontal bone. The tendon of the superior oblique passes through it. You will often hear the trochlear referred to as a "pulley," but it is more like a sling. This arrangement enables the specific muscle actions unique to the SO.

---

* Note that we are only discussing a nerve's effect *on the eye*. CNs V and VII are complex and affect other parts of the head in different ways.
** "Sensory" in the case of CN II refers to vision. When referencing other nerves, the term refers variously to the sensations of pressure, touch, temperature, and pain.

21.   d) The extraocular muscles are striated muscle, like the other moveable parts of your body that are under your control. Smooth muscle is under the autonomic ("automatic") nervous system, and are not under your voluntary control, such as the iris. (The lining of the stomach and intestines is another example).

22.   d) The episclera overlies the sclera. The conjunctiva lies over the episclera. The choroid is the interior, vascular coat of the eye. Dua's layer is a "new" layer of the cornea.

23.   b) The ophthalmic artery (which has 9 branches, by the way) supplies the eye. From the heart, the aorta branches into the left and right common carotid arteries. The internal and external carotids spring from the common carotids. The ophthalmic artery comes from the internal carotid.

24.   d) The orbital fat provides cushioning and volume and helps the extraocular muscles to move smoothly. It plays no role in the growth of an infant's eye socket.

25.   c) Tenon's capsule (or sheath) is a thin membrane that encapsulates the eyeball from the nerve to the limbus. The conjunctiva does not extend to the nerve; it lines the inner lids then folds over to cover the visible sclera. The Annulus of Zinn is a fibrous ring at the back of the orbit and serves as the origin for the 4 rectus muscles. The sclera is the tough wall of the eyeball itself.

26.   d) The skin of the lids is among the thinnest in the body: about 1 mm thick. There is essentially no fat just under the surface. Because the skin is so thin, the lids are one of the first places that swell when a person is retaining water. Lids also help regulate incoming light in a rudimentary way, squinting or closing in bright, noxious light.

27.   a) The goblet cells are found in the conjunctiva, not the eyelid. The other glands (Moll producing sweat, Zeis and meibomian producing oil) are found in the eyelids. If you missed this because you thought of the bulbar conjunctiva as being part of the eyelid, that's okay! The "real" test won't be that literal.

28.   a) The orbicularis oculi muscle, innervated by CN VII, is the muscle that closes the eye. The superior tarsal is part of the opening mechanism. The superior rectus is an extraocular muscle. And, of course, there is no such thing as the blinkus superiorus, but I hope I made you smile.

29.   a) CN VI, the abducens nerve, has a motor function to activate the lateral rectus muscles, which abducts the eyeball. The CN involved in opening the eye is CN III. The levator and superior tarsal muscles, which attach to the tarsus (tarsal plate) all take part in opening the eye.

30.   c) The tarsus (or tarsal plates) are dense connective tissue in the upper and lower lids. They give the lids a measure of rigidity, contain the meibomian glands, and serve as an attachment to the levator and superior tarsal muscles. The sclera is part of the eyeball itself, the bulbar conjunctiva covers the eyeball, and the limbus is where the cornea and sclera meet.

31.   a) CN III controls movement of the orbicularis oculi muscle. CN VII innervates the levator and superior tarsal muscles.

32.   c) Epicanthal folds are "extra" folds of skin at the nasal canthus that pretty much cover the caruncle. Some children who have them, because of the wide nasal bridge found in the very young, can look as if they have esotropia. Testing, however, reveals their eyes to be in alignment. Thus the apparent strabismus is false: pseudostrabismus.

33.   b) Each set of lids has an upper and lower punctum (singular).

34.   a) The corners of the eyes are the canthi (plural; canthus is singular). There is a temporal (or lateral) canthus and a nasal (or medial) canthus. The fornix is the pocket formed where the palpebral and bulbar conjunctiva join. The fissure is the distance between the upper and lower lid margins when the eye is opening naturally. The angle is found in the anterior chamber where the iris meets the cornea.

35.   d) The opening between the upper and lower lids when the eye is opened is the fissure. You may also see this referred to as the palpebral fissure/aperture. The upper lid fold is the skin between the eyebrow and the upper lid. The inferior lid crease is below the lower lid. The term visual margin is made up.

36. b) Mucous membranes are found throughout the body. In addition to the conjunctiva, they are also found lining the mouth, nasal cavity, and various passageways and organs. They are generally smooth and moist, designed to reduce friction.

37. a) The cilia are the lashes; there is no conjunctiva involved here. The bulbar conjunctiva covers the eyeball, the palpebral the inner lids; the fornix is the pocket created where the 2 join.

38. d) The conjunctiva envelopes the globe all the way around. While the upper fornix is deep, there is no way that a soft contact lens can get behind the eye. It is not an emergency, and a patient should never use a contact lens plunger to fish around in the eye trying to find a "lost" lens.

39. c) The conjunctiva contains accessory lacrimal glands that contribute to the tear film. The bulbar conjunctiva lines the eye lids. The bulbar conjunctiva covers the sclera/episclera and extends to the limbus. The arcus senilis is a cholesterol deposit in the cornea and has nothing to do with the conjunctiva.

40. a) There are no such thing as trabecular glands. The goblet cells (found in the conjunctiva epithelial cells) secrete mucin, and the glands of Wolfring and Krause (found in the palpebral conjunctiva) secrete the watery portion of the tears (see also Answers 45 and 46).

41. c) We usually instill eye medications by gently pulling down the lower lid and placing the medication in the little "pocket" or cul-de-sac. You may also see this referred to as the lower/inferior fornix. (There is an upper fornix as well; this is usually where contact lenses get "lost.")

42. b) The plica (also called plica semilunaris, because of its somewhat half-moon shape) is a tiny fold in the bulbar conjunctiva, right in front of the caruncle. The punctum is the opening in the nasal canthus (corner of the eye next to the nose) where the tears drain off the eye. The cul-de-sac is the lower "pocket" created where the bulbar and palpebral conjunctiva blend.

43. b) There is no outlet for aqueous in the lacrimal system. The other statements are true. The cornea is part of the visual system and must be clear. The tears assist this function by supplying oxygen to the cornea, as well as lubricating the cornea's anterior surface.

44. c) The 3 layers of the tear film are mucin, water (sometimes called the aqueous layer, not to be confused with the aqueous humor), and oil (you may see this referred to as the lipid layer). The mucin directly coats the corneal epithelium, the water layer overlies the mucin, and the oil layer is on top, exposed to the environment. One reference suggests that the mucin and water combine to form a gel-like substance that forms the first layer.[1]

45. d) Surprisingly, the glands that make the watery portion of basal tear production are Wolfring and Krause. The main lacrimal gland functions in the watery reflex tearing.

46. a) The goblet cells, found in the conjunctiva, contribute mucin to the tear film. The Glands of Moll and Zeis are modified sweat glands associated with the follicles of the lashes. The meibomian glands supply an oily over-film.

47. c) The mucin layer of the tear film coats the corneal surface and fills in any uneven areas of the epithelium.

48. b) The average blink rate is 5 to 10 times per minute.

49. a) The tears are swept down and across the eye by the lids and toward the inner canthus where they collect before going through the punctum. This pool of tears at the nasal canthus is called the lacrimal lake. Reflex tears are the watery tears (secreted by the main lacrimal gland) in response to irritation or emotion. The caruncle is the little pink triangle of flesh in the nasal canthus. The plica is a little fold of bulbar conjunctiva just in front of the caruncle.

50. c) CN V, the trigeminal nerve, has 3 branches as you would expect. The ophthalmic branch further divides. One of its branches is the lacrimal nerve, which stimulates the lacrimal gland to produce reflex tearing.

51. b) During blinking, the orbicularis oris muscle squeezes the puncti and creates a negative pressure that "sucks" the tears into the puncti, down the canaliculi, and into the nasolacrimal sac. This phenomenon is known as the lacrimal pump.

52. c) The tears move off the eye via the punctum, canaliculus, nasolacrimal sac, nasolacrimal duct, and thence into the nasal cavity.

53. b) The episclera is highly vascular and as such nourishes the largely avascular sclera.

54. d) The cornea and sclera are actually composed of the same type of fibers. The sclera is opaque (and light-blocking) because it is hydrated. In contrast, the cornea must maintain a dehydrated state (accomplished by the corneal endothelium) in order to remain clear. The sclera's color may vary somewhat with age (bluish in the young and slightly yellow in older adults), as well as other factors.

55. d) The sclera meets the cornea at the limbus. The trabeculum is the meshwork located in the angle of the anterior chamber. For info on the lamina cribrosa and scleral spur, see Answers 56 and 57.

56. a) A small horn (spur) of the sclera juts into the trabecular meshwork of the angle. The ora serrata is where the retina meets the ciliary body (which lies behind the iris).

57. c) At the place where the optic nerve meets the sclera, the sclera is perforated, allowing passage of nerve and circulatory tissues. This is the lamina cribrosa. Disc is another name for the nerve head. The ora serrata is where the retina meets the ciliary body (which lies behind the iris). There is no such thing as the sieve of Orbiculum; I made that up. Sounds pretty genuine, though, doesn't it?

58. c) The average central corneal thickness is 551 to 565 μm.[2] (References vary; elsewhere in this book you will also see 540 to 560.) Did you notice the mistake in units of measurement in Answer b)? It gave millimeters, instead of micrometers.

59. c) About 2/3 of the refracting power of the eye is in the cornea. The average is 40 to 44 diopters (references vary).

60. a) Both the cornea and sclera are largely composed of collagen fibers. But those in the cornea are precisely aligned to allow transparency. Those in the sclera, however, are arranged haphazardly. Crystallins are the highly organized, structural proteins that make up the lens.[3] Neurons are nerve cells; tendons attach muscle to bone.

61. b) The highly sensitive cornea is innervated by the nasociliary branch of the first division (ophthalmic) of the trigeminal nerve (CN V). The frontal is also a branch of the ophthalmic nerve but supplies the forehead, upper lid. The maxillary is the third division of CN V and provides sensation to the lower lid, cheek, and sinuses. The optic nerve, CN II, is the nerve of vision.

62. d) The cornea is pretty much the only avascular tissue of the body. It gets oxygen and waste removal from the tear film exteriorly and the aqueous interiorly. Neovascularization is abnormal and occurs when the cornea is oxygen deficient. The lymphatic system's role is part of the immune system. The ophthalmic artery supplies much of the orbit and globe but does not directly supply the cornea.

63. b) The junction of the cornea (specifically, Descemet's membrane) and the trabecular meshwork is called Schwalbe's line. It can often be seen with gonioscopy. Schlemm's canal is in the angle, as is the scleral spur. The limbus is where the sclera meets the cornea externally.

64. b) The layers of the cornea are (from external to innermost): epithelium, Bowman's membrane, stroma, Descemet's membrane, endothelium. Some references may add Dua's layer between the stroma and Descemet's. The pigment epithelial cells are found in the retina.

65. c) The approximate thickness of the corneal tissues are: endothelium 5 μ thick, Descemet's 7 μ, stroma 490 μ, Bowman's 12 μ, and epithelium 50 μ.[2] The "mu", or μ as used in the metric system, means "micro," or 10^{-6}. You may also see μm to designate micrometers.

66. a) The cells of the epithelium can regenerate; the tissue is among the fastest-healing tissue in the body.

67. c) The corneal epithelium rests on Bowman's layer.

68. a) Of those listed, the epithelium (tissue exposed to the environment) is capable of regeneration. If only the most superficial cells are abraded, healing may occur within 24 hours. Descemet's membrane and the stroma can also regenerate to some degree, but usually form scar tissue. Bowman's membrane does not regenerate, nor does the endothelium.

69. d) The inner, endothelial layer's function is to prevent the rest of the corneal tissues from become hydrated. (You may also see the term *endothelial pump*.) This is key to corneal clarity, because if the stroma gets hydrated it becomes hazy and more opaque. The canaliculi and nasolacrimal sac are part of the lacrimal (tear) system of the eye.

70. b) The cells in the single-layer endothelium are hexagonal in shape, resembling a honeycomb.

71. d) The endothelium of the cornea is only one cell layer thick.

72. d) The endothelial cells rest on Descemet's membrane, not the stroma or Bowman's. The cornea has no nucleus.

73. d) Cataract surgery involves removal and insertion of materials through the anterior chamber. This can involve some "bumping" into the inner cornea: the nonregenerative endothelium that is responsible for corneal clarity. If this layer is already compromised (eg, by corneal dystrophy), the surgery may be deemed too risky. An endothelial cell count will help determine the health of the layer, and whether it is robust enough to withstand the rigors of the procedure.

Part II

74. b) The epithelium of the ciliary processes (part of the ciliary body) is responsible for aqueous production.

75. a) The aqueous humor is most like blood plasma (ie, the liquid of the blood without the cells). Cerumen is ear wax.

76. d) The aqueous flows out of the posterior chamber, through the pupil, into the anterior chamber, and then through the angle.

77. c) Once the aqueous reaches the angle, it flows through the trabecular meshwork, into Schlemm's canal, and is then carried away by veins in the episclera. This is called the *conventional* pathway, and about 90% of the aqueous drains this way. The other 10% leaves the eye via the *uveoscleral* pathway, where the aqueous seeps through the sclera.

78. b) Intraocular pressure results from the combination of the amount of aqueous produced over time and its ability to drain out of the eye.

79. a) Intraocular pressure varies during the day ("diurnal"). It is usually higher early in the morning and lower during the afternoon. (In monitoring glaucoma, many physicians will vary the time of day that a patient comes in for intraocular pressure checks, to get a clearer idea of how treatment is affecting the pressure.)

80. c) Since the ocular media must be clear, there cannot be any blood vessels. However, the structures still require nutrition (eg, oxygen, glucose, amino acids) in order to function. The aqueous provides the needed nutrients with a constant flow, bathing the lens and cornea. The aqueous is internal, not external, and is confined to the anterior chamber. (The retina is in the posterior segment.) The aqueous has only minimal refractive power.

81. a) Like blood, the aqueous functions to transport cells and certain chemical mediators to the anterior chamber. It also provides a vehicle for medications to reach the anterior chamber structures. Waste products are physically removed by the aqueous, not detoxified by it. While the aqueous does have refractive properties, the cornea and lens far outclass it in this area.

82. d) Just like blood, the aqueous also flushes away the waste products of metabolism (eg, carbon dioxide, lactic acid), which would be toxic to the tissues if they were to remain. If outflow is impeded then there can be increased intraocular pressure, but it would not be the purpose of the aqueous to increase intraocular pressure. The aqueous is confined to the anterior chamber, and the retina is in the posterior segment. The back of the lens is faced by the vitreous.

83. b) The muscles of the iris are the sphincter, responsible for closing the pupil, and the dilator, which opens the pupil. *Note*: Some references call the iris muscles the *circular* and *radial* muscles (the sphincter and dilator muscles, respectively).

TABLE 16-2
MOTOR INNERVATION OF THE PUPIL

CN III (oculomotor nerve) → parasympathetic fibers of long ciliary nerves = stimulation of pupillary sphincter muscle = miosis
CN V (trigeminal nerve) → ophthalmic nerve branch → nasociliary branch → sympathetic fibers of short ciliary nerves = stimulation of pupillary dilator muscle = dilation

---

84. a) The iris sphincter muscle, which makes the pupil smaller (miosis) is part of the parasympathetic system.

85. c) A sympathetic response is "fight or flight"; the dilator muscle is stimulated, and the pupil dilates.

86. b) See Table 16-2.

87. c) The collarette is the junction between the dilator (innermost) and sphincter (outermost) muscles of the iris. (In some people it may look frilly.) *Fundus* is a general anatomic term for the inside of a hollow organ; in eye care it usually means the part of the eye's interior that is visible with the ophthalmoscope. The ora serrata is the frilly-looking edge where the ciliary body meets the retina.

88. b) Melanin is the dark pigment found on the posterior iris surface. This helps prevent light from coming through the iris tissue. Visual purple is found in the photoreceptor cells of the retina. Cyanin and chlorophyll are found in plants.

89. b) The lens does not get thinner over the years. Instead, it puts down more layers and the center hardens.

90. c) The post-birth lens is basically avascular, so there are no lenticular blood vessels. The anterior capsule is part of the lens, so it is likewise avascular. The aqueous, which bathes the anterior capsule, brings oxygen and nutrients to the lens, and removes waste products. The ciliary body generates the aqueous.

91. d) The lens (technically, the lens capsule) is suspended behind the iris by fibrils called zonules. The zonules attach to the ciliary muscle.

92. b) The zonules of the lens are firmly attached to the ciliary muscle. When the muscle is relaxed, the zonules are taut and the lens is pulled a little flatter. If more "plus" is needed for clear vision (usually at near), the ciliary muscle contracts, relaxing the zonules and allowing the lens to "plump up" a little. "Orbicularis lenticuli" is a made-up term. CN II is the optic nerve; it is not a motor nerve.

93. d) Presbyopia occurs when the nucleus of the lens has hardened to the point where it can no longer change shape (ie, thicken) enough to give the necessary boost of plus power that is required to focus at near. While there is probably some reduction in the muscle tone of the ciliary muscle, that would not be the main cause of presbyopia. Sustained accommodation (as in reading a lot) does not cause presbyopia.

94. c) Lamination is the process of putting down layers, which is what happens in the lens throughout life. Syneresis (liquefaction) is usually spoken of in relation to the vitreous. In rare cases a hypermature cataract may cause the lens material to liquefy. Matriculation means you're going to college!

95. c) See Answer 92. There is no such thing as the orbicularis lenticuli.

96. a) Focusing at near requires the ciliary muscle to contract, which relaxes the zonules and allows the lens to thicken, adding plus power.* (Convergence also occurs, but this question was regarding the lens.)

97. b) Although not a true reflex (strictly speaking), the threesome of accommodation, miosis, and convergence in response to viewing a near object is known as the accommodative reflex. You may see the terms *near-vision triad* and *the near triad* in some references.

98. b) The root of the iris inserts into the ciliary body, which is continuous with the choroid. The ciliary muscle controls the shape of the crystalline lens and is not a part of the uvea proper.

99. b) The uveal tissues are highly vascular, hence another name for it is "vascular tunic."

100. a) The choroid extends from the ciliary body and lies between the sclera and the retina.

101. c) The choroid is the blood supply to the outer and middle layers of the retina, as well as the macula. The inner layer of the retina (ie, the part closest to the vitreous) is supplied by what is called the retinal circulation. (Remember in fluorescein angiography you first see the choroidal vessels fill in the choroidal flush phase. Then you see the retinal circulatory system appear.)

102. b) The vitreous adheres to the *posterior* lens capsule, as well as the macula, optic nerve, and retinal blood vessels. The other statements are true.

103. d) The vitreous, filling the largest cavity in the eye, helps maintain the shape of the eyeball. It does not regenerate. The vitreous, while avascular itself (and thus incapable of supplying nourishment to anything), receives nourishment from the retinal blood vessels and the ciliary body.

104. c) If a concussive force is applied to the eye, the vitreous acts as a shock absorber. This is also the case in forceful movements of the head.

105. b) The term for the liquefaction of the vitreous is *syneresis*. This may result in the patient noticing floaters, which are particles of proteins that can now swish around in the collapsed gel. Cyclitis is inflammation of the ciliary body. Presbyopia is the natural loss of accommodation that occurs with age.

106. a) The use of intravitreal injections (eg, anti-VEGF for macular degeneration) turns the vitreous into a drug reservoir. It is interesting to note that the vitreous in younger persons, still being a gel, may not be as good a drug reservoir as the semi-liquid, collapsed gel state of the vitreous in older persons.

107. b) The term fundus is a general anatomy word that means the inside of a curved organ, especially that part of it that is farthest from the opening. Besides the eye, other organs that have a fundus are the stomach and uterus. The posterior *chamber*, remember, is between the iris and lens.

108. d) The posterior pole is generally meant to be the area between the nerve head and the macula, so both of these features will be visible in the photo.

109. d) The retina is sandwiched between the vitreous and the choroid.

110. a) Because the film and the retina both receive incoming light impulses and use them to create an image, they are often compared.

111. c) When light hits the retina, it is converted into electric impulses that can travel along the nerve fibers to the brain. The choroid provides blood supply to the retina, not the other way around. Stereopsis is a complex function of vision, extraocular muscle alignment, and brain power. The retina's job is to convert light, not reflect it. In any case, the optic nerve has no photoreceptors, so any light that hits it falls onto a blind spot.

112. b) The macula is the area of fine, central, and color vision.

113. d) The external limiting membrane overlies the photoreceptor cell layer.

114. b) The foveola (you may see this referred to as the *foveal pit*) is in the center of the fovea, which is in the center of the macula. There is no vision at the optic nerve.

115. c) The macula normally has no blood vessels; blood vessels in this area would impede incoming light. Most of the cone cells are in the macula. See also Answer 127.

---

*For more accommodation, see Chapter 7, Questions 45 to 48; Chapter 9, Questions 4 to 7; and Chapter 17, Questions 62 to 65.

116. a) The choroid supplies the majority of the blood supply to the retina. Also contributing, to a lesser extent, is the central retinal artery.
117. a) CN II is the optic nerve (whose ganglion fibers are a specific retinal layer) is the sensory nerve associated with the retina. See Table 16-1 for information on the other CNs.
118. c) After the vitreous, light passes first through the inner limiting membrane (not listed as a possible answer) and then the nerve fiber layer. After that, it passes through the ganglion cells to the rods and cells, and then to the pigment epithelium. (There are some other layers in between.)
119. d) The axons of nerve cells are the "stem" of the nerve. In this case, the nerve fibers are coming from the optic nerve and into the retina.
120. b) Because the fibers of the RNFL are so specifically arranged, it is possible to identify the location of a lesion that is causing a visual field defect (see also Chapter 3, Questions 8 to 10).
121. a) The fibers coming from the area of the disc that is directly opposite the macula go straight across to the macula. The further away you get around the disc, the fibers arc above and below the macula and meet at the horizontal raphe (see Figure 3-1). The equator is just an imaginary line around the largest circumference of the globe. The angle is in the anterior chamber (between iris and cornea). There is no vertical raphe. (*Raphe* is a general anatomic term referring to a ridge or line where 2 halves are fused.)
122. d) The rods and cones (photoreceptor cells) do not attach directly to the NFL. They attach to the horizontal and bipolar cells, which connect to the ganglion cells, which then connect to the NFL. The remainder of the statements are true.
123. d) Rod cells are scattered throughout the retina, but not evenly. Most are about 4 to 5 mm from the macula. The fovea is in the center of the macula, where the cones are concentrated. There are no photoreceptor cells around the optic nerve.
124. a) The cones actually are outnumbered by the rods (about 1 cone for every 20 rods.) The other statements are true. *Note*: Rhodopsin is a biochemical protein (photopigment) that is sometimes referred to as *visual purple*.
125. b) Bright light causes the breakdown of rhodopsin in a process known as *bleaching*.
126. a) Full dark adaptation takes 20 to 40 (30) min, depending on how bright it was before you went into the dark. It takes that long for the rods to get enough rhodopsin, which is depleted in bright light and must be resupplied by the RPE. "Twilight vision" is vision in light dim enough to activate the rods but still light enough for the cones to be activated to some degree. (During dark adaptation, the cones turn off before the rods are fully functional.) Photomacular stress is a test of how long it takes vision to recover to normal levels after the macula is "dazzled" with a bright light.
127. c) There are 3 types of cones with *variations* of the same photosensitive pigment (photopsin). A single cone cell "specializes" in a specific wavelength, although there is some overlap. There are short (s-cones), medium (m-cones), and long-wavelength (l-cones) cones that are variously sensitive to red (short), green (medium), and blue (long) regions of the spectrum. See also Answers 140 to 142 regarding color vision.
128. b) While full dark adaptation takes about 30 minutes, light adaptation takes only about 1 minute.
129. d) The cells of the RPE have tight junctions. In this way they are able to provide a blood-retinal barrier to prevent access to the rods and cones by any toxic material. The pigments in the RPE protect the rest of the retina from harmful light frequencies that cause toxins to build up and damage the other tissues. The RPE also absorbs nutrients from the blood and provides them to the rods and cones. The RPE functions in a garbage-removal capacity as well: the rods and cones "shed," and the shed materials are engulfed by the RPE cells that recycle anything useful in the garbage and send it back to the photoreceptors. The junk that is left is digested in the RPE.
130. b) The RPE lies on Bruch's membrane, which separates the RPE from the choroid.
131. d) There are no photoreceptor cells where the optic nerve enters the eye, so it is an area of *blindness*. We don't normally notice it for several reasons, including overlapping vision between the 2 eyes, and the brain "filling in" the empty area.

TABLE 16-3
RETINAL LAYERS

Layer Name	Function
Inner limiting membrane	Basement membrane; contacts the vitreous
Nerve fiber layer	Contains axons of the ganglion cell nuclei
Ganglion cell layer	Contains nuclei of the ganglion cells
Inner plexiform layer (amacrine cells)	Contains the synapse layer between the dendrites of the ganglion cells and the bipolar cell axons
Inner nuclear layer (bipolar cells)	Contains the nuclei of the bipolar cells
Outer plexiform layer (horizontal cells)	Contains the synapse layer between the bipolar cells and the rods and cones
Outer nuclear layer (Müller cells)	Contains the cell bodies of the rods and cones
Outer/external limiting membrane	Separates the photoreceptors from their cell nuclei
Photoreceptor layer	Contains the rods and cones
Retinal pigment epithelium	Contains a single layer of pigmented epithelium; overlies the choroid

Reproduced with permission from Beck CA. Ocular anatomy. In: Ledford JK, Lens A, eds. *Principles and Practice in Ophthalmic Assisting: A Comprehensive Textbook.* SLACK Incorporated; 2018:21.

132. c) The optic disc is easily visible on fundus examination. You may also see it referred to as the *optic nerve head*. The fovea is the center of the macula; the lamina cribrosa is the portion of sclera that the retinal nerve axons pass through; the chiasm is beyond the optic nerve, in the brain.

133. b) The average size of the optic disc in an adult is 2 x 1.5 mm.

134. a) In roughly the center of the optic disc is a depression known as the physiologic cup. The disc rim is the outer edge of the nerve head. The macula is the most sensitive part of the retina. Fossa is a general anatomic term meaning a depression, usually in bone.

135. b) Estimating the cup-to-disc ratio is an important part of every fundus exam. This ratio is a comparison of the total size of the disc as compared to the size of its inner cup. This is a key factor in the diagnosis and managing of glaucoma. Axial length, if required, is measured using ultrasound. There is no call for an estimate of the disc-to-macula distance or fundus curvature.

136. b) The nerve fibers that meet at the optic nerve head are actually the axons (extensions) of the retinal ganglion cells. The rods and cones (photoreceptors) are found between the RPE and the external limiting membrane (see Table 16-3). The optic radiations are found in the brain (not the eye), as is the brain stem.

137. c) The lamina cribrosa is a perforated, sieve-like area of the sclera through which the nerve axons pass, as well as capillaries. The trabecular meshwork is in the angle of the anterior chamber (between iris and cornea). The ora serrata is where the ciliary body meets the retina. The limbus is where the sclera meets the cornea.

138. c) After the optic nerve, light impulses traverse the chiasm, optic tract, lateral geniculate body, and occipital cortex in that order. The brain stem, cerebral cortex, and cerebellum do not receive light impulses.

139. d) Genetics plays a role, too.
140. c) There are short (s-cones), medium (m-cones), and long-wavelength (l-cones) cones that are variously sensitive to red (short), green (medium), and blue (long) regions of the spectrum. They are not differentiated by shape or color. There are no cones in the retinal periphery.
141. b) There are normally 3 different types of cone cells (see also Answer 140). It is reported that some women have 4.[4]
142. d) If you remembered that the human retina has 3 types of cones, you probably guessed correctly (if you had to guess) that this gave rise to the trichromatic theory of color vision. The other answers are all made up. (Some references assert that some of us have more than 3, but that is not the norm.)
143. d) If all of the 3 types of cones are equally stimulated, then you will perceive the color as white.

Part III

144. b) An infection is always caused by invasion of tissues by microorganisms (including bacteria, fungi, and viruses). Trauma in and of itself does not *cause* an infection, although it might predispose to one.
145. d) All of the answers could have associated inflammation. Inflammation occurs when there is a threat to tissues, whatever the cause. That cause does not have to be infectious, although infections cause inflammation.
146. c) The hallmarks of inflammation are swelling, redness, pain, and heat/fever. You may read these in the classic Latin: *tumor, rubor, dolor,* and *calor,* respectively. Some references also include loss of function.
147. c) Any time you see the suffix -itis, inflammation is implicated. The papillomacular bundle is a group of nerve fibers running from the disc to the macula, there is no "bundling" phenomenon. A papilloma is a skin lesion usually on the lids. A papilla is any small, elevated area of tissue. Papillitis, however, is an inflammation of the optic disc.
148. **a) cranial nerves II, III, IV, V, VI, VII**
afferent or efferent pupillary defect (CN II)
Bell's palsy (CN VII)
corneal or facial numbness (CN V)
ptosis (CN III)
strabismus (CN III, IV, VII)
tonic pupil (CN II)
b) orbit
blow-out fracture
cellulitis
c) extraocular muscles
Brown syndrome
Duane's syndrome
myasthenia gravis
strabismus (see Chapter 7: Ocular Motility Testing)
d) globe
anophthalmos
buphthalmos
exophthalmos
microphthalmia
sympathetic ophthalmia

e) lids
blepharitis
blepharospasm
cellulitis
chalazion
coloboma
dermatochalasis
entropion/ectropion
lagophthalmos
meibomian gland deficiency/disease
molluscum contagiosum
ptosis
sty
trichiasis
xanthelasma
f) lacrimal
canaliculitis
dacryocystitis
duct obstruction
epiphora
prolapsed lacrimal gland

149.　**a) conjunctiva**
ophthalmia neonatorum
pinguecula
prolapsed lacrimal gland
trachoma
b) sclera/episclera
episcleritis
scleritis
subconjunctival hemorrhage
c) cornea
arcus senilis
buphthalmos
dry eye syndrome
erosion
Fuchs' dystrophy
keratitis
Krukenberg's spindle
pannus
pterygium
synechea (anterior)
ulcer
d) anterior chamber/angle/aqueous
angle closure
cells/flare
hyphema
hypopyon
narrow angle

e) iris and ciliary body
albinism
aniridia
coloboma
cyclitis
exfoliation
heterochromia
iritis
prolapse
synechea (anterior/posterior)
f) pupil
anisocoria
Marcus Gunn
g) lens
cataract
Mittendorf's dot
subluxation
synechea (posterior)

150. **a) uvea**
prolapse
uveitis (anterior/posterior)
b) vitreous
asteroid hyalosis
detachment
floaters/scoots
hemorrhage
prolapse
c) retina (*not* including macular or optic nerve)
albinism
coloboma
color vision deficiencies
cotton wool spots
degenerations
detachment
diabetic retinopathy
drusen
hypertensive retinopathy
presumed ocular histoplasmosis syndrome
RP
retinoblastoma
retinopathy of prematurity
tears/holes
toxoplasmosis
vascular occlusion
d) macula
age-related degeneration
central serous chorioretinopathy
epiretinal membrane
macular hole

e) optic nerve (CN II)
coloboma
cupping
drusen
glaucoma
papilledema
papillitis (inflammation of disc)
f) visual pathway (*not* including retina or optic nerve)
pituitary tumor
quadrantanopsia visual field defect
traumatic brain injury

151. c) Nystagmus is a neurological disorder that causes repeated, involuntary jerking of the eyes. The movement may be horizontal, vertical, or in a circular/pendular motion. Saccades are the normal, rapid "following" movements the eyes make, for example when riding by a line of fence posts. Strabismus is misalignment of the eyes. There is no "CN II palsy."

152. a) The second cranial nerve is the optic nerve. Its function is vision (sensory), not movement. CN III innervates the inferior obliques and recti, as well as the superior recti. CN IV controls the superior obliques and CN VI the lateral recti.

153. d) Orbital cellulitis in an inflammation involving the tissues around the eye. It is usually associated with infection of the sinuses.[5] Sepsis (a potentially lethal condition where infection is in the blood stream) and meningitis (inflammation of the sheath that surrounds nerves and the brain, also may be deadly) can result. Even more tragic, this type of cellulitis is most common in children.[5] Preorbital cellulitis has not advanced into the orbital tissues. Molluscum contagiosum is a skin/lid disorder. A corneal abrasion is not considered life-threatening.

154. d) Officially called the Von Graefe sign, this phenomenon is also known simply as lid lag. It can be a sign that the patient has Graves' disease. Other symptoms/signs of Graves' disease are exophthalmos, lid swelling, and double vision. Sarah's palsy is something I made up.

155. b) The terms exophthalmos and proptosis are pretty much interchangeable. However, the term *proptosis* can be used to indicate any body part that is bulging abnormally. *Exophthalmos* refers specifically to the eye.

156. **Matching:**

blepharitis	lid infection
blepharospasm	lid twitch
cellulitis	infected, inflamed tissues of lid/orbit
chalazion	blocked meibomian gland
dermatochalasis	sagging skin of upper lid
ectropion	out-turned eyelid
entropion	in-turned eyelid
hordeolum	infected hair follicle
lagophthalmos	incomplete lid closure
ptosis	drooped eyelid
trichiasis	inward-growing eyelash
xanthelasma	yellow lipid skin deposit

157. c) Anywhere from 6% to 20% of newborns show some symptoms of NLD obstruction, which occurs when the membrane across the NLD opening fails to disappear by birth.[6]

158. d) Because tears can't flow through the lacrimal drainage system, the tears flow down the face. Also, stasis of the system is a prime situation for infection to set up, accompanied by mattering, redness, and swelling. Eye movement is not an issue.

159. c) Most cases of NLD obstruction in an infant will resolve on its own by age one. However, many practitioners advocate massaging the NLD area, as well as use of an antibiotic drop to treat any infection. If not cleared by age 1, or if the situation warrants, the obstruction can be opened manually by inserting a probe into the canaliculus and pushing through the offending membrane. In some cases a stent might be placed to hold the canaliculus open.

160. c) *Dacry-* tears, *cyst-* sac, *-itis* infection = dacryocystitis. Infection of the canaliculus would be canaliculitis. Blepharitis is an infection of the lids, and a chalazion is an infected lid gland.

161. a) The proper term for excessive tearing is epiphora. Trichiasis is an errant eyelash; entropion is an in-turned lid. I made up the term contralacrimation.

162. d) The most common cause of halos around lights is cataracts. Corneal edema can do it, too. The other symptoms are all associated with dry eye.

163. d) Having a humidifier in the bedroom would add moisture to the environment, exactly what's needed for dry eye. The other scenarios are associated with contributing to dry eye.

164. d) The meibomian glands make the oil layer of the tear film. They can get plugged, in which case the oil is not there to help prevent tear evaporation. In addition, if the glands aren't free-flowing, infection can set up and cause chalazia.

165. c) See Answer 164.

166. c) The purpose of plugging or permanently sealing the puncti is to keep what tears that are produced on the eye. It does not cause the eye to make more tears.

167. b) Tear osmolality is a test that indicates the salt content of tears. The lower the amount of tears, the higher the salt content. Meibography is a photographic technique to evaluate the meibomian glands in real time.

168. c) Meibomian gland dysfunction removes the oily part of the tear film, leaving the watery component exposed to the environment. Evaporation occurs and the eye becomes dry.

169. a) A pinguecula is a small, noncancerous growth on the conjunctiva. A pterygium is a fibrous growth that extends onto the cornea. A nevus (benign) and melanoma (malignant) are both pigmented.

170. c) Antibiotics are for bacterial infections. Fungal, viral, and allergic conjunctivitis would each be treated with other, appropriate medications. An antibiotic might be added to this later if a secondary bacterial infection sets up.

171. d) *Kerato-* cornea, *conjunctiv-* conjunctiva, *-itis* inflammation/infection = keratoconjunctivitis. Epidemic conjunctivitis is a very contagious viral infection but does not indicate that the cornea is involved. Keratoconus is where the cornea becomes cone-shaped and is not an infection. Episcleritis means an inflammation of the episclera.

172. b) GPC, the cause of such lesions, is thought to be an allergic reaction to deposits on contact lenses (opinions vary).

173. d) An SCH is like a bruise anywhere else on the body, but instead of looking black and blue because it's under the skin, it looks a startling blood-red against the white sclera. The patient often finds out it's there when someone else mentions it. Patients taking blood thinners (including aspirin) are more prone to get them.

174. a) SCH is not generally associated with any kind of infection. Any of the other factors listed can cause an SCH.

175. c) When the liver is not filtering the blood properly, urea can build up causing a yellow tint to the sclera, mucosa, and skin. Hope the lemonade answer made you smile!

176. d) If the collagen of the sclera degenerates, it becomes more transparent and the underlying dark, choroid shows through a little, giving the sclera a blue tinge. This might be associated with collagen disorders as seen in osteogenesis imperfecta and Marfan's syndrome.

177. a) The episclera lies between the conjunctiva and the sclera. If it is inflamed, there may be some redness and discomfort, as well as a raised area under the bulbar conjunctiva.

178. c) Actually, women are more prone to developing scleritis, which often accompanies autoimmune diseases (notably RA, lupus, inflammatory bowel disease, and Sjögren's syndrome). The pain can be severe, worsening when the eye is moved. Worst case scenario, it can cause necrosis (death) of the tissues and blindness.

179. d) Precipitates are inflammatory cells that clump and stick to the innermost surface of the corneal endothelium. They look yellowish-white, roundish, and pearly (they are sometimes called mutton-fat deposits) and may become darker with time. Corneal edema, causing the cornea to appear cloudy, is not usually a find in iritis. Punctate keratopathy and corneal ulcer are external, and not specific to iritis.

180. c) Corneal neovascularization in the superior limbal area (under the upper lid) is most often associated with contact lens wear. It is an indication that the cornea is not getting enough oxygen.

181. b) Anterior basement membrane dystrophy has the appearance of lines (like fingerprints or the outline of a map) and dots. Keratitis and corneal abrasions are external, Fuchs' dystrophy occurs in Descemet's and the endothelium.

182. c) Krukenberg's spindle is actually pigment, usually associated with pigment dispersion syndrome. Since the pigment can also block the trabecular meshwork, this finding is an alert that the patient has a higher risk for developing glaucoma.

183. d) See Answer 182.

184. c) One of the first symptoms of Fuchs' dystrophy is blurred vision in the *morning*, not the evening. Descemet's membrane gets thicker, and the endothelial cells are damaged and distorted. This affects their ability to "pump" fluid out of the cornea, so the cornea becomes edematous. Eventually the edema causes blurry vision. If the endothelium is severely damaged, this becomes a risk factor in the successful outcome of cataract surgery.

185. c) When the cornea bulges out far enough to bow the lower lid margin in downgaze, it is known as *Munson's sign*: a sign of keratoconus.

186. b) Topical steroids are not used to treat keratoconus. Corneal cross-linking serves to strengthen the corneal collagen using Vitamin B and UV light. Intracorneal rings are tiny arcs of plastic that are implanted into the corneal tissue. They cause the periphery of the cornea to steepen and the center to flatten. Corneal transplant replaces the cone with donor tissue from a normal eye.

187. a) Bell's palsy is also known as facial palsy and is a paralysis of CN VIII. This means (in the scenario given) that the left upper lid may not close completely, leaving the cornea exposed. Without the blink, the tears don't get swabbed over the eye and dryness occurs. In some cases, the patient may have to tape the eye shut. A tic is an involuntary twitch.

188. b) Over-wear syndrome (OWS) occurs when contacts are worn past the point that the eye can tolerate. Some patients may have problems after just a few hours of over-wear; others may not run into trouble until a few days.

189. d) The white, creamy ring (or arc, if not 360 degrees) is a lipid deposit. In older adults, it is not a significant finding. In younger persons (age 45 or younger) it can be associated with high cholesterol.[7]

190. d) I have never, in all my years of practice, seen an infantile pterygium, but they can occur. They are, however, very rare. The remainder of the statements are true.

191. c) If the epithelium migrates into a space under the flap, it will grow and invade the space. A viral dendrite is on the corneal surface, a pinguecula on the conjunctiva. Stromal rejection can occur in keratoplasty, not LASIK.

192. c) White blood cells react to inflammation and infection. If enough of these collect in the anterior chamber, gravity may pull them into a puddle at the bottom of the chamber. It is then visible as white material. Hyphema is blood in the anterior chamber; arcus senilis is on the outside of the cornea at the limbus; pigment dispersion is seen on the back of the cornea.

193. b) The cells (minute round particles) are actually white blood cells, and the flare (looks like dust) are clumps of protein. Both are common when there is inflammation present in the eye, as in the case of uveitis. Floaters are in the vitreous, lashes are external, and you can't objectively see the patient's flashes.

194. d) The aqueous actually circulates inside the anterior chamber, but unless there are cells/flare in the aqueous you can't see it. The iris gives off heat, so some of the circulation is like a convection current. There is also the natural flow of aqueous from the posterior chamber to the anterior, through the pupil.

195. a) When inflamed, there can be pain when the iris moves. Dilating the pupil keeps the iris immobile and prevents spasms, rather like putting a splint on a sprained wrist. This decreases pain and aids in healing. It also helps prevent formation of senechia (adhesions between the iris and cornea or lens).

196. a) The iris is most anterior part of the uvea; another name for iritis is anterior uveitis. Posterior uveitis would be inflammation of the choroid, the most posterior part of the uvea. Panuveitis (*pan-* meaning *all*) means all layers of the uvea are involved. *Shipyard eye* is an old term for epidemic keratoconjunctivitis.

197. b) When the circle of the iris does not completely fuse (and this usually occurs in the inferior segment of the iris), there is a gap or coloboma. Thus the pupil looks key-hole shaped.

198. d) The hallmark of albinism is lack of pigment, so their iris will be very pale. The lack of pigment also predisposes the albino to sensitivity to light.

199. a) The aqueous is made by the ciliary body, so it is implicated in glaucoma in cases where there is an excessive amount of aqueous present. The other structures mentioned are not implicated.

200. c) If the iris bunches up into the angle (perhaps because the iris has contact with the crystalline lens at the margin of the pupil), this can close off the aqueous' access to the trabecular meshwork. Intraocular pressure can build up quickly, resulting in an angle closure glaucoma attack.

201. **Matching:**

congenital	lens opacity present at birth
cortical	opacity between the epithelium and nucleus
hypermature	whitish cataract with breakdown of the cortex
incipient	early; just beginning
nuclear sclerotic	opacity in the hardened center of the crystalline lens
posterior subcapsular	opacity in the membrane behind the crystalline lens

202. c) Inflammation of the uvea (uveitis) is usually accompanied by pain, redness, and light sensitivity, as well as decreased/blurry vision.

203. c) Iritis (inflammation of the iris) is also called anterior uveitis, because the iris is the anterior portion of the uvea (iris, ciliary body, choroid).

204. b) The prefix *pan-* means "affecting everything" (as in pandemic). So panuveitis means that all parts of the uvea are inflamed.

205. b) A melanoma of the choroid is the most common type of intraocular cancer in adults and can occur anyplace in the uvea.[8] A choroidal nevus is a harmless "freckle," although these are periodically monitored for changes. Neurofibroma are tumors associated with neurofibromatosis (a genetic neurological disorder) and are not usually malignant. Retinoblastoma is usually found in the young.

206. d) Lung and breast cancers are the most common types of cancer that spread to the choroid.[9]

207. d) Asteroid hyalosis is the presence of tiny deposits of calcium and phospholipids (fatty acids with phosphates) in the vitreous. The patient usually has no symptoms, but when you look inside the eye it resembles a snow globe. An aura is a visual disturbance, often associated with ocular migraine. A TIA is considered to be a "prestroke." Amaurosis fugax (a temporary loss of vision, usually associated with impeded blood flow to the retina) is a symptom of TIA.

208. d) A posterior vitreous detachment (PVD) is often associated with floaters (clumps of cells and protein in the vitreous that cast a shadow on the retina and appear in the patient's vision) and flashes (caused when the detaching vitreous tugs on the retina).

209. a) The symptoms of a PVD and retinal detachment can be the same (ie, floaters and flashes).

210. c) The Amsler grid might be called a "checkerboard" by some patients, referring to the squares. It is commonly used as a home-screening device for patients with macular degeneration.

211. b) The wet form of AMD is, fortunately, the more rare kind. With the advent of anti-VEGF intra-ocular injections, treatment is possible. It is the second leading cause of blindness in developed countries, and the most common cause of blindness in the United States in those over 65 years of age.

212. b) Because AMD affects the central vision, distortion may be one of the first symptoms. A gritty sensation is a symptom of ocular surface problems. Tunnel vision is not seen in macular degeneration; it's the central vision that is lost. Floaters are in the vitreous, unrelated to AMD.

213. a) The classic cherry red spot is associated with central retinal artery occlusion.

214. c) In wet AMD, the formation of subretinal fluid may cause swelling of the macula and macular scarring. The choroid may develop neovascularization: weak, abnormal blood vessels that can leak and hemorrhage. Macular hole is not necessarily associated with AMD.

215. d) ERM is most commonly seen in older adults. The remaining statements are true.

216. b) In RP, there is a degeneration and loss of photoreceptors in the retina. See Answer 217.

217. b) RP is usually diagnosed in the teen and early adult years; onset varies from person to person. It usually starts with loss of the rod cells and worsens with time. The patient is usually blind by age 40. It is a genetic disorder.

218. b) There is currently no treatment for RP. Vision aids such as telescopes, magnifiers, and special lighting may be helpful.

219. a) Cardiac arrest is not associated with the presence of retinopathy of prematurity. However, there have been cases where premature infants went into cardiac arrest after being dilated for the fundus exam. The other factors are definitely associated with retinopathy of prematurity.

220. c) Because the child is born before development is complete, a release of vascular growth factors occurs. This can cause the periphery of the retina, where there are not yet blood vessels, to be triggered into forming trying to form blood vessels. Unfortunately, these new blood vessels are weak and can leak. The abnormal blood vessels can also pull on the retina, possibly causing a detachment.

221. d) Advances in medicine have worked toward the survival of younger and younger preemies. This increase has been coupled with a rise in the incidence of ROP.

222. d) When the retina detaches, the tissue become oxygen deprived due to being separated from its blood supply. If the macula is still attached, the patient should retain central vision. The vitreous is not destroyed, nor is the optic nerve. But light signals won't be getting through in the area where the detachment is.

223. c) The most common type of retinal detachment occurs when fluid seeps through a tear in the retina, distancing the retinal tissue from its blood supply. This is known as a rhegmatogenous detachment.

224. d) Other factors include age, poorly controlled diabetes, retinal detachment in the fellow eye, and even heredity. But not cataracts.

225. c) Tractional detachment occurs when scar tissue (as may be seen in diabetic retinopathy) pulls the retinal off. A macular pucker will cause distorted vision. Macular degeneration is not generally associated with flashes and floaters, nor is iritis (which is painful).

226. b) In a case where detaching vitreous remains attached at the macula, the vitreous puts traction on the macula. A macular hole may result. Hypertensive changes are due to high blood pressure. The retina does not get ulcers, and this scenario is not associated with glaucoma.

227. b) Any time you hear the word *stroke*, the association is that blood is not getting to some part of the body (usually the brain). This can be caused by anything that reduces or blocks the blood supply: a hemorrhage, a clot, or thinning of the blood vessels. A "stroke in the eye" usually refers to an occlusive event.

228. d) An obstruction in a branch artery or vein will often cause a loss of peripheral vision, where a central occlusion generally affects both central as well as peripheral vision loss. Acute angle closure is painful, and vision loss with cataracts is generally gradual.

229. d) All 4 entities can cause sudden, painless loss of vision and constitute an emergency. But the central retinal artery occlusion (which affects the entire blood supply to the retina) is the most dire, as the treatment window is the first 2 to 4 hours after onset.

230. c) The classic fundus finding in a central retinal artery occlusion is a bright-red spot at the macula. The rest of the retina is pale, making the macula stand out. In addition, the retina is thinnest at the macula, and the red blood vessels of the choroid "shine" through.

231. c) Vein occlusions affect the *drainage* of blood *from* the retina, not the supply to it.

232. b) Intraocular pressure results from the combination of the amount of aqueous produced over time and its ability to drain out of the eye.

233. c) While slight, the aqueous *does* exert a refractive influence on light entering the eye. Answer a) refers to the diurnal curve of intraocular pressure, where intraocular pressure tends to be higher in the morning than in the evening. (In monitoring glaucoma, many physicians will vary the time of day that a patient comes in for intraocular pressure checks, to get a clearer idea of how treatment is affecting the pressure.) The intraocular pressure is slightly higher in the posterior chamber because the aqueous meets some resistance as it encounters the margin of the pupil. The circulating aqueous also acts to bring nutrients to and remove wastes from the eye's internal structures.

234. b) There normally is a small depression, known as the physiologic cup, where the optic nerve enters the eye through the sclera, and through which the optic fibers pass.

235. c) In glaucoma, the pressure is transferred to the back of the eye where it can "excavate" the optic nerve. This causes the cup to be enlarged and caved-in, known as *cupping*. The blood vessels may dip over the cup's edge, but this in itself is not referred to as cupping.

236. b) The cup-to-disc ratio compares the size of the outer nerve rim to the size of the cup. (Like comparing the size of the donut to the size of the donut hole.)

237. b) A large cup would be 0.9. In this case, 90% of the disc has been cupped out.

238. d) The normal disc is slightly oval in the horizontal direction. A cup that is vertical is very suspicious of glaucoma.

239. a) Because of the pattern of nerve fibers, optic nerve fiber damage is correlated to specific patterns of loss on the visual field.

240. d) In order to lower the intraocular pressure (theoretically, at least), decrease the amount of aqueous being produced and/or increase the draining of it.

241. d) The classic hallmarks of glaucoma are increased intraocular pressure, loss of peripheral vision, and damage to the optic nerve head.

242. a) A normal cup might withstand elevated pressures for years without field loss. Conversely, some eyes (especially if nerve damage has already occurred) experience further damage even if the intraocular pressure is in the normal range. (Once damage has occurred, it seems to take much less pressure to cause further damage. Thus, in the presence of a large c/d, some patients will experience field loss even with low intraocular pressures.)

243. c) Retinoscopy is used to evaluate refractive errors, not glaucoma. Corneal thickness (as measured with pachymetry), evaluation of the angle (as seen with a gonio lens), and visual field testing (perimetry) are all pieces of the diagnostic puzzle that is glaucoma. Patients with a central corneal thickness of 555 μm or less have a 3 times *greater* chance of developing open-angle glaucoma.[10]

244. a) Gonioscopy uses a goniolens (a contact lens utilizing several mirrors) and a slit lamp to view the angle structures.

245. d) Unfortunately, vision lost due to glaucoma is not recoverable even once the condition is controlled or treated.

246. b) The diurnal curve of the intraocular pressure in a patient with glaucoma may vary up to 10 mm, being higher in the morning. The average (nonglaucomatous) eye varies only by about 4 mm. Thus, this larger fluctuation is a factor in both diagnosis and treatment of glaucoma. See also Answer 233.

247. c) Open-angle glaucoma is the most common type of glaucoma. (Depending on your source there are over 40 different types of glaucoma.)

248. a) The incidence of open angle glaucoma rises with age, especially after age 60. For Blacks the risk begins rising at age 40. Answers b) through d) *do* indicate an increased risk.

249. b) Open-angle glaucoma cannot be cured; it can only be controlled. (In this respect, it resembles diabetes and high blood pressure.) Answers a), c), and d) are true.

250. c) Because open-angle glaucoma has no physical symptoms, the patient is not driven to seek care. The loss of peripheral vision occurs over a long period of time, often escaping the patient's notice. (Signs are perceptible to the examiner, such as optic disc cupping or an elevated intraocular pressure reading.)

251. d) As its name implies, the angle structure in open-angle glaucoma is open. Generally, it looks normal.

252. d) A patient with open-angle glaucoma needs an annual full exam including dilation, gonioscopy, and formal visual fields testing. Of course, they also need periodic intraocular pressure checks during the year. The air-puff tonometer is not accurate enough to monitor glaucoma. Likewise, confrontation fields are not sensitive enough to monitor for field loss in glaucoma. Generally, it is safe to dilate a patient with open-angle glaucoma.

253. a) In advanced open-angle glaucoma, often the patient retains a small temporal island of vision. Eventually that is lost as well.

254. d) A patient with glaucoma who misses a pressure check undoubtedly should be contacted to reschedule. The importance of the exam and the gravity of the disease should be stated. Answers a) and c) border on neglect. Answer b) is a breach of patient confidentiality.

255. d) Steroids do not cause a rise in intraocular pressure in every patient, but if a patient does experience an intraocular pressure increase while on steroids this is known as steroid responder.

256. d) The infant with photophobia, blepharospasm, and epiphora should be seen and evaluated for glaucoma. The manifestations of isolated congenital glaucoma are usually present at birth but may become evident during the child's first 2 years.

257. b) The key in the definition of ocular hypertension is that no nerve or visual field damage has occurred at all, *not* where it has remained stable.

258. a) The patient with ocular hypertension is often labeled a "glaucoma suspect." The Ocular Hypertension Treatment Study found that over a 5-year period, 9.5% of their glaucoma suspect study subjects who were *not* treated with intraocular pressure–lowering medications developed glaucoma.[11] (Only 4.4% of the treated suspects developed glaucoma.)

259. d) An attack of angle-closure glaucoma can include signs and symptoms as follows: redness, hazy cornea, mid-dilated pupil (not miotic), pain, vomiting, nausea, headache, eye ache, halos around lights, and decreased vision.

260. c) A subconjunctival hemorrhage is red, but not painful.

261. a) When ACG occurs, the iris is pushing against the lens and angle. Aqueous production continues, but the fluid is not drained out, causing a rise in intraocular pressure. If the pupil were miotic, as suggested in Answer c), the iris would be pulled *away* from the angle, increasing drainage.

262. a) The pupil in ACG is mid-dilated. Miotics are used in an effort to constrict the pupil and pull the iris out of the angle. Mydriatics would keep the pupil dilated. Antibiotics would have no effect, nor

would corticosteroids. (Steroids can elevate the pressure when used for a period of time.)

263. c) Answers a), b), and d) all act to dilate the pupil, creating a potential for the iris to block the angle. A sudden bright light would cause the pupil to constrict.

264. a) The eye of a person with high hyperopia is short, meaning there is not much room for the angle. This increases the chances of iris obstruction. It is also the reason that we check angle depth prior to dilation, to make sure the angle is not going to occlude during mydriasis or cycloplegia.

265. b) Corneal edema has a prismatic effect, breaking light into its component colors, and thus creating halos around lights. Pressure build-up during an attack causes a breakdown in the pumping function of the corneal endothelium, and edema results.

266. a) Optic nerve pallor is not a disease itself; rather, it is a sign that there is a problem somewhere in the ganglion cells and axons of the retinal ganglion cells. It may be associated with inflammation, elevated intracranial pressure, genetic disorders, trauma, inadequate blood supply, toxins, and other entities. It can extend along the visual pathway from nerve to chiasm to tracts and the lateral geniculate body, but not beyond (ie, to the optic radiations or visual cortex).

267. a) When you see a pale nerve, you can expect decreased vision and probably an afferent pupillary defect as well. Visual field defects may also occur.

268. b) Strictly speaking, the term *papilledema* is reserved for optic nerve swelling caused by increased intracranial pressure. This may be caused by tumor, trauma, or anything that can result in an increase in the amount of cerebrospinal fluid or a decrease in its absorption. A papilloma is a benign growth that usually appears on the skin or mucosa.

269. c) Oddly enough, papilledema is not accompanied by eye pain or redness.

270. b) In physiologic cupping, the cup-to-disc ratio is higher than normal but there is no sign of glaucoma. Intraocular pressure, visual fields, and other associated factors are normal. In a case such as this, the cupping is considered normal for this person.

271. d) Optic neuritis is inflammation of the optic nerve. It can damage the retinal nerve fibers. In addition, the myelin sheath (a fat + protein covering over the nerve fibers) can also be at risk. I made up Jacob's retinopathy. Graves disease is an autoimmune disorder that causes inflammation in the tissues and muscles around the eye. Uveitis is inflammation of the uvea (iris, ciliary body, and choroid).

272. a) Optic neuritis is usually associated with some type of autoimmune disease, especially multiple sclerosis. In fact, it may be the first sign that a person has the disease.

273. c) In optic neuritis, there is vision loss. It may become noticeable in a period of hours and decrease over time (1 to 2 weeks). The patient may notice that: vision seems gray, distorted, or washed out; there is a loss of contrast; and colors may not be as vivid. There is eye pain which may increase when the eye is moved. (Interestingly, pain may also increase with heat or exercise.) A scintillating aura is associated with ocular migraine.

Part IV

274. d) Protanomaly is a deficiency in the "red" or l-cones, so this person would have difficulty to distinguish red.* This can be a factor in some professions, especially where one must distinguish between red and green signal lights. The suffix *-omaly* denotes a deficiency; *-opia* (or *-opsia*) means a complete lack. Thus protanopia and tritanopia are a complete lack of functioning "green" or m-cones and "blue" or s-cones, respectively. Monochromatism is a rare situation in which only one type of cone is functioning.

---

* See Questions 113 to 115 and 118 in this chapter, regarding the anatomy of rods and cones. See Questions 139 to 143 in this chapter, regarding the physiology of color vision.

275. a) Deuteranomoly (so-called "red/green color blindness") is the most common type of genetic color vision deficiency, affecting some 6% to 10% of males (references vary). Rod monochromatism (ie, no functioning cones) and blue cone monochromatism (ie, *only* the "blue" cones are functioning) are extremely rare. Protanopia means that *none* of the "green" cones are functioning, occurring in about 1% of the male population.[12]

276. c) The most common type of color vision deficiency is not acquired but genetic, linked to the X chromosome. Acquired means that the deficiency is due to nongenetic causes, such as age or medication. The other statements are true. The term "color blindness" is a misnomer, since most people with deficiencies *can* see colors, just not in full spectrum.

277. c) When a medication is causing a color vision defect, there is a chance that color vision will improve once the drug is stopped. Answers a) and b) represent a condition present at birth and will not improve.

278. c) Sympathetic ophthalmia occurs in the noninsulted eye following trauma (or sometimes surgery) of the other eye. It is a bilateral uveitis and may occur 10 days to years after the original injury (though most cases occur within 1 year). Blindness in both eyes can occur in months (or sometimes years) if the disorder is allowed to progress untreated. Once the scenario has begun, enucleating the insulted eye will not stop the disorder's progression in the fellow eye; this is why a severely damaged eye is enucleated within 10 days of the injury.

279. c) Snow blindness occurs when the UV rays of the sun are reflected into unprotected eyes. The result is a "sunburn" of the cornea, a very painful condition where the corneal epithelium is scorched. The same thing can happen when sun is reflected off sand or water.

280. b) The sclera is thinnest at the points where the lateral and medial rectus muscles attach. These attachment sites are near the limbus, ie, at the front of the eye. This makes blunt trauma the injury most likely to cause a globe rupture.

281. d) If you break down the word *lachrymatory*, it means causing lacrimation, or tearing. The chemical reaction on the eye causes excessive irritation to the conjunctiva and other exposed tissues. This causes pain, tearing, and at least temporary incapacitation.

282. b) A first-degree burn is superficial and marked by redness. Blistering indicates a second-degree burn, which has gone just beyond the surface. In third-degree burns, deeper tissues are affected. Fourth degree involves muscle and bone.

283. d) A concussive blow to the orbit, as may be seen after an air bag to the face, can fracture the paper-thin bones in the floor of the orbit. This is called a blow-out fracture. If any of the extraocular muscles herniated through the opening, then diplopia can result.

284. c) Recurrent erosion syndrome (also called recurrent corneal erosion) occurs when the corneal epithelium is stripped off the site of a previous wound. The usual scenario is that the patient wakes up in the middle of the night and feels like there's something in the eye. What probably happens is that the eye dries a little during sleep, and the epithelium adheres to the back of the lid. When the eye opens, the epithelium is stripped off, causing a foreign body sensation. For some reason, the epithelium that grew back after the original injury does not adhere to the underlying layer properly, predisposing it to being torn away. This can happen years after the original injury.

285. a) If a hyphema fills up the entire anterior chamber, the area behind the cornea can look completely black. That's why another name for this is *8-ball hyphema*. Hypopyon is pus in the anterior chamber. An SCH is just under the conjunctiva. A corneal ulcer would be on the surface and does not look black.

286. c) A metallic foreign body can rust directly on the eye and cause a rust "stain" to leach into the corneal tissue. The rust must then be removed with a drill. A foreign body per se does not cause elevated intraocular pressure.

287. b) If a foreign body perforates the eye, then uveal tissue may prolapse through the opening. The uveal tissue contains melanin, so the exposed material looks dark brown or black. If you suspect that there is any chance of a perforated globe, do not apply pressure or instill anything into the eye. Put a shield over the eye and alert the practitioner at once. The longer the uveal tissue is exposed to the environment, the poorer the prognosis.

288. b) Any sport where there are small projectiles ejected at a high velocity (paintball, BB gun, air rifle) has a high risk of eye injury. The list, in decreasing risk, is fencing, golf, then swimming.

289. b) The exam findings so far can be seen in cases of shaken baby syndrome. The most telling evidence, however, will be inside the eye: retinal hemorrhages (perhaps multiple, at various stages of healing) occur in over 80% of cases.[13] Other testing may be ordered at another time, but for today the dilated fundus exam is the most important thing.

290. c) In shaken baby syndrome, the baby's brain is "sloshed" back and forth, often causing neurological brain damage. Vision loss in these children is most often due to brain damage affecting the visual cortex.[13]

291. **Matching:**

A-V crossing	c)
cataracts	a) (steroid usage), d), g) (malnourishment)
dry eye	a), e) (AIDS), g) (Vitamin A deficiency)
emboli	c)
exophthalmos	h)
herpes zoster	e) (AIDS)
Kaposi's sarcoma	e) (AIDS)
keratitis sicca	a), e) (AIDS), g) (Vitamin A deficiency)
melanoma	b)
"night blindness"	g) (Vitamin A deficiency)
nystagmus	f)
ptosis	f)
retinoblastoma	b)
retinopathy	c), d), e)
Sjögren's syndrome	a)
squamous cell of the lid	b)
strabismus	f), h)
uveitis/ocular inflammation	a), e) (AIDS, TB), h)

292. a) Vitamin A deficiency in the eye can cause night blindness and retinopathy, as well as dryness and ulceration of the cornea. In its final stages, it progresses to death of the corneal tissues. Vitamin A deficiency is most common in developing countries. "An estimated 250,000–500,000 children who are Vitamin A–deficient become blind every year, and half of them die within 12 months of losing their sight. Deficiency of Vitamin A is … the world's leading preventable cause of childhood blindness."[14]

293. a) The Age-Related Eye Disease Study found that certain vitamins and supplements (found in "eye vitamins") may slow the progression of macular degeneration.

294. d) While smoking has the effects listed in every answer, the most common problem is chronic irritation caused by exposure to smoke, with about 67% of smokers in one study experiencing dry eye.[15]

295. c) The main factor in the occurrence of retinopathy related to diabetes is the duration of the diabetes. Other factors include poor glucose control, hypertension, and smoking.[16]

296. c) Cataracts occur earlier and more often in diabetics. Changes in the patient's refraction occur in cases where the blood sugar level is not well controlled. In theory, diabetes works like this. First, the patient's blood sugar becomes elevated. In an effort to try to equalize the sugar content of the body tissues, water is taken out of the tissues and added to the blood stream. (One sign of diabetes is frequent urination, a result of this added fluid.) The lens of the eye is not exempt from this tissue dehydration. This dehydration of the lens causes an increase in the curvature of the lens surfaces, which is responsible for the shift toward myopia. Finally, nerve palsies can occur. CNs III, IV, and VI may be affected; the patient complains of diplopia.

297. c) In Graves' disease (associated with an overactive thyroid), the extraocular muscles become inflamed and swollen. This swelling forces the eyeball outward, causing exophthalmos. Exophthalmos may progress to the point where the upper lid can no longer close over the globe, creating problems with exposure. (The most common cause in children is orbital cellulitis.)[17]

298. a) Severe dry eye as well as dry mouth, known as Sjögren's syndrome, is often associated with rheumatoid arthritis (RA). Other ocular manifestations associated with RA are scleritis and episcleritis. Medications used to treat RA (such as steroids) can also cause ocular problems. RA is not causative in corneal dystrophy, subconjunctival hemorrhages, or hypopyon (pus in the anterior chamber).

299. c) The most common ocular findings in HIV are changes in the retinal blood vessels (with hemorrhages and areas of tissue death) and changes in the conjunctival blood vessels (the appearance of tiny, curved vessels as well as hemorrhages).[18] H. zoster infection is seen, but in only 5% to 15% of those with HIV.[18]

300. c) Damage to blood vessels in hypertension is the most common source of vision impairment. The vessels may twist and thicken, or clots may cause a vessel occlusion and the death of retinal tissue.

301. a) In atherosclerosis, fat builds up in the arteries, including the arteries of the eye. This could build up to the point of obstructing an artery. Or, a piece of fatty plaque (from anywhere in the body) might break free, travel to the eye, and become lodged in an artery, blocking it off. (It might be worth noting that the term *atherosclerosis* refers to this fatty build-up in larger arteries [larger than 300 microns]. In smaller vessels [including the retinal arterioles, which are less than 30 microns], the disorder is called *arteriosclerosis*. The central retinal artery is large enough to be involved in atherosclerosis. In addition, arteriolosclerosis is characteristically associated with hypertension, while atherosclerosis is not.)

302. d) A neurological disorder affects the "wiring" or nervous system of the body. When any of the cranial nerves associated with the eye are involved, there may be a corresponding change in vision, eye movement, lid position, pupils, etc.

303. a) Because the brain is encased in the skull with little room for expansion, many of the symptoms caused by brain tumors are due to an elevation in the pressure inside the head (intracranial pressure).

304. d) These symptoms are due to increased intracranial pressure caused by the tumor. (Did you notice that the items in Answer c) were *signs*, not *symptoms*? Reading a question carefully can help you rule out certain answers.)

305. d) The papilloma is an area of thickened epithelium. They are sometimes pigmented, but they are the most common of the benign lid tumors.

306. c) Retinoblastoma is a congenital (and genetic) malignant tumor of the photoreceptor cells. It is often undiagnosed in its early stages; however, it is usually found by age 3. Leukocoria ("white pupil") and strabismus are often the presenting *symptoms*.

307. b) Herpes zoster virus (also called shingles) occurs in people with a history of previous infection with chicken pox (varicella-zoster). Shingles occur on one side of the body and are often quite painful. Episcleritis and uveitis may also occur with the infection. If there is a lesion on the tip of the nose, corneal involvement is certain. While Answer d) is possible, contact dermatitis is not necessarily painful, nor does it respect the midline of the face.

Part V

308. **Matching:**

all	pan-
around	para-
bad	mal-
behind	retro-
blue	cyano-
bones	osteo-
brown	bruno-
cornea	kerato-
different	aniso-
eye lids	blepharo-
false	pseudo-
green	chloro-
in	en-, endo-, entero-, eso-
life	bio-
muscles	myo-
out	ab-, abo-, e/ex-, exo-
over	hyper-
red	rubeo-
respiration	pulmo-
self	auto-
under	hypo-, infero-, infra-
up	supra-
white	leuko-
without	a/an-
yellow	xanth-

309. **Matching:**

condition of	-osis
deficient vision	-opsia/-opia
inflammation	-itis
measurement	-ometry
move	-duct
pain	-algia
study of	-ology
tumor	-oma
turn	-tropia

310. c) *Kinetic* refers to motion. *Static* refers to stationary, or nonmoving. *Transient* means something "comes and goes."

311. a) *Latent* means that something isn't readily seen until something is done to reveal it, such as a phoria (which is not evident until fixation is disrupted). *Patent* means something is open and working, such as a laser iridotomy that is open and allowing the aqueous to flow through. *Idiopathic* means that the cause is unknown.

312. d) *Manifest* means that a condition or entity is visible, such as a large exotropia. *Occult* means hidden.

313. c) A *symptom* is something the patient notices and describes to you, for example pain or redness or decreased vision. Sometimes a symptom is also a *sign*, which is something you can also observe yourself, such as redness. Other times, a sign is something that you discover through testing or your own observations, such as elevated intraocular pressure.

314. b) *Objective* testing does not involve any response by the patient, such as retinoscopy. (I remember this by the thought that in objective testing, I am regarding the patient as an object, no human response required.) *Subjective* testing requires a response from the patient, such as refraction or vision testing.

315. a) *Pseudo-* means false. *-phakic* refers to the crystalline lens. So pseudophakic means that a false lens (intraocular lens) has been put in place of the natural crystalline lens. Aphakic (*a-* without) means that there is no lens present. Phakic means that the natural lens is in place. Pseudophoric is a term I made up.

316. d) *Endocrine* refers to the hormonal system of the body. *Lymphatic* refers to the lymph system, part of the immune and circulatory systems. *Sympathetic* and *parasympathetic* refer to divisions of the nervous system.

317. a) You may use abbreviations (and acronyms, symbols, and codes) in patient records *only* as long as your clinic maintains a list of office-approved abbreviations. Every employee who has access to records and makes notes in them must be given this list. Periodic audits can help assure that everyone is using the abbreviations appropriately.

318. a) The concept of a "do not use" list was initiated by the Joint Commission and requires accredited facilities to formulate such list of abbreviations. These are the most frequently used abbreviations that carry the highest risk of patient harm if misinterpreted. Even clinics not requiring accreditation should have this list.

319. c) Did you notice that all the choices except the correct one involved written communication *given to the patient*? Abbreviations are never appropriate in patient education material or legal documents.

320. **Matching:**
    AMD- age-related macular degeneration- deterioration of the macula associated with aging
    AT- applanation tonometry- method of checking eye pressure (also used for artificial tears, which wasn't given as a possible answer here)
    c̄- *cum* (Latin)- with
    COAG- chronic open angle glaucoma- most common form of glaucoma
    DME- diabetic macular edema- thickening/swelling of the macula associated with diabetes
    EOM- extraocular muscles- muscle(s) responsible for eye movement
    gtt- *guttae* (Latin)- drops
    IOP- intraocular pressure- pressure inside the eye
    NLP- no light perception- patient has no vision; can't even see light
    NSAID- nonsteroidal anti-inflammatory drug- anti-inflammatory drug that doesn't have steroids in it
    NTG- normal tension glaucoma- glaucoma that is present in a patient with normal pressures
    OWS- over-wear syndrome- painful condition resulting from wearing contact lenses longer than recommended
    PD- pupillary distance- the distance between one pupil and another
    PH- pinhole- disk with tiny hole(s) in it
    PI- peripheral iridotomy- laser treatment to help prevent angle closure
    prn- *pro re nata* (Latin)- as needed
    PRP- panretinal photocoagulation- laser procedure for diabetic retinopathy
    PVD- posterior vitreous detachment- jelly inside the eye has pulled away from the retina
    s̄- *sine* (Latin)- without
    SCH- subconjunctival hemorrhage- bloody-looking area on the white of the eye
    SPK- superficial punctate keratopathy- fine dots of corneal staining
    ung- *unguentum* (Latin)- ointment
    W4D- Worth four dot- test for binocular vision or suppression
    YLC- YAG laser capsulotomy- laser treatment to remove cloudy area of posterior capsule

321. b) Batteries are considered *hazardous* waste, which poses a threat to the environment. Hazardous waste generally originates from industry/manufacturing sources (eg, gasoline and similar products, brake fluid, aerosol cans). *Biohazards* are potentially hazardous to humans and/or other forms of life, and originate from living sources. Examples include excised tissue, bacteria cultures, body fluids and products, used needles and sharps.

322. a) The cotton swab used to obtain material for culturing is considered biohazardous. Disposal of biohazardous waste is regulated. Not all medical waste is biohazardous, however.

323. a) Contaminated sharps (needles, blades, disposable forceps) must be disposed of in red, clearly marked, puncture-proof containers. Most have a "fill line" marked on the container; do not fill beyond the line. Approved disposal carriers must remove containers from the premises.

324. b) Contaminated broken glass should be placed into a sharps container. (In fact, any glass should be placed in a sharps container. Even a corrugated biohazard container might be punctured by broken glass.)

325. b) Any *tissue* removed from the patient that isn't sent for biopsy must be disposed of as pathological biohazardous waste. Technically, pathological waste *is* a type of biohazardous waste, but is generally considered to *originate from the patient's tissues* (thus ruling out the needles). The biopsy specimen, once evaluated by the pathologist, becomes pathologic biohazardous waste that must be disposed of by incineration, chemicals, autoclaving, or other approved method.

326. c) If blood is considered to be *THE* potentially infectious material, anything else is "other." That said, the "other" must have (or be suspected of containing) blood in order to be considered OPIM. Thus, tears or aqueous alone are *not* considered potentially infectious; bloody tears or aqueous *are*, and would be designated as OPIM. The same is true of non-bloody vomitus.

327. b) Bloodied items go into the red biohazard bag if there is a potential for contact. The word "soaked" is key here. A cotton ball with a little dot of dried blood (as following a blood draw) is not considered hazardous. The #10 blade goes in a sharps container. Saliva, tears, sweat, nasal secretions are not considered hazardous unless blood is present. So the gloves you used when performing a routine eye exam can go in the regular trash as well.

References

1. Nerad JA. Clinical Anatomy. In: *Techniques in Ophthalmic Surgery.* 2nd ed. Accessed June 2, 2021. http://ed.sciencedirect.com/topics/medicine-and-dentistry/tear-film

2. Sridhar MS. Anatomy of cornea and ocular surface. *Indian J Ophthalmol.* 2018;66(2):190-194. doi:10.4103/ijo.IJO_646_17

3. Cvekl A, McGreal R, Liu W. Lens development and crystallin gene expression. *Progress in Molecular Biology and Translational Science.* 2015;134:129-167. doi:10.1016/bs.pmbts.2015.05.001

4. Jameson KA, Highnote SM, Wasserman LM. Richer color experience in observers with multiple photopigment opsin genes. *Psychonomic Bulletin & Review.* 2001;8:244-261. doi:10.3758/BF03196159

5. Eske J. What is orbital cellulitis? MedicalNewsToday website. Accessed March 18, 2023. www.medicalnewstoday.com/articles/324460

6. Perez Y, Patel BC, Mendez MD. Nasolacrmal duct obstruction. Accessed March 18, 2023. www.ncbi.nlm.nih.gov/books/NBK532873/

7. Lopez-Jimenez F. Arcus senilis: a sign of high cholesterol? Mayo Clinic Website. Accessed March 18, 2023. www.mayoclinic.org/diseases-conditions/high-blood-cholesterol/expert-answers/arcus-senilis/faq-20058306

8. American Society of Clinical Oncology (ASCO). Eye cancer: an overview. Cancer.Net, website of ASCO. Accessed July 10, 2021. www.cancer.net/cancer-types/eye-cancer/overview

9. Finger PT. Choroidal metastasis. New York Eye Cancer Center website. Accessed March 18, 2023. https://eyecancer.com/eye-cancer/conditions/choroidal-tumors/choroidal-metastasis/

10. Gordon MO, Beiser JA, Brandt JD, et al. The ocular hypertension treatment study: baseline factors that predict the onset of primary open-angle glaucoma. *Arch Ophthalmol.* 2002;120:714-720. doi:10.1001/archopht.120.6.714

11.   Kass MA, Heuer DK, Higginbotham EJ, Johnson CA, Keltner JL, Miller JP, Parrish RK 2nd, Wilson MR, Gordon MO. The Ocular Hypertension Treatment Study: a randomized trial determines that topical ocular hypotensive medication delays or prevents the onset of primary open-angle glaucoma. *Arch Ophthalmol*. 2002;120(6):701-713; discussion 829-30. doi:10.1001/archopht.120.6.701

12.   Simunovic M. Colour vision deficiency. *Eye*. 2010;24:747-755. doi:10.1038/eye.2009.251

13.   Kivlin JD, Simons KB, Lazoritz S, Ruttum MS. Shaken baby syndrome. *Ophthalmology*. 2000;107(7):1246-1254. doi:10.1016/s0161-6420(00)00161-5

14.   Vitamin A deficiency. World Health Organization (WHO). Accessed March 18, 2023. https://www.who.int/data/nutrition/nlis/info/vitamin-a-deficiency

15.   Shah S, Jani H. Prevalence and associated factors of dry eye: our experience in patients above 40 years of age at a tertiary care center. *Oman J Ophthalmol*. 2015;8(3):151-156. doi:10.4103/0974-620X.169910

16.   Mandal A. Diabetic retinopathy risk factors. News-Medical February 26, 2019. Accessed March 18, 2023. www.news-medical.net/health/Diabetic-Retinopathy-Risk-Factors.aspx

17.   Butt S, Patel BC. Exophthalmos. [Updated 2022 June 27]. In: StatPearls [Internet]. StatPearls Publishing; 2021 Jan. Accessed March 18, 2023. https://www.ncbi.nlm.nih.gov/books/NBK559323/

18.   Feroze KB, Wang J. Ocular Manifestations of HIV. [Updated 2022 July 18]. In: StatPearls [Internet]. StatPearls Publishing; 2021 Jan. Accessed March 18, 2023. https://www.ncbi.nlm.nih.gov/books/NBK441926/

Bibliography

Kolb H. Simple anatomy of the retina. Webvision, Web Site of the University of Utah School of Medicine. Accessed March 18, 2023. https://webvision.med.utah.edu/book/part-i-foundations/simple-anatomy-of-the-retina/

Osaguona VB. Differential diagnoses of the pale/white/atrophic disc. *Community Eye Health*. 2016;29(96):71-74. Accessed March 18, 2023. www.ncbi.nlm.nih.gov/pmc/articles/PMC5365044/

Rubin M. Overview of neuro-ophthalmologic and cranial nerve disorders. In: Merck Manual professional version website. Modified September 2022. Accessed March 18, 2023. www.merckmanuals.com/professional/neurologic-disorders/neuro-ophthalmologic-and-cranial-nerve-disorders/overview-of-neuro-ophthalmologic-and-cranial-nerve-disorders#v1042095

Chapter 17

Optics and Spectacles**

* The author wishes to acknowledge the assistance given by Aaron Shukla on this chapter. (See also Reference.)
** Transposition and vertex distance are covered in Chapter 9: Refraction, Retinoscopy, and Refinement.

Ledford JK.
Certified Ophthalmic Technician Exam Review Manual, Third Edition (pp 391-414).
© 2023 Taylor & Francis Group.

ABBREVIATIONS USED IN THIS CHAPTER

- BD   base down
- BI   base in
- BO   base out
- BU   base up
- cm   centimeter
- D   diopter
- F   focal length (in meters)
- IR   index of refraction
- M   meter
- P   power
- PAL   progressive add lens
- PD   prism diopter
- Rx   prescription (glasses)
- SE   spherical equivalent

Optics and Spectacles*

1. Matching, one answer:

    Term
    candela
    foot candles
    intensity
    light ray
    wave length

    Definition
    _____ brightness
    _____ distance between the crests or troughs of a wave
    _____ measurement of light at a given distance from the source
    _____ measurement of light at its source
    _____ representation of the path of light in a given direction

2. The range of light waves detectible by the human eye is termed the:
    a) electromagnetic spectrum
    b) visible spectrum
    c) micro-spectrum
    d) polarized spectrum

3. The range of wavelengths in the visible spectrum is:
    a) 100 to 400 nanometers
    b) 400 to 800 nanometers
    c) 450 to 650 nanometers
    d) 400 to 800 meters

---

* Although not listed as a separate topic, the IJCAHPO® flash cards include questions on optical physics as well as geometric and ophthalmic optics.

4.   **Which color has the longest wavelength?**
      a) red
      b) yellow
      c) green
      d) blue

5.   **Immediately on either side of the visible spectrum are the invisible light segments of:**
      a) infrared and ultraviolet
      b) X-rays and radio waves
      c) gamma rays and laser
      d) microwaves and radar

Geometric Optics

6.   **Matching, one answer:**
      Term
      aberration
      converge
      diffraction
      diopter
      diverge
      index of refraction/refractive index
      medium
      reflection
      refraction

      Definition
      _____ bending of light as it passes an edge or corner
      _____ bending of light as it passes through a medium
      _____ having multiple focal points due to diffraction
      _____ light bounces off the surface of an object
      _____ light rays brought together to a point
      _____ light rays spread apart
      _____ measuring unit of lenses and prisms
      _____ designation of speed of light through a substance
      _____ substance that light can pass through

7.   **Geometric optics includes:**
      a) the origin of light waves and particles
      b) the effects of media on the path of light
      c) how light travels through the eye
      d) physics of the visible light spectrum

8.   **When light bounces back from an object, this is known as:**
      a) reflection
      b) refraction
      c) transmission
      d) index of refraction

9. **In reflection, the light rays that hit the object or interface between media with different indices of refraction are called:**
    a) incident rays
    b) reflected rays
    c) refracted rays
    d) transmitted rays

10. **In optics, a *medium* (or *media*, plural) is:**
    a) an object that refracts light
    b) an object that emits light
    c) an object that reflects light
    d) an object through which light passes

11. **When light passes through a transparent medium, it may travel straight through (transmission) or its path may be altered. This altering or bending property of a medium is known as:**
    a) reflection
    b) refraction
    c) absorption
    d) tropism

12. **The ray of light that enters a transparent medium is termed:**
    a) incident ray
    b) divergent ray
    c) emergent ray
    d) parallel ray

13. **A comparison of the speed of light in air to the speed of light through a substance is:**
    a) index of refraction
    b) angle of refraction
    c) internal reflection
    d) optical interference

14. **The denser the substance, the more slowly light passes through it, and:**
    a) the lower the IR
    b) the higher the IR
    c) the more transparent it is
    d) the more suitable it is for use as an ophthalmic lens

15. **The IR of crown glass is:**
    a) 0
    b) 1.00
    c) 1.33
    d) 1.50

16. **When light is filtered so that only parallel rays are allowed through, this is an example of:**
    a) polarization
    b) stereopsis
    c) virtual imaging
    d) illumination

17. **Light traveling through a prism will be bent toward the prism's:**
    a) apex
    b) base
    c) center
    d) smallest angle

18. **The image of an object viewed through a prism:**
    a) is real and shifted toward the base
    b) is virtual and shifted toward the base
    c) is real and shifted toward the apex
    d) is virtual and shifted toward the apex

19. **A 1.00-D prism bends light:**
    a) 1 cm at a distance of 1 cm from the prism
    b) 1 m at a distance of 1 cm from the prism
    c) 1 cm at a distance of 1 m from the prism
    d) 1 m at a distance of 1 m from the prism

20. **A 2.00-D prism displaces an object 1 cm at a distance of:**
    a) 0.2 m
    b) 0.5 m
    c) 1.5 m
    d) 5.0 cm

21. **The displacement of an object 5 cm at a distance of 1 m would require prism of:**
    a) 0.5 diopters
    b) 1.0 diopters
    c) 2.0 diopters
    d) 5.0 diopters

22. **If light passes through a lens and the rays are spread *apart* on exiting, this is known as:**
    a) IR
    b) convergence
    c) zero vergence
    d) divergence

23. **If light passes through a lens and the rays are bent *toward* each other on exiting, this is known as:**
    a) IR
    b) convergence
    c) zero vergence
    d) divergence

24. **A spherical lens refracts light:**
    a) not at all
    b) in one direction only
    c) equally in every direction
    d) at 90 degrees from its axis

25.   **Designate each as an attribute of a + plus or - minus lens.**
___ concave
___ convergent
___ convex
___ correction of aphakia
___ correction of hyperopia
___ correction of myopia
___ correction of presbyopia (in the emmetrope)
___ divergent
___ magnification
___ minification
___ real image
___ thicker in the center
___ thinner in the center
___ 2 prisms apex-to-apex
___ 2 prisms base-to-base
___ virtual image

26.   **All of the following regarding the optical center of a lens is true *except*:**
a) it should coincide with the geometric center of the lens
b) light rays passing through it are not refracted
c) it also is known as the nodal point
d) it should be centered in line with the patient's visual axis

27.   **A 1.00-diopter spherical lens focuses light at:**
a) 1/2 m
b) 1 m
c) 1 cm
d) 1 yard

28.   **The point at which a lens forms an image (whether real or virtual) is the:**
a) nodal point
b) conoid of Sturm
c) focal length
d) focal point

Focal Length

29.   **The focal length of a lens is:**
a) the distance between the lens and the focal point
b) the dioptric power of the lens
c) the point where light is focused
d) related to the axis of the cylinder

30.   **Which of the following is the formula for finding focal length?**
a) IR = speed of light in air/speed of light in substance
b) P = C/D
c) P = 1/F
d) U + P = V

31. **What is the focal length of a 5-diopter lens?**
    a) 5 m
    b) 0.5 m
    c) 2 m
    d) 0.2 m

32. **A lens has a focal length of 33 cm. What is its dioptric power?**
    a) 0.03 diopters
    b) 0.3 diopters
    c) 3 diopters
    d) 30 diopters

33. **All of the following regarding cylindrical lenses are true *except*:**
    a) they are used to correct astigmatism
    b) they have power in one axis, but no power in the axis 90 degrees away
    c) they focus light in a line
    d) they are plus power lenses

34. **The direction of the line of light as focused by a plus power cylindrical lens:**
    a) is virtual and cannot be placed
    b) is 90 degrees from the axis
    c) is aligned with the axis
    d) is 45 degrees from the axis

35. **Light passing through a cylindrical lens is focused in 2 lines perpendicular to each other and separated by an area known as:**
    a) induced interval
    b) Sturm's interval
    c) anterior focal interval
    d) posterior focal interval

36. **The light rays in the previously-mentioned interval are projected in the shape of a:**
    a) circle
    b) prism
    c) curve
    d) cone

37. **Within the conoid of Sturm, the area where the image would be most clearly focused is:**
    a) the circle of least confusion
    b) the cone of least confusion
    c) the focus of least confusion
    d) the secondary focal point

38. **Magnification functions as a low vision aid by:**
    a) shortening the viewing distance
    b) shortening the working distance
    c) increasing the size of the retinal image
    d) using only one lens

39. **A magnifying glass with the designation 10X has a dioptric power of approximately:**
    a) +4
    b) +10
    c) +25
    d) +40

40. **A magnifying glass with a dioptric power of +20 is designated by:**
    a) 4X
    b) 5X
    c) 10X
    d) 20X

Induced Prism/Prentice's Rule

41. **Prentice's rule for induced prism is:**
    a) multiplying vertex distance by millimeters of decentration
    b) multiplying millimeters of decentration by pupillary distance
    c) dividing centimeters of decentration by lens power
    d) multiplying centimeters of decentration by lens power

42. **A +4.25 sphere lens is decentered *in* by 0.50 cm. What is the prismatic effect?**
    a) 2.125 base in
    b) 2.125 base out
    c) 8.5 base in
    d) 8.5 base out

43. **Which lens is *least* likely to cause its wearer grief if decentered horizontally?**
    a) +12.00 sphere
    b) –6.00 sphere
    c) +4.00 sphere
    d) –2.00 sphere

Physiological and Ophthalmic Optics*

44. **The primary goal of the eye's components is to:**
    a) interpret what is seen
    b) focus incoming light onto the lens
    c) focus incoming light onto the retina
    d) maintain proper intraocular pressure

45. **A theoretical "mathematical" eye used to describe the numeric values of various ocular components as a way of evaluating the optics of the eye is the:**
    a) schematic eye
    b) Snellen eye
    c) natural eye
    d) Sturm's eye

---

* The term *physiological optics* refers to how the eye refracts light. *Ophthalmic optics* covers the use of lenses to correct refractive errors.

46. The ocular media consist of:
a) the lens correction for ametropia
b) contact lenses and intraocular lenses
c) the eyelid, sclera, uvea, and optic nerve
d) the tear film, cornea, humors, and lens

47. Which of the following is *true* regarding the ocular media?
a) each component has its own refractive index
b) the tear film is the only variable component
c) the aqueous and vitreous can be discounted
d) transparency remains the same throughout life

48. Which of the following ocular structures has the *highest* refractive power?
a) tear film
b) cornea
c) lens
d) aqueous and vitreous (combined)

Refractive Errors*

49. The "power" of a myopic eye itself is:
a) minus
b) plus
c) neutral
d) irrelevant

50. If a spectacle lens is determined to be spherocylindrical, one can deduce that the patient has:
a) myopia
b) hyperopia
c) astigmatism
d) presbyopia

51. Which refractive error would indicate that the patient had compound hyperopic astigmatism?
a) −3.00 + 2.00 x 088
b) +3.00 + 2.00 x 176
c) Plano + 3.50 x 023
d) −0.25 − 0.25 x 019

* See also *Prescriptions*, in this chapter.

52. **Which situation is depicted by the following progression of figures (Figures 17-1A through 17-1C)?**
    a) correction of simple myopic astigmatism with minus sphere and plus cylinder
    b) correction of simple hyperopic astigmatism with minus sphere and plus cylinder
    c) correction of simple myopic astigmatism with plus sphere and minus cylinder
    d) correction of compound myopic astigmatism with minus sphere and plus cylinder

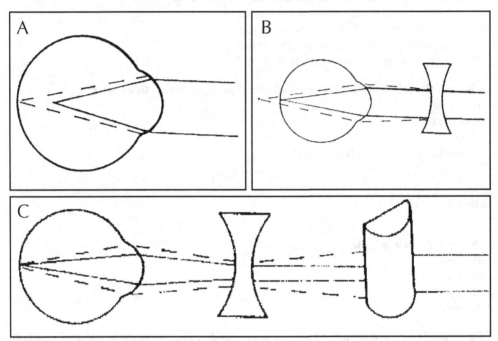

Figure 17-1. (Illustrations by Holly Hess Smith.)

53. **Which situation is depicted by the following progression of figures (Figures 17-2A and 17-2B)?**
    a) correction of myopia with minus sphere
    b) correction of simple myopic astigmatism with minus sphere
    c) correction of simple myopic astigmatism with minus cylinder
    d) correction of myopia with minus cylinder

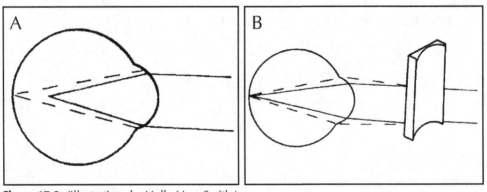

Figure 17-2. (Illustrations by Holly Hess Smith.)

54. **Which situation is depicted by the following progression of figures (Figures 17-3A through 17-3C)?**
    a) correction of simple myopic astigmatism with minus sphere and plus cylinder
    b) correction of mixed astigmatism with minus sphere and plus cylinder
    c) correction of compound myopic astigmatism with minus sphere and plus cylinder
    d) correction of compound myopic astigmatism with plus sphere and minus cylinder

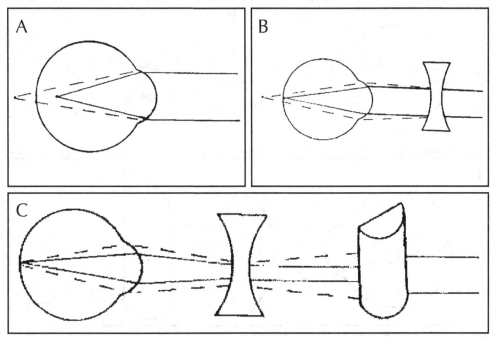

Figure 17-3. (Illustrations by Holly Hess Smith.)

55. Which situation is depicted by the following progression of figures (Figures 17-4A through 17-4C)?
    a) correction of simple hyperopic astigmatism with plus sphere and plus cylinder
    b) correction of compound hyperopic astigmatism with plus sphere
    c) correction of compound hyperopic astigmatism with plus sphere and plus cylinder
    d) correction of compound hyperopic astigmatism with plus sphere and minus cylinder

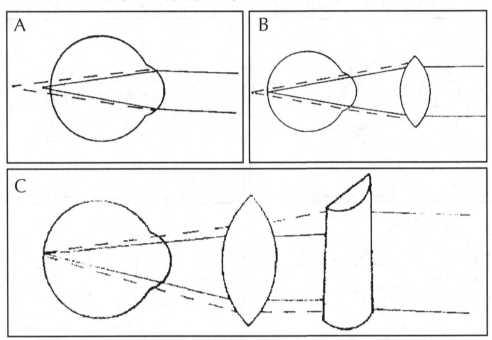

Figure 17-4. (Illustrations by Holly Hess Smith.)

56. The patient's single vision Rx is +2.25 OD and –1.25 OS. This is an example of:
    a) antimetropia
    b) refractive amblyopia
    c) anisocoria
    d) compound vision

57. The conoid of Sturm is a way of visualizing:
    a) myopia
    b) hyperopia
    c) astigmatism
    d) aphakia

58. At the center of the conoid of Sturm is the _____, which represents the _____.
    a) circle of least confusion, spherical equivalent
    b) optical cross, near point
    c) refractive error, transposed Rx
    d) far point, distance Rx

59. **Given a lens with the power +3.00 - 1.00 x 080. When a parallel light ray passes through it, where is the circle of least confusion?**
    a) 20 cm
    b) 33.3 cm
    c) 40 cm
    d) 50 cm

60. **In the case of astigmatism, the goal is to collapse the conoid of Sturm. This is done using spherical lenses and:**
    a) contact lenses
    b) polarized lenses
    c) hand-held magnifiers
    d) cylindrical lenses

61. **When correcting refractive errors, the goal is to use lenses that:**
    a) move the focal point as little as possible
    b) move the focal point created by the eye's optics
    c) move the focal point as much as possible
    d) obliterate the focal point

Accommodation

62. **All of the following are true regarding the accommodative reflex** *except*:
    a) it is stimulated by a blurred image
    b) it is not a true reflex
    c) it is required for viewing distant objects
    d) it includes convergence, miosis, and focusing

63. **When the ciliary muscle relaxes:**
    a) close objects become clear
    b) there is more focusing power
    c) the lens is pulled thinner
    d) the zonules go limp

64. **The main reason one's accommodative ability decreases with age is due to:**
    a) one's arms becoming shorter
    b) laxity of the ciliary muscle
    c) laxity of the zonules
    d) hardening of the crystalline lens

65. **Decreased near vision associated with lack of accommodation associated with age is known as:**
    a) antimetropia
    b) presbyopia
    c) amblyopia
    d) proximity blindness

66. **With accommodation fully relaxed, what is the patient's point of clearest vision?**
    a) the far point
    b) the near point
    c) accommodative amplitude
    d) range of accommodation

67. **What is the far point of a non-accommodating patient with an uncorrected refractive error of –2.50?**
    a) 40 mm
    b) 40 cm
    c) 50 cm
    d) infinity

68. **The distance between the near point and the far point is the:**
    a) SE
    b) accommodative amplitude
    c) range of accommodation
    d) visual morbidity

Prescriptions*

69. **If a lens is determined to be spherocylindrical, one can deduce that the patient has:**
    a) myopia
    b) hyperopia
    c) astigmatism
    d) presbyopia

70. **Label the parts of the following Rx using the provided terms:**
    +3.00   - 2.00   x 037   ADD: 2.25
       a)   b)   c)   d)

    __ bifocal power
    __ cylinder axis
    __ cylinder power
    __ sphere power

71. **An optical cross is a means of:**
    a) marking the optical center of a lens
    b) calculating the amount of induced prism
    c) determining whether or not a lens is polarized
    d) indicating the dioptric power of a lens

* See also Chapter 8: Lensometry.

72. **What is the Rx of the lens represented by the following optical cross (Figure 17-5)?**
    a) +3.00 sphere
    b) +3.00 + 3.00 x 090
    c) +3.00 + 3.00 x 180
    d) +3.00 + 6.00 x 090

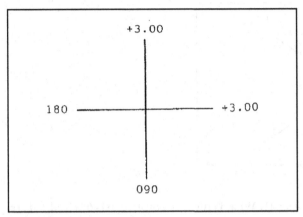

Figure 17-5.

73. **What is the Rx of the lens represented by the following optical cross (Figure 17-6)?**
    a) Plano – 2.25 x 180
    b) –2.25 – 2.25 x 180
    c) Plano + 2.25 x 090
    d) Plano – 2.25 x 090

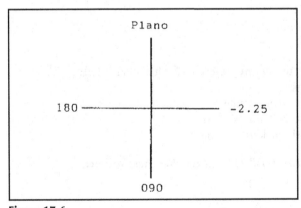

Figure 17-6.

74. **What is the Rx of the lens represented by the following optical cross (Figure 17-7)?**
    a) –1.25 + 2.00 x 135
    b) + 2.00 – 1.25 x 135
    c) +2.00 – 3.25 x 045
    d) –3.25 + 2.00 x 045

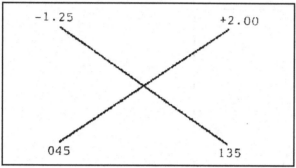

Figure 17-7.

75. **You have read a lens as +1.75 – 2.50 x 041. What is the lens power at axis 041 and 131, respectively?**
    a) –4.25 at 041, +1.75 at 131
    b) –0.75 at 041, +1.75 at 131
    c) +1.75 at 041, –2.50 at 131
    d) –2.50 at 041, +1.75 at 131

76. **A spectacle Rx has the notation "ADD: 2.25, 2.50 if PAL." This means that:**
    a) a trifocal should be ordered
    b) a "no-line" lens may be dispensed
    c) the optician may choose what add to use
    d) the patient may choose what add to use

77. **A glasses Rx has the notation "Tint to patient preference." This means that:**
    a) the patient should receive sunglasses
    b) the patient wants lenses that get darker outside
    c) the patient may choose how dark the lenses should be
    d) the optician may choose how dark the lenses should be

78. **A glasses Rx has the notation "2PDBU OD." This means that there will be:**
    a) 2 diopters of base up prism in the right lens
    b) 2 prisms in the right lens
    c) 2 prism bars bisecting the pupil in the right lens
    d) a 2-diopter bifocal at the top of the right lens

79. **The glasses Rx for a 4-year-old has a bifocal with the notation "split pupil." This means that:**
    a) the horizontal placement of the bifocal is crucial
    b) the patient has coloboma of the iris
    c) the upper edge of the bifocal should be in the center of the lens
    d) the upper edge of the bifocal should be at the center of the pupil

80. **A glasses Rx has the notation "single vision near." Which of the following is *least* likely to receive such an Rx?**
     a) a 64-year-old person who can see 20/20 at distance
     b) a 52-year-old who cannot tolerate bifocals
     c) a 72-year-old person with myopia
     d) a 32-year-old person with hyperopia

Study Notes

Suggested reading in *Principles and Practice in Ophthalmic Assisting: A Comprehensive Textbook:*
      Chapter 4: Optics (pp 39-53)
      Chapter 11: Retinoscopy and Refractometry (*Refractive Errors* and *Correcting Refractive Errors* pp 179-180, *Using the Optical Cross* Sidebar 11-2 pp 186-187)
      Chapter 19: Optical Procedures (*Lens Power* and *Optical Center of a Lens* pp 347-348, *The Format of a Spectacle Prescription* p 348, *Calculating Induced Prism* p 357, Sidebar 19-6 p 358)
      Chapter 20: Eyewear: Spectacles and Lenses (*Spectacle Lenses* p 369, *Lens Forms* pp 369-374, *Position of Multifocal Segments* p 374)

Explanatory Answers

1.   **Matching:**
candela	measurement of light at its source
foot candles	measurement of light at a given distance from the source
intensity	brightness
light ray	representation of the path of light in a given direction
wave length	distance between the crests or troughs of a wave

2.   b) The electromagnetic spectrum is made up of all light rays, and includes gamma rays, X-rays, infrared, the visible spectrum, ultraviolet, microwaves, radar, and radio waves. The portion that humans can see is, sensibly, called the visible spectrum.

3.   b) Depending on which reference is consulted, visible light is in the range of 400 to 750 nanometers. Be sure to watch the units of measurement given in an answer. "Meters" in Answer d) should have indicated that it was incorrect.

4.   a) Red has the longest wavelength: 650 nanometers.

5.   a) Infrared light borders the visible color red and ultraviolet light borders the visible color violet. All of the other answers are invisible components of the electromagnetic spectrum, but do not directly abut red or violet.

6.   **Matching:**

aberration	having multiple focal points due to diffraction
converge	light rays brought together to a point
diffraction	bending of light as it passes an edge or corner
diopter	measuring unit of lenses and prisms
diverge	light rays spread apart
index of refraction/refractive index	designation of speed of light through a substance
medium	substance that light can pass through
reflection	light bounces off the surface of an object
refraction	bending of light as it passes through a medium

7.   b) Geometric optics involves the reaction of light as it passes through media (any transparent object) or strikes a surface. Answers a) and d) refer to optical physics. Physiologic optics defines Answer c).

8.   a) When light strikes an object or an interface between media with different indices of refraction and bounces back, this is called *reflection*.

9.   a) The light that hits the object or interface is termed incident. Those rays that bounce back from the object or interface are called *reflected*.

10.   d) A medium is a transparent object through which light can pass. It is not a light source (ie, does not emit light). It does not necessarily refract light, either (see Answer 11).

11.   b) The quality of a medium to bend light is called *refraction*. In reflection, the rays are bounced off of the surface. Absorbed light does not pass through a medium. Tropism actually refers to the phenomenon of plants bending toward a light source.

12.   a) The incident ray is the ray that first strikes and enters a medium. A divergent ray has been refracted outward. The emergent ray is the ray as it exits the medium. A parallel ray is straight.

13.   a) The IR of a substance is found by dividing the speed of light in air by the speed of light through the substance. This is known as Snell's Law.

14.   b) A substance with a high IR is more dense and slows down the light passing through it.

15.   d) Depending on which reference is consulted, the IR of crown glass is 1.50. Light traveling through a vacuum is zero, through air is 1.0, and through water is 1.33.

16.   a) Polarization blocks all light rays except those traveling in a specific orientation. This reduces the amount of "scattered" rays and reduces glare (as seen in polarized sunglasses).

17.   b) Light traveling through a prism is bent toward the prism's base.

18.   d) Because light is bent toward the base, the image *appears* to be shifted toward the apex. Since the object doesn't really move, this is a virtual image.

19.   c) A 1.00-diopter prism bends light 1 cm at a distance of 1 m from the prism.

20.   b) The formula for figuring prism displacement is $P = C/D$, where P is the prism power, C is the displacement of the object in cm, and D is the distance from the prism in meters. To plug in this problem: $2 = 1/D$. Do algebra and multiply both sides by D/1, yielding $2D = 1$. Now divide both sides by 2: $D = 1/2$. 1/2 equals 0.5 m.

21.   d) Plug in again: $P = 5/1$. Thus $P = 5.0$ diopters.

22.   d) If the light is spread apart by the lens, the rays are said to be divergent.

23.   b) Convergence occurs when light rays are brought together (bent inward) by the lens.

24.   c) A spherical lens refracts light equally in every direction. This is evidenced by the fact that you can shine a light through a plus lens and focus it to a point.

25.   Attributes of plus and minus lenses:

concave	−
convergent	+
convex	+
correction of aphakia	+
correction of hyperopia	+
correction of myopia	−
correction of presbyopia (in the emmetrope)	+
divergent	−
magnification	+
minification	−
real image	+
thicker in the center	+
thinner in the center	−
2 prisms apex-to-apex	−
2 prisms base-to-base	+
virtual image	−

26.   a) The optical center does not always coincide with the geometrical center of a lens. The other statements are true.

27.   b) A 1.00-diopter lens focuses light at 1 m. (Technically, the light entering the lens must be parallel for this to hold true.)

28.   d) The focal point is the place where the lens focuses incoming light. The focal point may be real (can be projected onto a screen) or virtual (exists in theory but cannot be projected).

29.   a) Measure the distance between the lens and the focal point, and you will have measured the focal length. It is related to the dioptric power of the lens in that the stronger the lens, the shorter the focal length.

30.   c) The formula for focal length is P = 1/F. Answer a) is the formula for IR, b) is for prism displacement, and d) is for finding the vergence of light rays.

31.   d) P is 5 diopters. 5 = 1/F. Multiply each side by F/1 and get 5F = 1. Now divide each side by 5 and get F = 1/5 = 0.2 meters.

32.   c) This time it's done backward. F is 33 cm. The formula calls for meters, so change cm to m before doing the math. There are 100 cm in a meter, so 33 cm = 0.33 m. F is 0.33. Now plug into the formula: P = 1/0.33. Simple math, and you end up with 3.0 diopters.

33.   d) Cylindrical lenses can be plus or minus power.

34.   c) The line of light projected by a lens lines up with the axis. To prove it, get the strongest plus cylinder lens you have in your trial set. Shine a pen light through it onto the wall. Move the lens and light back and forth a bit until the line focuses.

35.   b) Between the anterior focal line and the posterior focal line is an area known as Sturm's interval.

36.   d) The light rays in Sturm's interval are arranged in a cone shape and are called Sturm's conoid or the conoid of Sturm (Figure 17-8).

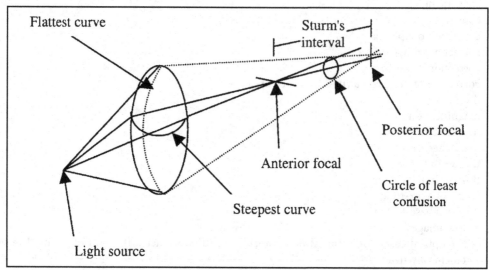

Figure 17-8. Conoid of Sturm formed by a spherocylindrical lens. (Reproduced with permission from Lens A. *Optics, Retinoscopy, and Refractometry*. 2nd ed. SLACK Incorporated; 2006.)

37.   a) The circle of least confusion is at the midpoint between the 2 focal lines of a spherocylindrical lens. While the image is not perfectly focused here, it is the most clear image available. (The goal in using a cylinder to correct astigmatism is to collapse the conoid of Sturm and place both focal lines on the retina, which gives a sharper focus than that at the circle of least confusion. See Answers 57 to 60.)

38.   c) Any type of magnifying system enlarges the image that falls on the retina.

39.   d) To find the approximate dioptric power of a magnifier, multiply the "X" power by 4 (10X x 4 = +40 D). *Note*: The "X" system of designating magnifiers can be confusing, and you can find all sorts of formulae and reasonings on the internet and in various texts. The method used here is what you'll find in most texts for ophthalmic medical personnel.

40.   b) To convert the dioptric power of a magnifier to the "X" system, divide by 4: in this case 5X.

41.   d) Prentice's rule says that displacement (in cm) X lens power (in diopters) = power of induced prism.

42.   a) The induced prismatic effect of a lens in prism diopters equals the power of the lens (in diopters) multiplied by the displacement of the optical centers (in cm). Thus, 4.25 x 0.50 = 2.125. As to base placement, a plus lens is like 2 prisms placed base to base. A plus lens that is decentered horizontally "in" has had the optical center moved toward the nose. (This holds true for left or right eye.) This moves the prism base nasal to the pupillary center of the eye, resulting in base in. If it had been a *minus* lens that had been decentered nasally, the answer would have been base *out*.

43.   d) The weaker the lens, the less induced prism there is if it is decentered (regardless of direction). For example, 0.50 cm decentration will induce 6 prism diopters in the +12.00 lens, 3 diopters in the −6.00 lens, 2 diopters in the +4.00 lens, and 1 diopter in the −2.00 lens.

44.   c) Incoming light is focused on the retina in the healthy eye. (Interpretation occurs in the occipital cortex of the brain.)

45. a) The schematic eye is a theoretical eye comprised of measurements and features of the "average" eye. It is used as a mathematical model for explaining and learning about the optics of the eye. There are several types, but the one you'll probably read about most is Gullstrand's. The model eye used to teach retinoscopy is sometimes called a schematic eye as well.

46. d) The ocular media are the transparent structures of the eye through which light passes. Some references might not include the tear film. The term "the humors" refers to the aqueous humor and vitreous humor.

47. a) Each component of the ocular media (see Answer 46) has its own refractive index. Any of the elements might be considered variable, but most notably the crystalline lens (think accommodation); even the aqueous and vitreous cannot be discounted because any material in them can affect the entering image. Transparency can vary, the most common problem being cataracts.

48. b) The cornea has more refractive power than even the lens. The average crystalline lens has 15 diopters of plus power. The cornea has 43.0 D.

49. b) This was a tricky question. Your first impulse probably was to say "minus" since that is the type of lens that myopia is neutralized with. But in order to neutralize with minus, logically the eye must be plus. A myopic eye has too much plus power.

50. c) Spherocylindrical means the lens has sphere combined with cylinder. Cylinder is used to correct astigmatism, so the correct answer is c).

51. b) In compound hyperopic astigmatism, both focal lines are in front of the retina. The only refractive error given that fits the bill is b). In a) and d), both focal lines are behind the retina. In c), one of the focal lines is on the retina while the other is in front of it. (*Note:* The type of astigmatism always remains the same even if you transpose the Rx. Try it!)

52. a) Figure 17-1A shows simple myopic astigmatism. Figure 17-1B depicts the corrected myopic portion with a minus sphere. But that pushes the originally emmetropic point back beyond the retina. So in Figure 17-1C, a plus cylinder is used to pull that segment back onto the retina.

53. c) Figure 17-2A again shows simple myopic astigmatism. But this time, in Figure 17-2B, it is corrected with a single minus cylinder. The cylinder moves only the myopic portion of the error, leaving the emmetropic section on the retina.

54. b) Figure 17-3A depicts mixed astigmatism. In Figure 17-3B, the myopic portion is corrected with a minus sphere. This pushes the hyperopic segment even further from the retina. Figure 17-3C pulls the hyperopic rays forward onto the retina using plus cylinder, while leaving the previously corrected portion undisturbed.

55. c) Figure 17-4A shows compound hyperopic astigmatism. Figure 17-4B shows a plus sphere pulling one meridian onto the retina. The other meridian is closer, but still not focused on the retina. So a plus cylinder is used, as in Figure 17-4C, to pull that meridian the rest of the way onto the retina.

56. a) You may have been looking for the term "anisometropia." If listed, it would have been a correct response. However, *antimetropia* means that one eye is plus and the other minus; it does not designate how many diopters difference there has to be between one eye and the other (as does anisometropia, usually >2 D although some references say >1 D). Thus, while +0.50 OD and –0.25 OS would not be anisometropic, it would still be noted as antimetropic.

57. c) The conoid of Sturm is a graphic way of visualizing astigmatism in the eye. On one end it represents the focal point of the most posterior foci, on the other end the focal point of the most anterior (See Figure 17-8). See also Answers 35 to 37.

58. a) At the middle of Sturm's interval, midway between the anterior focal point and the posterior focal point, is the circle of least confusion (see Figure 17-8). It represents the SE.*

---

* For more on SE, see section of that name in Chapter 9: Refraction, Retinoscopy, and Refinement.

59.   c) Remember, the circle of least confusion represents the SE. The SE of this lens is +2.50 (sphere power +3.00 plus half the cylinder power [–0.50]). Now find the focal distance of a +2.5 lens using the equation f(m) = 1/D. Thus f(m) = 1/2.50 = 0.4 m. To convert m to cm, move the decimal to the right 2 places: 40 cm.

60.   d) Cylinders bring light to focus in one meridian only and are used to move one end of the conoid of Sturm into focus on the retina. If this moves the other end of the conoid off the retina (as is the case in mixed astigmatism), a spherical lens is used to move this focal point back onto the retina.

61.   b) We use lenses to correct (or neutralize) the eye's refractive error. When a refractive error exists, the focal point(s) created by the optics of the eye fail to place the image on the macula. We use lenses to move this focal point (or points, if astigmatism exists) onto the retina by appropriately converging or diverging the light rays before they enter the eye.

62.   c) The accommodative reflex (which actually is not a true physiologic reflex) operates for near vision, not distant.

63.   c) When accommodation is relaxed, the ciliary muscle relaxes. This pulls the zonules tight, which stretches the lens out (thinning it). Distant objects become clear and the focusing power is decreased (Figure 17-9).

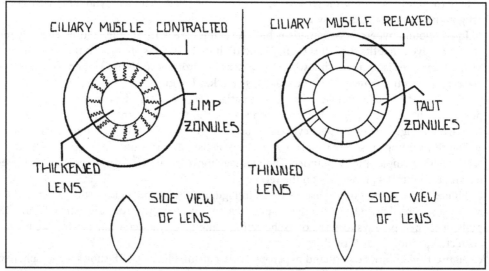

Figure 17-9. The lens and ciliary body in accommodation (left) and relaxation (right). (Illustration by Holly Hess Smith.)

64.   d) No matter how many of your patients swear that a) is the correct answer, the *best* explanation is that the lens loses its elasticity. There may be some laxity of the ciliary muscle, but this is not the major contributing factor.

65.   b) Presby- (meaning "old man") and -opia (referring to vision) is the term used to describe the loss of near vision associated with aging. Antimetropia is where one eye is near sighted and the other farsighted. Amblyopia is reduced vision in one eye from childhood. Proximity blindness is a phenomenon where we fail to see what's close to us because we are concentrating on something else ("can't see the trees for the forest").

66.   a) The far point is that place where the vision is clearest with accommodation totally relaxed. The near point is the closest place where the patient can focus using full accommodation. The range of accommodation is the area between the near and far points. Accommodative amplitude is the dioptric value of the near point (ie, the amount of accommodation, in diopters, that the patient has available).

67. b) This is a focal length question. Remember, a myopic eye actually has too much plus (see Answer 49). So use the equation f(m) = 1/D. Thus f(m) = 1/+2.5. f(m) = 0.4 m = 40 cm. (And 40 cm = ~16" Remember, in order to convert cm to inches, divide cm by 2.54 [in this case, 40/2.54].)

68. c) The far point is the point beyond which vision begins to blur. The near point is the closest an object can be before beginning to blur. Between the 2 is the accommodative range. SE combines the spherical portion of a spectacle lens with half of its cylinder power.* Accommodative amplitude is the dioptric value of the near point of accommodation. Visual morbidity is a general term referring to disorders of vision.

69. c) Spherocylindrical means the lens has sphere combined with cylinder. Cylinder is used to correct astigmatism, so the correct answer is c).

70. a) sphere power, b) cylinder power, c) cylinder axis, d) bifocal power

71. d) An optical cross is a way of diagramming the power of a lens in the 2 principal meridians (which are always 90 degrees from each other). *Note:* Some confusion has arisen in the past regarding the optical cross. The *true* optical cross is a representation of the effective power of a lens system. That is what is being discussed here. However, some clinicians use a cross to represent the patient's refractive error as measured on the phoropter. In this case, the power readings are taken right off the phoropter, representing the meridians where the patient's refractive error was neutralized, *not* where the lens system's effective power lies.

72. a) Since the power in each meridian is the same, this is a spherical lens of +3.00 power.

73. d) Remember this rule: whatever meridian you choose to start with when figuring the power, that also is going to be the axis of the answer. In this example, start with the zero (Plano). It is in the 90-degree meridian, which will be the axis of your answer. So far you have Plano +/– _____ x 090. (You can't decide on the cylinder sign until you move to the next step.) For the next step, imagine that you are on a number line and have gone from zero to –2.25. How many steps from zero to –2.25? –2.25. That is your cylinder sign and power. The answer: Plano –2.25 x 090. Of course, this could be transposed to –2.25 + 2.25 x 180. Or you could have arrived at the plus cylinder answer by starting the process at the 180 meridian.

74. c) You can start in either meridian. Let's use –1.25. Now you know most of the answer: –1.25 +/– _____ x 135. How many steps to get from –1.25 to + 2.00? + 3.25. Finish it off: –1.25 + 3.25 x 135. However, this doesn't appear as an option in the answers listed. Instead, just transpose: + 2.00 – 3.25 x 045.

75. b) Remember that the power of a lens is 90 degrees away from its axis. If you draw this out on an optical cross (as I did), you'll see that the power reading at axis 041 is +1.75; that means the power is at 131. If you then subtract +1.75 from –2.50, you get –0.75. This goes on the optical cross at 131, and the power of –0.75 is actually at 041.

76. b) The initials PAL mean progressive add lens, or a "no-line" lens. When written this way, the Rx means that if the patient wants a standard bifocal, then the add power should be 2.25. If the patient elects the no-line, then the add should be 2.50. Raising the add by 0.25 when using a PAL is commonly done in order to give the patient a bit more leeway for near viewing. This Rx is NOT for a trifocal, nor may the patient or optician choose the power without consulting the prescriber.

77. c) "Tint to patient preference" means that the patient can choose the degree of tint they want. This may be to the extent of sunglasses, but not necessarily. Lenses that get darker when outside are photochromic, not a tint. The optician may suggest a specific degree of tint, but the patient makes the decision.

---

* SE is covered in Chapter 9: Refraction, Retinoscopy, and Refinement.

78.   a) The translation of the acronym is 2-prism diopters base up; this would be put into the right lens.

79.   d) Bifocals in an adult are aligned so that the upper edge of the segment is in line with the top of the lower lid. However, bifocals prescribed for children are usually for ocular motility issues. It is very important, in such cases, that the child look *through* the bifocal for near, and not over it. So the prescriber will ask the optician to place the upper edge of the bifocal so that the line bisects ("splits") the pupil. This is a vertical placement issue, not horizontal. In addition, the geometric center of a lens is not necessarily the optical center. Thus, putting the bifocal in the physical center of the lens may not align it properly.

80.   d) The 32-year-old person with hyperopia will need glasses to wear at all times, if accommodation is to be relaxed. A separate pair of reading glasses would not be needed. In the other 3 cases, separate reading glasses may be desired; remember, even a 72-year-old person with myopia may need glasses for close-up at specific focal lengths.

Bibliography

Shukla A. *Clinical Optics Primer for Ophthalmic Medical Personnel*. SLACK Incorporated; 2009.

Chapter 18

Contact Lenses

Ledford JK.
*Certified Ophthalmic Technician Exam
Review Manual, Third Edition* (pp 415-442).
© 2023 Taylor & Francis Group.

ABBREVIATIONS USED IN THIS CHAPTER

- CAB   cellulose acetate butyrate (a GPCL material)
- GPC   giant papillary conjunctivitis
- GPCL   gas-permeable contact lens
- HCL   hard contact lens
- HEMA   hydroxyethylmethacrylate (most common SCL material)
- LARS   left add/right subtract
- OD   right eye
- OS   left eye
- OU   both eyes
- OWS   over-wear syndrome
- PMMA   polymethyl methacrylate ("old timey" HCL material)
- SAM/FAP   steeper add minus/flatter add plus
- SCL   soft contact lens

Part I*

Contact Lens Types

1. **The actual amount of oxygen that gets through a contact lens and reaches the cornea is a product of:**
    a) lens material and design, plus central and edge thickness
    b) the cylinder axis and movement on blinking
    c) a Schirmer's tear test and the water content of the lens
    d) wearing time, lens solutions, and patient compliance

2. **The oxygen permeability of a contact lens is its:**
    a) base curve
    b) fluid resistance
    c) osmotic value
    d) Dk value

3. **The characteristic of soft lens material that is responsible for most of a contact lens's advantages (and disadvantages) is its:**
    a) tear exchange under the lens
    b) ability to absorb water
    c) resistance to deposits
    d) larger diameter

4. **The advantages of soft contact lenses include all of the following *except*:**
    a) they are more comfortable than rigid lenses
    b) they provide crisper vision than rigid lenses
    c) they can be worn intermittently
    d) there is less lens loss

---

* Sections have been inserted into this lengthy chapter for ease of study, to allow for a logical "break" point.

5. **One of the main risks of wearing soft contact lenses is:**
    a) modifications are impossible
    b) residual astigmatism
    c) infection
    d) lens discoloration

6. **Soft lens material includes all of the following polymers *except*:**
    a) hydrogel
    b) silicone
    c) CAB
    d) HEMA

7. **The lower the water content of a soft lens:**
    a) the more durable the lens
    b) the greater oxygen permeability
    c) the less frequently it needs to be cleaned
    d) the smaller the diameter

8. **A soft contact lens with a high water content will:**
    a) be more stable if lens dehydration occurs
    b) allow for greater oxygen transmission
    c) need to be disinfected by thermal methods only
    d) be more durable if it is made of HEMA

9. **Extended wear soft lenses should generally be replaced:**
    a) every month
    b) every 3 to 6 months
    c) annually
    d) only when ruined by deposits

10. **The PMMA rigid lens essentially has no permeability. How does oxygen reach the cornea in PMMA lens wearers?**
    a) through the eyelids
    b) through the tears
    c) through the choroidal blood vessels
    d) through the conjunctiva

11. **The fact that gas-permeable material allows more oxygen to the eye means that:**
    a) the lens can be larger than a PMMA lens
    b) the lens is more comfortable than a PMMA lens
    c) lens movement is not an important factor
    d) the lens can be allowed to rest on the lower lid margin

12. **Advantages of the gas-permeable lens include all of the following *except*:**
    a) reduced spectacle blur
    b) no deposit formation
    c) better centration
    d) adaptation to full time wear in about 1 week

Contact Lens Specifications/Parameters

13.   **Radius can be defined as:**
   a) the distance around a sphere
   b) the distance from the center of a sphere to its edge
   c) the distance from one edge of a sphere to the other through the sphere's center
   d) the distance from the center of one sphere to another

14.   **The longer the radius of curvature of a contact lens:**
   a) the steeper the lens
   b) the flatter the lens
   c) the larger the diameter
   d) the greater the vault

15.   **The radiuscope is used to:**
   a) measure the curvature of the peripheral cornea
   b) measure the base curve of a rigid lens
   c) check the calibration of the keratometer
   d) help fit toric lenses with greater precision

16.   **If you place a contact lens on a flat surface, the distance of the drop from the center of the lens to the flat surface would be a measurement of the lens's:**
   a) base curve
   b) diameter
   c) vault
   d) radius

17.   **A line through the center of the contact lens from one edge to the other would be a measure of the lens's:**
   a) sagittal depth
   b) radius
   c) base curve
   d) diameter

18.   **Increasing the diameter of a lens acts to:**
   a) loosen the lens
   b) tighten the lens
   c) improve vision
   d) increase oxygen transmission

19.   **The portion of a contact lens that is intended to position in front of the patient's line of sight is the:**
   a) pupillary distance
   b) optic zone
   c) peripheral zone
   d) pupillary aperture

Wearing Schedules

20. Which lens type has a slower schedule for building up wearing time?
a) rigid lens
b) daily wear soft lens
c) extended wear soft lens
d) disposable lens

21. Using a proper wearing schedule, a soft lens wearer can build up to full-time wear in approximately:
a) 1 week
b) 3 to 4 weeks
c) 6 to 8 weeks
d) 10 to 12 weeks

22. Using a proper wearing schedule, a rigid contact lens wearer will work up to full-time wear in about:
a) 1 to 2 weeks
b) 3 to 5 weeks
c) 8 to 10 weeks
d) 12 to 15 weeks

23. In general, the recommended upper limit wearing time for daily wear rigid or soft lenses is:
a) 8 hours
b) 10 hours
c) 15 hours
d) 20 hours

Contact Lens Care Systems

24. The difference between cleaning and disinfecting is:
a) cleaning is mandatory; disinfecting is optional
b) cleaning removes film and debris; disinfecting kills germs
c) cleaning kills germs; disinfecting removes film and debris
d) cleaning is optional; disinfecting is mandatory

25. The "all-in-one" (soaking and wetting) solutions are convenient due to all of the following *except*:
a) the cleaning step is eliminated
b) one can insert the lenses right from the case
c) one less bottle of solution is required
d) lens comfort is increased

26. When cleaning the lens after removal, one should apply one-step solution to the lens and:
a) rub it hard between the thumb and index finger
b) place the lens in the palm and gently rub with a fingertip
c) place the lens in one palm and rub it with the other palm
d) rinse the cleaner right off again so it does not penetrate the lens

27. **Soft lenses should be cleaned immediately after removal because:**
    a) grunge is easier to remove at body temperature
    b) the patient might forget to do it later
    c) grunge is harder to remove once the lens has dried out
    d) otherwise enzymes are needed

28. **A surfactant cleaner:**
    a) is rubbed over the lens surface
    b) is used to soak the lens
    c) is used to rewet the lens
    d) is put in the eye for redness

29. **Enzymatic cleaners are sometimes recommended weekly for daily wear soft lenses and gas-permeable lenses in order to:**
    a) sterilize the lenses
    b) prolong the life of the lens material
    c) remove protein deposits
    d) reduce splitting and chipping

30. **"Jelly bumps" on a soft contact lens are actually:**
    a) areas where the lens has dehydrated
    b) dried mucus
    c) calcium and lipid deposits
    d) dried eye ointment

31. **There is some evidence that as deposits form on a lens:**
    a) there is a decrease in its water content
    b) there is a decrease in its oxygen transmission
    c) there is an increase in lens dehydration
    d) there is a decrease in lens dehydration

32. **Wetting solutions for rigid lenses are used to:**
    a) keep lenses sterile while stored in the case
    b) enable tears to spread evenly on the lens surface
    c) make the lens resistant to deposit build-up
    d) prevent scratches on the lens surface

33. **Which of the following is the *least* sterile of these nonapproved, ill-advised, and dangerous rewetting fluids?**
    a) saliva
    b) tap water
    c) urine
    d) water from a swimming pool

34. **Patients should be told that regarding contact lens solution types and brands:**
    a) they can buy whatever is on sale
    b) all brands are mix and match
    c) they should only buy from your practice
    d) some chemicals react negatively with others

35. **Which of the following has been associated with *Acanthamoeba* infections in contact lens wearers?**
    a) enzymatic cleaners
    b) thimerosal preserved solutions
    c) homemade saline
    d) sample bottles of solutions

36. **If the lenses are not going to be worn for a few days:**
    a) add more soaking solution periodically to keep the lenses covered
    b) screw the case lid on tight to prevent evaporation
    c) use only non-preserved saline as a soak
    d) change the soaking solution every day to maintain disinfection

37. **All of the following are true regarding a contact lens case *except*:**
    a) It can be boiled in water.
    b) It should be washed weekly with hot water and soap.
    c) It should be replaced every month or so.
    d) The interior is disinfected along with the contacts.

Contraindications*

38. **Which patient is a poor candidate for soft lenses?**
    a) a patient with dry eye
    b) a patient with a spherical refractive error
    c) an infant or child
    d) a recreational basketball player

39. **All of the following are poor candidates for extended wear lenses *except*:**
    a) those who work in a dusty environment
    b) those with chronic blepharitis
    c) those taking blood thinners
    d) those with pre-existing GPC

40. **Which of the following makes a patient a poor candidate for gas-permeable contact lenses?**
    a) history of GPC
    b) exophthalmos
    c) corneal irregularity
    d) neovascularization from soft lenses

41. **Patients who work around smoke, dust, and chemical fumes should be told:**
    a) they are not good candidates for contact lenses
    b) they should wear rigid lenses, which will not absorb fumes
    c) they should not wear contacts at work
    d) they should change jobs if they want to wear contacts

---

* Currently, the criteria list this item as "Contraindications, symptoms, and fitting." I have elected to move the symptoms and fitting part to a position following "Perform contact lens fitting" in this chapter.

42. **A rigid lens might be contraindicated in a patient who:**
     a) plays contact sports
     b) is presbyopic
     c) has mild problems with manual dexterity
     d) is compulsive about their vision

43. **Which patient might you logically want to discourage from wearing contact lenses?**
     a) a 65-year-old patient with aphakia who has worn glasses for 12 years
     b) a 35-year-old patient with emmetropia who wants to change their eye color
     c) a 50-year-old patient with emmetropia
     d) a teen with moderate myopia

44. **All of the following might contraindicate contact lens wear *except*:**
     a) history of herpetic keratitis
     b) history of episcleritis
     c) pinguecula with history of inflammation
     d) pterygium

45. **All of the following are associated with dry eye and may render a patient a poor contact lens candidate *except*:**
     a) rheumatoid arthritis
     b) diabetes
     c) menopause
     d) use of allergy medications

Part II

Perform Contact Lens Fitting

46. **For most contact lens fitting purposes, it is acceptable to measure corneal diameter:**
     a) using an ophthalmoscope set on +10.0 and a millimeter rule
     b) by measuring the visible iris with a millimeter rule
     c) by using a pachymeter
     d) by anesthetizing the eye and using calipers

47. **The general rule about corneal diameter is:**
     a) neither a rigid nor a soft lens should touch the limbus
     b) a soft lens should cover the cornea to the limbus, but not beyond
     c) the diameter of a rigid lens should exceed the corneal diameter by 1 mm
     d) corneal diameter does not figure into the fit of any contact lens

48. **If the cross hairs of the keratometer* are *not* centered during the initial reading for contact lens fitting:**
     a) you may select a lens that is too strong
     b) the resulting fit may be too tight
     c) the resulting fit may be too loose
     d) you may select a lens that is too small

*Keratometry in general is covered in Chapter 6.

49. **Which of the following statements about vertex distance is *correct*?**
    a) persons with myopia may require more minus power in a soft lens than in spectacles
    b) persons with hyperopia may require less plus power in a soft lens than in spectacles
    c) persons with aphakia may require less plus power in a soft lens than in spectacles
    d) persons with hyperopia may require more plus power in a soft lens than in spectacles

50. **At what power threshold should you begin adjusting the contact lens power for vertex distance?**
    a) 1.00 diopter
    b) 2.00 diopters
    c) 4.00 diopters
    d) 6.00 diopters

51. **Over-refraction of a contact lens is useful in fine tuning:**
    a) lens power
    b) lens diameter
    c) lens centration
    d) lens base curve

52. **When performing over-refraction of a contact lens, it is important to:**
    a) check for residual astigmatism first
    b) check for a reading add first
    c) subtract the least amount of sphere that you can
    d) reduce plus power as much as possible

53. **When refracting over the contact lenses of a patient over 40 years old:**
    a) first find out how the patient is corrected for presbyopia
    b) measure each eye for distance only
    c) measure each eye for near only
    d) measure the right eye for distance and the left eye for near

Soft Spherical

54. **Selecting the power of a soft spherical contact lens is based on:**
    a) the spherical element found on refraction
    b) the cylindrical element found on refraction
    c) the spherical equivalent of the refraction
    d) the refraction and keratometry measurements

55. **To obtain the spherical equivalent:**
    a) add half of the sphere to the cylinder algebraically, keeping the cylinder
    b) add half of the cylinder to the sphere algebraically, keeping the cylinder
    c) add half of the sphere to the cylinder algebraically, deleting the cylinder
    d) add half of the cylinder to the sphere algebraically, deleting the cylinder

56. **You want to fit a spherical soft contact. The refraction is –3.00 + 1.00 x 180. Your lens choice is:**
    a) –3.00 sphere
    b) –3.50 sphere
    c) –2.00 sphere
    d) –2.50 sphere

57. **Fitting soft lenses steeper than K usually will result in:**
    a) good lens movement
    b) a minus tear layer under the lens
    c) fluctuations in vision following the blink
    d) excellent comfort and visual acuity

58. **Slit lamp examination in the case of a loose soft lens may reveal:**
    a) no movement, decentration, and conjunctival drag
    b) multiple deposits and "jelly bumps"
    c) limbal injection, corneal edema, and vascularization
    d) excessive movement, decentration, edge puckering, and edge standoff

59. **A loose soft lens may be tightened by:**
    a) decreasing the base curve or decreasing the diameter
    b) steepening the base curve or increasing the diameter
    c) removing deposits and instructing the patient on proper lens care
    d) increasing the power to compensate for vertex distance

60. **A good general rule for fitting extended wear lenses is to:**
    a) fit the highest water content possible
    b) fit the loosest lens possible
    c) fit gas-permeable whenever possible
    d) fit the smallest diameter possible

61. **An eye is considered "dry" if the tear breakup time is:**
    a) 10 seconds or less
    b) 15 to 25 seconds
    c) 30 to 40 seconds
    d) over 45 seconds

62. **A soft lens will react to a dry eye:**
    a) by drying it further as the lens draws moisture into itself
    b) by restoring the tear balance
    c) by releasing water content from the lens onto the eye
    d) with excessive movement

63. **Fitting a dry eye with a soft lens can be difficult because:**
    a) tear supplements cannot be used with soft lenses
    b) the lens will move excessively
    c) the diameter of the lens will change as it dries
    d) the optical properties of the lens will change as it dries

64. **The patient with excess tear secretion may experience:**
    a) "sucked on" lens syndrome
    b) increased risk of neovascularization
    c) excess lens movement
    d) indentation around the limbus

65. **Under the slit lamp a tight soft contact lens might exhibit all of the following** *except*:
 a) conjunctival drag
 b) redness at the limbus
 c) edge standoff
 d) scleral indentation

66. **A patient with a tight soft lens will notice that their vision:**
 a) is stable
 b) is clearer in the evening than in the morning
 c) is clearer just after a blink, then blurs
 d) is blurred just after a blink, then clears

67. **A tight soft lens can be loosened by:**
 a) decreasing the diameter or flattening the base curve
 b) increasing the diameter or steepening the base curve
 c) increasing the lens vault
 d) compensating for vertex distance

68. **When adjusting the physical fit of the lens, one must also make adjustments to the lens power. The rule to follow in such cases is:**
 a) compensate for cylinder changes by changing sphere
 b) steeper add minus, flatter add plus
 c) left, add; right, subtract
 d) transpose the prescription

Rigid

69. **In addition to the refractive error and residual astigmatism, when selecting the power for rigid contact lenses, one must also consider the:**
 a) axial length
 b) tear film
 c) size of the fovea
 d) endothelial cell count

70. **Current fitting philosophy for gas-permeable lenses dictates that:**
 a) the upper lid should control lens movement
 b) the lens should rest on the lower lid
 c) there should be as little movement as possible
 d) the lens should float down below the upper lid after each blink

71. **You want to fit a rigid contact lens, and the patient's K reading is 43.50/44.75. What base curve will you select to fit the patient "on K"?**
 a) 43.50
 b) 44.12
 c) 44.25
 d) 44.75

72.   **Patients with large pupils who are being fit for rigid lenses will require:**
a) miotics to reduce pupil size
b) larger optical zone and larger lens diameter
c) smaller optical zone and smaller lens diameter
d) larger optical zone and smaller lens diameter

73.   **Which adaptation may need to be made when fitting rigid lenses on a patient with dry eyes?**
a) insertion and removal with a plunger only
b) enzyme cleaning twice every week instead of once
c) less frequent blinking
d) longer period to build up to full-time wear

74.   **In calculating the power for a rigid lens, one must:**
a) first transpose the prescription into plus cylinder form
b) first transpose the prescription into minus cylinder form
c) calculate the spherical equivalent
d) always compensate for vertex distance

75.   **The power of a spherical rigid lens (under 4.0 diopters) fit on K:**
a) must be adjusted according to the K reading
b) is the spherical element of the refraction
c) is the spherical equivalent of the refraction
d) varies according to the lens diameter

76.   **You are using the slit lamp to evaluate a patient with rigid contacts. When the patient blinks, sometimes the upper lid grabs the lens so that the lens rides too high. At other times, the upper lid pushes the lens down. What may cause this to happen?**
a) the lens diameter is too small
b) the lens diameter is too large
c) the lids are too tight
d) the lids are too lax

Astigmatism/Toric

77.   **The amount of astigmatism that is present after the patient is fitted with lenses is referred to as:**
a) residual astigmatism
b) corneal astigmatism
c) lenticular astigmatism
d) irregular astigmatism

78.   **The most common cause of residual astigmatism in contact lens wearers is:**
a) the tear lens
b) the cornea
c) the crystalline lens
d) the retina

79.   With spherical soft lenses, a small amount of corneal astigmatism is:
       a) masked
       b) eliminated
       c) tolerated
       d) a reason to fit toric lenses

80.   The patient with astigmatism may tolerate spherical soft contact lenses up to the point that the
       astigmatism is:
       a) less than 1/3 of the total refractive error
       b) less than 1/2 of the total refractive error
       c) lenticular
       d) with the rule

81.   If the refraction over a spherical soft contact shows uncorrected astigmatism of 0.50 D or less:
       a) a toric lens should be tried
       b) refit, using spherical equivalent
       c) a rigid lens should be recommended
       d) in general this can be ignored

82.   The patient with astigmatism may tolerate a spherical rigid contact lens if the astigmatism is:
       a) with the rule
       b) against the rule
       c) 3.00 diopters or more
       d) 3.00 diopters or less

83.   The major difficulty with fitting toric lenses is:
       a) patient discomfort
       b) lens stability on the eye
       c) arriving at the correct prescription
       d) obtaining accurate over-refractions

84.   An aid in evaluating the stability of a soft toric lens is:
       a) the movement gauge
       b) etch or laser marks on the lens
       c) a protractor in the slit lamp ocular
       d) the contact lens gauge

85.   If toric lens rotation is to the left, one should add the number of degrees of rotation to the:
       a) axis of the contact lens
       b) axis of the steepest K reading
       c) axis of the flattest K reading
       d) axis of the patient's refraction

86.   The major factor(s) influencing toric soft lens stability is(are):
       a) the weighting and truncating of the lens
       b) the contour, position, and tightness of the lids
       c) the patient's K readings
       d) the thickness and water content of the lens polymer

87. **You plan to fit a soft toric contact lens. Which of the following is true regarding the refraction?**
    a) It must be converted to plus cylinder.
    b) You will use the spherical equivalent.
    c) You want the patient to accept the most cylinder power possible.
    d) You want the patient to accept the least cylinder power possible.

88. **Truncation is a method used to:**
    a) increase comfort of a toric lens
    b) increase oxygen supply to the cornea
    c) provide stability to a toric lens
    d) decrease corneal dehydration

89. **Toric rigid lenses may be required by patients:**
    a) whose refractive and corneal astigmatism agree in power but not in axis
    b) with spherical corneas and lenticular astigmatism
    c) whose corneal astigmatism is greater than their refractive astigmatism
    d) all of the above

Bifocal

90. **Simultaneous vision bifocal contact lenses:**
    a) involve fitting one eye for distance and the other eye for near
    b) are not available with progressive power
    c) have a reading segment at the bottom of the lens
    d) have distance correction in the center and near correction in an outer ring

91. **The most common visual complaint with simultaneous bifocal contacts is:**
    a) ghost images
    b) loss of depth perception
    c) loss of binocularity
    d) inability to coordinate the eyes

92. **Monovision contact lens fitting for presbyopia involves:**
    a) fitting both eyes for distance and using reading glasses for near
    b) fitting one eye (usually the dominant eye) for distance, and the other eye for near
    c) fitting one eye (usually the dominant eye) for near, and the other eye for distance
    d) fitting both eyes for near and using glasses for distance

93. **Which of the following probably would be a poor candidate for the monofit technique?**
    a) a public speaker
    b) a teacher
    c) a bookkeeper
    d) an actor

94. **Patients using the monovision technique might experience problems:**
    a) taking the driver's license vision test
    b) in very bright light
    c) looking from the desk to the board in classroom situations
    d) when their peripheral vision is checked by confrontation

Part III

Patient Instruction: Handling*

95. **A good rule of thumb when instructing patients regarding contact lenses is to:**
   a) provide a training session offering oral and written instruction
   b) provide written instruction and instruct the patient to call with questions
   c) provide a training session and oral instruction
   d) develop a support group where successful lens wearers teach others

96. **The first rule to teach patients about handling contact lenses is:**
   a) always use a mirror
   b) work over a clean surface
   c) always wash hands first
   d) never touch the lens itself

97. **Before inserting a soft lens, the patient should make sure it is not inverted. This can be done by:**
   a) visual inspection or the taco test
   b) visual inspection or the jelly roll test
   c) placing the lens in an inversion tester
   d) viewing the lens's reverse image in the mirror

98. **To insert a soft lens:**
   a) the lens should be dry and the finger wet
   b) the lens and finger should be dry
   c) the lens should be wet and the finger dry
   d) the lens and finger should be wet

99. **When first learning to insert contact lenses, it is helpful for the patient to use the nondominant hand:**
   a) to immobilize the upper lid
   b) to insert the contact
   c) to pull down the lower lid
   d) the right hand should always be used to insert the lens

100. **The patient should be instructed to place the lens:**
   a) directly on the cornea
   b) on the inferior sclera, then slide it up
   c) on the margin of the lower lid
   d) on the nasal sclera, then slide it over

101. **Use of lotion or moisturizer before handling lenses, or use of makeup, hair spray, or face cream after inserting lenses can cause:**
   a) lens film
   b) corneal edema
   c) degradation of the lens
   d) GPC

---

* In the criteria, patient instruction for contact lenses is listed under Ophthalmic Patient Services and Education. My sources suggest that the criteria refers to medically indicated therapeutic contact lenses.

102. **Soft lenses are most easily removed by:**
    a) using a plunger cup
    b) blinking them out
    c) squeezing them out
    d) pinching them out

103. **Damage to soft contact lenses is frequently caused by:**
    a) pinching them out
    b) rolling them between the fingers
    c) long fingernails
    d) defective materials

104. **Every patient who wears extended wear contact lenses should be told to:**
    a) remove the lenses and clean them daily
    b) allow the lenses to remain in the eye for up to 1 month
    c) use lubricating drops every morning and during the day
    d) endure occasional pain and redness as a matter of course

105. **Patients who sleep in their extended wear lenses should be told to:**
    a) removed weekly and leave out for one night
    b) remove every other night
    c) remove and leave out for one night once every month
    d) sleep in lenses nightly as long as comfortable

106. **Rigid lenses are often removed by blinking them out. For this technique to work:**
    a) the lens should be moved onto the sclera first
    b) the lens must be centered on the eye
    c) the patient must flip the edge of the lens with the finger
    d) the patient must squint and look up

107. **All of the following are helpful/proper techniques for using a plunger to remove a rigid lens**
    except:
    a) locate the lens on the eye before applying the plunger
    b) wet the plunger with wetting solution first
    c) run the plunger over the cornea and sclera to locate a "lost" lens
    d) carry an extra plunger in pocket or purse for emergency removal

108. **The patient asks what they should do if they drop the contact lens into the sink while trying to insert the lens. You tell them:**
    a) rinse the lens with saline and insert
    b) rinse the lens with rewetting drops and insert
    c) clean and disinfect the lens as per solution instructions
    d) replace the lens

109. **The contact lens patient should be told that if the eye ever becomes red or painful, they are to:**
    a) try another lens
    b) irrigate the eye
    c) bear with it
    d) remove the lens

Follow-Up Appointments

110. **Of the following, which is the *most* important reason for follow-up contact lens appointments?**
    a) check the vision
    b) check patient comfort
    c) check the fit
    d) check intraocular pressure

111. **Once the patient has been successfully fit with contacts, the prescriber must:**
    a) provide the patient with a contact lens prescription
    b) provide the patient with back-up glasses prescription
    c) provide the patient with 1 year's worth of lenses
    d) protect against release of the contact lens prescription

112. **You are looking at a contact lens patient with the slit lamp at a 1-month recheck appointment. You notice deposits on the 2-week replacement, daily wear lens. During this visit, you will:**
    a) make sure the deposits don't interfere with vision
    b) make sure the deposits aren't causing discomfort
    c) question the patient about compliance
    d) tell the patient to stop wearing the lenses

Problems

113. **The most common symptom of contact lens deposits is:**
    a) foreign body sensation
    b) corneal edema
    c) vascularization
    d) itching and watering

114. **Corneal edema, sensations of soreness, injection, foggy vision, and ghost images usually indicate:**
    a) a tight-fitting lens
    b) decentration and corneal exposure
    c) allergy to soft lens solutions
    d) that the lens is too small and too flat

115. **Your patient complains that they can constantly feel their soft lens in their eye. They also experience some blurred vision, especially when they move their eyes around a lot. These are symptoms of:**
    a) a tight lens
    b) a loose lens
    c) inadequate power
    d) poor hygiene

116. **Corneal edema is caused by:**
    a) excess oxygen permeability
    b) insufficient oxygen
    c) excess carbon dioxide
    d) excess tear production

117. **Symptoms of corneal edema include:**
    a) blurred vision
    b) rainbows around lights
    c) injection and burning
    d) all of the above

118. **A common problem associated with thicker (higher power) contact lenses is:**
    a) poor durability
    b) poor optical quality
    c) hypoxia
    d) conjunctival drag

119. **Blurred vision due to hypoxia usually:**
    a) fluctuates throughout the day
    b) starts as soon as the lenses are inserted but clears later
    c) starts several hours after the lenses are inserted
    d) is continuous from the time of insertion to removal

120. **A patient wearing extended wear contact lenses who develops corneal edema might be managed by:**
    a) increasing the lens diameter
    b) trying different water contents
    c) fitting on K
    d) switching to a different cleaning system

121. **Vascularization can result from chronic:**
    a) hypoxia
    b) solution sensitivity
    c) conjunctival injection
    d) GPC

122. **The area of the cornea that most commonly becomes vascularized is the:**
    a) inferior limbal area
    b) superior limbal area
    c) 9 o'clock limbal area
    d) 3 o'clock limbal area

123. **In a soft lens patient with vascularization, the problem might be remedied by all of the following *except*:**
    a) a looser lens
    b) a change in solutions
    c) a thinner lens
    d) a higher water content

124. **A rigid lens may stimulate vascularization if it:**
    a) is not cleaned weekly with enzymatic cleaner
    b) lifts, then slides down a little after each blink
    c) habitually rides on the central cornea
    d) habitually rides on the limbus

125. *Pseudomonas* ulcers are seen more frequently in patients wearing:
    a) gas-permeable lenses
    b) extended wear soft lenses
    c) daily wear soft lenses
    d) daily wear soft toric lenses

126. A corneal ulcer associated with contact lens wear can be caused by all of the following *except*:
    a) chemical sensitivity
    b) infection
    c) trauma
    d) hypoxia

127. Corneal ulcers are usually unrelated to use of:
    a) daily wear soft lenses
    b) extended wear soft lenses
    c) extended wear soft lenses removed on a daily basis
    d) gas-permeable rigid lenses

128. GPC is suspected to be:
    a) an allergic response
    b) an infection
    c) a response to mechanical irritation
    d) a sign of over-wear

129. In addition to mucus formation, itching, and lens intolerance, the hallmark of GPC is:
    a) corneal ulcers
    b) inflamed pinguecula
    c) papillae on the palpebral conjunctiva of the upper lid
    d) papillae on the bulbar conjunctiva under the upper lid

130. GPC usually can be managed by:
    a) switching the patient to a heat disinfection system
    b) refitting the patient with extended wear lenses
    c) dispensing new lenses and using surfactant and enzymatic cleaners regularly
    d) continuing lens wear while using vasoconstrictor drops

131. Symptoms of rigid contact lens over-wear include all of the following *except*:
    a) moderate to severe pain and photophobia
    b) lid swelling
    c) discomfort starts immediately after removing lenses
    d) tearing

132. The most obvious slit lamp finding in OWS is:
    a) apical fluorescein staining
    b) corneal edema
    c) corneal neovascularization
    d) corneal ulceration

133. Some patients experience reduced vision with their glasses after removing their contact lenses. This can last from several minutes to several weeks, and is known as:
    a) contact lens blur
    b) spectacle blur
    c) over-wear syndrome
    d) corneal dryness

134. Spectacle blur is due to:
    a) corneal edema
    b) corneal molding
    c) contact lens over-wear
    d) both a) and b)

135. The best solution for spectacle blur is to fit the patient with:
    a) PMMA rigid lenses
    b) gas-permeable lenses
    c) daily wear soft contact lenses
    d) extended wear soft contact lenses

136. Blurred vision associated with a tight or loose lens:
    a) fluctuates throughout the day
    b) fluctuates with blinking
    c) starts several hours after the lenses are inserted
    d) is always accompanied by redness and discomfort

137. Vision that is clear initially after a blink but then blurs may be associated with:
    a) incorrect power
    b) excessive lens movement
    c) sucked-on lens syndrome
    d) too large an optical zone

138. Blurred vision that occurs after prolonged reading may be due to:
    a) presbyopia
    b) lack of tearing
    c) excessive blinking
    d) an out-of-date prescription

139. In soft lens wearers, the most common cause of blurred vision is:
    a) an inverted lens
    b) a chemical allergy
    c) excessive movement
    d) lens dehydration

140. A 25-year-old patient was prescribed a –1.75 sphere contact lens for the right eye and a –2.50 sphere contact lens for the left. They come in complaining that the vision in the left eye is blurry. You measure their visual acuity at 20/20 OD and 20/40 OS. Slit lamp exam is clear. Over-refraction shows +0.75 sphere OD = 20/20 and –0.75 sphere OS = 20/20. What happened?
    a) The patient was prescribed the wrong lenses.
    b) The patient has developed corneal edema in the right eye.
    c) The patient has developed a cataract in the left eye.
    d) The patient has switched (crossed) the lenses.

Study Note

Suggested reading in *Principles and Practice in Ophthalmic Assisting: A Comprehensive Textbook:*
   Chapter 21: Contact Lenses (pp 379-415)

Explanatory Answers

Part I

1. a) The oxygen that reaches the cornea is affected not only by the permeability of the material, but by lens design, and thickness (both of edges and periphery). An aphakic lens, for example, has a large central thickness and less oxygen transmissibility than a +3.00 lens. By contrast, a high minus lens is thicker at the periphery, which can also cut down on transmission of oxygen.

2. d) The Dk value of a contact is a measure of the material's oxygen permeability. The higher the Dk value, the more oxygen permeable the lens. The base curve is a geometric value. Fluid resistance and osmotic value are made-up terms.

3. b) The soft lens is hydrophilic, which means "loves water." The fact that it absorbs water is responsible for its entire nature. This includes comfort, flexibility, oxygen transmission, etc. There is very little tear exchange under a soft lens (as opposed to a rigid lens). These lenses are not resistant to deposits. A larger diameter is possible because of oxygen transmissibility, but the diameter in and of itself is not responsible for the lens's advantages and disadvantages.

4. b) As a rule, soft lenses (being soft and flexible) do not provide the crisp, sharp vision of rigid lenses.

5. c) The biggest risk listed is that of infection. The pores of soft lens material generally are too small for bacteria to penetrate. However, once the lens forms deposits, there is a rough surface on which bacteria may grow. In addition, the removal of a deposit may create a pit large enough to harbor bacteria. While it is true that modifications are impossible, residual astigmatism goes uncorrected, and the lenses can discolor, these hardly qualify as risks.

6. c) CAB is a gas-permeable material. HEMA is the most common soft lens material. Sometimes other polymers are added to HEMA to enhance lens characteristics. Soft lenses also can be made of silicone polymers. Hydrogel is another word for soft lenses made of HEMA.

7. a) The lower the soft lens's water content, the more rigid it is, and hence, the more durable. Still, the soft lens does not approach rigidity in the sense that a hard or gas-permeable lens does. A low water content lens has *less* oxygen transmissibility.

8. b) The higher the water content of a soft lens, the more oxygen can be transmitted to the cornea. Unfortunately, these lenses are sensitive to dehydration if the environment changes. They also are heat sensitive, and some types may not be disinfected using thermal methods. Given the same water content, a non-HEMA lens is more durable.

9. b) It is generally recommended that extended wear soft contacts be replaced every 3 to 6 months, even if there are no deposits.

10. b) Oxygen circulates under a PMMA lens via the tears.

11. a) Because a gas-permeable lens allows more oxygen to get to the cornea, the eye can tolerate a larger lens. True, it is more comfortable than a PMMA lens, but this is due to the fit (sliding under the upper lid vs bumping into it), not permeability. Lens movement still is important. The properly fit gas-permeable lens does not sit on the lower lid.

12. b) Gas-permeable lenses develop fewer deposits than soft lenses, but they still develop deposits. Answers a), c), and d) are true.

13.   b) Radius is a line drawn from the center of a sphere to the edge. The base curve of a contact lens is actually the radius of the sphere to which the lens corresponds. Answer a) describes circumference, and Answer c) defines diameter.

14.   b) A longer radius corresponds to a flatter base curve. The longer the radius, the bigger the sphere from which the lens was "sliced." A slice of a big sphere would be flatter.

15.   b) The radiuscope is used to measure the base curve of rigid lenses, as well as to provide information about the lens surface, including warpage.

16.   c) The vault of a lens describes the distance from the lens's center to a flat surface. A flatter lens would be closer to surface thus it would have a lower vault. Base curve and radius are the same thing and were defined previously. Diameter is a measurement from one side of the lens to the other, running directly across the center of the lens.

17.   d) See Answer 16. *Note*: Sagittal depth is another term for vault.

18.   b) Increasing lens diameter increases vault and acts to tighten the lens.

19.   b) The optic (or central) zone of a contact is generally in the center, designed to put the best optics of the prescription (which give the clearest vision) directly in front of the patient's line of sight.

20.   a) A rigid lens has a longer wearing time building schedule than a soft lens as in Answers b) through d).

21.   a) It takes about 1 week (barring problems) for a soft lens wearer to build up to full-time daily wear.

22.   b) Full wearing time for a rigid lens wearer can be achieved (in the absence of problems) in 3 to 5 weeks.

23.   c) The upper limit recommended for daily contact lens wear is 15 hours a day.

24.   b) Neither cleaning nor disinfecting is optional. A disinfectant can't reach all the surfaces of a dirty lens. Cleaning removes dirt, film, and deposits; a disinfectant kills germs.

25.   a) The combination soak and wet solutions *do not* eliminate the all-important first step of surface cleaning.

26.   b) The lens should be cleaned gently by a fingertip as the lens rests on the palm. The pressure between the thumb and forefinger is too great. In order for the cleaner to be effective, there must be some physical friction; little, if any, cleaning takes place when the cleaner is applied and rinsed off without any rubbing.

27.   a) Body temperature grunge is easier to remove. A soft lens should not be allowed to dry out.

28.   a) The surfactant acts to clean the surface of the lens, usually rigid contacts. It is not used to soak or rewet. It is toxic to the eye and should never be instilled directly into the eye.

29.   c) Enzyme cleaners are used to remove protein build-up on soft and gas-permeable lenses. They do not provide the advantages listed in Answers a), b), or d).

30.   c) "Jelly bumps" form when calcium and lipids (fat or oil) precipitate out of the tear film and onto the lens.

31.   b) As a lens becomes coated with deposits, its ability to transmit oxygen decreases.

32.   b) Wetting solutions, used with rigid lenses, cause the tear film to spread evenly over the lens. This increases comfort. Wetting solution does not sterilize, reduce deposits, or prevent scratches.

33.   a) Gross as it may be, urine is more sterile than saliva. (Telling your patients this may discourage the terrible habit of wetting a rigid lens in the mouth!) Saliva harbors all kinds of nasty, infection-causing bacteria. Tap water and pool water (although "cleaner" than saliva) are not the right solutions, either, and can cause the lens to adhere to the cornea as well as corneal edema.

34.   d) Patients should understand that contact lens solutions are chemicals that do not always mix well with each other and may even cause an undesirable chemical reaction. Although they need not buy only from your office, they should use one solution system and stick with it unless problems develop.

35.   c) *Acanthamoeba* has been linked with homemade saline made from salt tablets and distilled water. Thimerosal is a preservative that was associated with allergic reactions and is mostly no longer in use. Enzymatic cleaners and packaged samples have not been implicated in *Acanthamoeba* infections.

36. d) In order for disinfection to be maintained, the disinfecting solution should be changed daily. Adding a little active disinfectant to a chamber of old disinfectant ("topping off") dilutes the active solution, rendering it too weak for the purpose. Saline (preserved or otherwise) does not disinfect.

37. b) The contact lens case should *not* be washed with soap because residue could interfere with the disinfectant or cause a film on the lenses. The entire case should be replaced every month or so.

38. a) If a hydrophilic lens doesn't get the water it "wants" from the tear film, its thickness (and thus, optics) can change. However, soft lenses correct spherical errors more successfully than astigmatic errors. An infant and a child are good candidates because the soft lens provides more comfort and a low rate of lens loss on impact. Rigid lenses may pop out on impact, which makes the soft lens a good choice for the recreational basketball player as well.

39. c) There is no connection between taking blood thinners and wearing contact lenses.

40. b) An exophthalmic eye usually is fit better with a soft lens, which is more stable on the eye and doesn't interfere with the lids. Cases represented by the other answers are good candidates.

41. c) A patient who works around smoke, dust, and fumes still can wear contacts, just not at work!

42. a) Contact sports often involve blows to the head, which might pop out a rigid lens. Patients with presbyopia can wear soft or rigid lenses. A person with very mild dexterity problems probably can handle a rigid lens *more* easily. Rigid lenses generally give sharper, more stable vision, and would be ideal for a compulsive person.

43. b) Many practitioners agree that a person who wants contacts only for cosmetic reasons, and doesn't need them for improved vision, is taking more risk than the benefit is worth. The 50-year-old may be emmetropic, but they also are presbyopic, and may warrant a contact lens in one eye for near, or a set of bifocal contacts. The teen and person with aphakia probably will be very motivated.

44. b) A history of episcleritis does not make one a poor contact lens candidate. The patient with the pinguecula might get by with an intrapalpebral fit. The pterygium creates an irregular corneal surface. The patient in Answer a) is the poorest candidate of all. While the infection may clear, the virus itself is still there and can become active again.

45. b) Diabetes is not necessarily associated with dry eye.

Part II

46. b) The methods in Answers a), b), and d) are all accurate. But for most purposes, measuring visible iris is good enough. A pachymeter measures corneal thickness.

47. a) The edges of a rigid lens should fall within the corneal diameter without limbal contact. A soft lens should overlap the limbus.

48. c) If the crosshairs are not centered, you are not reading the corneal apex. Because the corneal periphery is flatter, the resulting fit will be too loose when placed on the steeper apex.

49. d) The closer you get to the retina, the more plus power it takes to converge and focus the image. So a patient with hyperopia may need more power in the contact than in the glasses. Patients with aphakia also have hyperopia. A patient with myopia might need more plus, too (translating to less minus).

50. c) Compensate for vertex distance if the spherical power is 4.00 diopters or more. *Note*: some references may say 3.00 diopters.

51. a) Over-refraction is used to refine the power of the contact lens, and has little application in Answers b) through d).

52. c) You always want to encourage the patient to take as much plus as possible to prevent accommodation. Translated, this means giving the most plus (or subtracting the least).

53. a) If the patient is presbyopic, find out how the lenses are fit before pulling the refractor forward. Are they wearing monofit? Bifocals? Maybe distance OU with reading glasses? Knowing what to expect before you start will make your job easier.

54. c) The power of a soft spherical contact is chosen by the spherical equivalent of the refraction. The K readings are not used for calculating the power.

55. d) To find the spherical equivalent, add half of the cylinder to the sphere, then drop the cylinder and axis.

56. d) The spherical equivalent is necessary since you are fitting a soft spherical contact. Half of the cylinder is +0.50. Add this to the sphere power: –3.00 + 0.50 = –2.50.

57. c) A soft lens fit steeper than K usually will have the effect of a steep lens: poor movement, a plus tear layer, fluctuations in vision when blinking, and discomfort. The vision usually is clearer right after the blink (when the apex of the lens is pushed onto the cornea) and blurs thereafter (when the apex of the lens pulls back off of the cornea).

58. d) A loose lens is a flat lens. There is often edge standoff, which can cause a foreign body sensation. A loose lens also exhibits excessive movement. If the lens slips off center when the patient moves their eyes, vision will blur.

59. b) A loose lens may be tightened by increasing lens diameter or steepening the base curve. Either of these measures will cause the curve of the lens to conform more to the curve of the eye. (A thinner lens also may work because it will adhere to the cornea better.)

60. b) Fit the loosest lens that will give good vision and comfort. Even if it looks like a "sloppy, floppy" fit, as long as the patient is comfortable and can see well, go with it.

61. a) If the tear breakup time is 10 seconds or less, the tear film is considered subnormal.

62. a) A hydrophilic lens (*hydro* = water, *philic* = love) wants water. If it doesn't get it, it will pull any available fluid off the eye, drying a dry eye even more. In this situation, the lens has a tendency to get stuck, not move excessively.

63. d) As a soft lens dries out, its base curve (not diameter) changes, altering its optical qualities and producing blurred vision. Selected tear supplement drops can be used with soft lenses in place. The dry lens moves little if at all.

64. c) Excessive tears equals excessive movement as the lens floats around on the extra fluid. Answers a), b), and d) are seen in a tight/dry lens situation.

65. c) Edge standoff is a sign of a *loose* lens.

66. c) A tight lens is a steep lens. When the patient blinks, the apex of the contact is pushed onto the apex of the cornea, clearing the vision. After 1 or 2 seconds, the lens apex pops back off the cornea and the vision blurs. The opposite is true of a loose, flat lens.

67. a) A tight lens can be loosened by decreasing the diameter or flattening the base curve. Either one of these solutions makes the lens flatter and looser. Doing the opposite would make the lens even tighter, as would increasing the vault. Vertex distance has nothing to do with the lens's physical fit.

68. b) Remember the mnemonic SAM/FAP: steeper add minus, flatter add plus. Answer a) applies in refraction. Answer c) refers to changing the axis of a toric lens. Transposition is not a factor.

69. b) The tear film may create a "lens" (referred to as the *lacrimal lens*) under a rigid contact. If the contact is fit steeper than K, it will have a high vault. The tears under the contact will form a plus tear lens, and the contact will need to have minus power added to adjust. A lens fit flatter than K has a low vault, creating a minus tear lens. Plus power will need to be added to the contact to compensate. Axial length is not used in determining contact lens power, nor is a cell count. The size of the fovea is not a factor, either.

70. a) The upper lid should control the movement of the gas-permeable lens. The lid should "grab" the lens, move it with each blink, and "hold" the lens up off the lower lid.

71. a) Fitting a lens "on K" means to match the base curve of the lens to the *flattest* corneal curve.

72. b) A patient with large pupils needs a larger optic zone and a larger lens for best vision. If the pupil dilates beyond the optic zone, then light is coming through the peripheral curves into the eye. This causes glare and light flares. The risks and side effects associated with miotics make that option unacceptable.

73. d) A patient with dry eyes needs to take longer to build up rigid lens wearing time. The word "only" in Answer a) should have identified it as incorrect.

74. b) Minus cylinder form is used for rigid lens power calculation. Spherical equivalent is used in soft lenses. See Answers 49 and 50 about vertex distance.

75. b) When fitting a low power spherical rigid lens on K, just use the spherical portion of the refraction. No other calculating is needed.

76. c) An upper lid that grabs or pushes is a tight lid. A lax lid may move the lens little, if any.

77. a) Astigmatism that is "left over" after the eye is fit with a contact lens is called *residual astigmatism*.

78. c) Residual astigmatism is most often caused by lenticular astigmatism, or irregular curvature of the crystalline lens (which doesn't show up on K readings).
c) Residual astigmatism (the amount of astigmatism that is not corrected by the contact lens) is usually due to lenticular astigmatism, or irregular curvature of the crystalline lens inside the eye.

79. c) A small amount of astigmatism in a spherical soft lens wearer is merely tolerated, not masked or eliminated. As long as the patient tolerates it, there is no reason to rush into fitting a toric lens.

80. a) As long as the astigmatism is less than 1/3 of the total refractive error, there is a good chance that the patient can tolerate the vision provided by a spherical soft contact lens.

81. d) You can generally ignore residual astigmatism of 0.50 or less when fitting a soft spherical contact.

82. d) If astigmatism is 3.00 diopters or less, it is generally adequate to fit a spherical rigid lens. The lens itself, by its position and tilt, may induce enough cylinder to compensate.

83. b) Keeping the cylinder properly aligned means keeping the lens aligned. A spherical lens normally is pushed around and rotated during blinking. This spells disaster for a toric lens fit.

84. b) Soft toric lenses have etch marks or dots either at the base or at the horizontal meridian. These can be observed with the slit lamp. The examiner looks for lens rotation as the patient blinks.

85. d) The degrees of rotation are added to the patient's refraction.

86. b) Stability of a soft toric lens is influenced by the contour, position, and tightness of the lids. Weighting and truncation are the techniques used to cope with lens instability but are not the cause of the instability. K readings are used to fit the lens but are not the cause of instability. The thickness and water content are not factors either.

87. d) When fitting a soft toric, you want the least amount of cylinder correction that the patient will accept, because the lens will rotate a bit on the eye. The higher the amount of cylinder, the more pronounced the visual problems caused by this rotation.

88. c) Truncation is removing a portion of the bottom of the lens to create a straight edge. This straight edge rides the lower lid margin and helps keep the soft toric lens from rotating, thus providing stability.

89. d) Rigid toric lenses might be the lens of choice when the K readings and refraction don't match either in power or in axis as in Answers a) and c), as well as when there is lenticular astigmatism.

90. d) Simultaneous vision bifocal contacts are concentrically designed. The inner "bull's-eye" is for distance vision, and the outer ring is for near vision. Each eye is fit with such a lens. They are available in progressive style.

91. a) Ghost images are a frequent complaint. First, this is due to the transition area between the segments. It is also due to the unfocused areas, or portions of what the patient is looking at (whether near or far) that fall into the "wrong" segment.

92. b) In the monovision technique, one eye (usually the dominant eye) is fitted for distance and the other eye is fitted for near. In some cases, the dominant eye might be fitted for near, but this is not the routine procedure.

93. c) Anyone who continuously works up close and requires "perfect" near vision all the time (eg, a bookkeeper, accountant) probably is not a good candidate for monovision. Monovision involves a trade-off. Both distance and near vision are somewhat compromised and binocular vision is sacrificed, but the patient doesn't have to cope with bifocals (glasses or contacts). Those people listed in the other answers do some up-close work, but also need to look frequently at a distance to see their audience.

94.   a) The test for the driver's exam is a distance vision test. Often the eye fit for near will fail to read the required distance figures. In this case, a letter or form may be required from the physician, explaining the situation.

Part III

95.   a) Patients should be given a training session that includes verbal instruction, plus written instructions to refer to at home. Providing only written instruction or no written material at all is an invitation to failure. Trusting patient instruction to other patients (who may or may not remember *their* instructions) is ill-advised.

96.   c) Patients should be taught to wash their hands before handling lenses. This is one of the rare times where "always" does not signal a wrong answer. Its use in Answer a) renders it incorrect, however.

97.   a) Patients can be taught to recognize an inverted lens by both visual inspection and the taco test. There's no such thing as the jelly roll test or an inversion tester.

98.   c) Inserting a soft lens is easiest if the lens is wet (not dripping) and the finger is dry (to prevent sticking).

99.   a) The nondominant hand is used to pin the upper lid to the brow to prevent blinking. The lens itself is best handled with the dominant hand.

100.   a) The lens should be placed directly on the cornea, bull's-eye style. Sliding isn't a good idea with a rigid lens, as this can cause a corneal abrasion. A lens on the lid margin is almost sure to be blinked out.

101.   a) To prevent a filmy build-up on the lens, only hand soap that is free of moisturizers and other additives should be used. Make up, face cream, and hair spray should be used before inserting lenses. Hand lotion should be used after.

102.   d) Soft lenses are pinched out with thumb and forefinger at the 9 and 3 o'clock positions. A plunger could tear a soft lens. Blinking and squeezing don't work.

103.   c) Long fingernails are the nemesis of soft contact lenses. A person who is unwilling to cut the nails can learn to adapt, however, by turning the fingers to keep the nails away from the lens and eye.

104.   c) Every patient who wears contact lenses on an extended basis needs to lubricate the lenses regularly, especially every morning. It is not necessary for every patient to remove and clean the lenses every day, although some do and should. Nor is it advisable to blithely allow every patient to wear them for a month at a time. Most physicians recommend weekly removal. If the eye is red or painful, the lens must always be removed.

105.   a) The FDA recommends that patients who sleep in extended wear lenses remove and clean (or dispose of, as appropriate) the lenses and leave them out for one night every week.

106.   b) Blinking out a rigid lens requires the patient to look down, open both eyes wide, and pull the temporal canthus with thumb or finger. The lens must be centered on the eye for this to work.

107.   c) Teach your patients never to apply the plunger to the eye unless they know exactly where the contact lens is. "Fishing" for a lost lens with the plunger is disastrous, and painful if the plunger adheres to cornea or conjunctiva. A drop of wetting solution helps the lens stick to the plunger, and carrying an extra plunger is always a good idea.

108.   c) A dropped lens should be cleaned and disinfected before wearing. No exceptions.

109.   d) Before the new contact lens wearer walks out the door, the final, cardinal rule to be emphasized is to remove a lens if the eye becomes red and/or painful. No exceptions.

110.   c) Of those listed, checking the fit is the most important. It is possible for the patient to have good vision and be comfortable in the lenses and still be developing corneal neovascularization. Intraocular pressure is not usually measured at a routine contact recheck, but would be at an annual exam.

111.   a) According to the Contact Lens Rule, the prescriber is required to give the patient a copy of their contact lens prescription once the patient is successfully fit.

112. c) There could be several reasons why a daily wear, 2-week replacement lens might have deposits. It is possible that the patient is just one of those people who form deposits quickly. But your main questions to the patient would be to ensure that the patient is cleaning the lenses properly and replacing them at the prescribed intervals.

113. a) A foreign body sensation is the most common symptom of lens deposits. The deposits rub on the cornea, creating discomfort and perhaps corneal abrasions

114. a) Problems associated with a tight lens include corneal edema, sensations of soreness, injection, foggy vision, and ghost images. Answers b) and d) go with a loose lens. Allergies to solutions don't affect the fit per se.

115. b) A loose lens is a flat lens. There is often edge standoff, which can cause a foreign body sensation. A loose lens also exhibits excessive movement. If the lens slips off center when the patient moves their eyes, vision will blur. Power and hygiene do not come into play.

116. b) Corneal edema is caused by a lack of oxygen to the cornea.

117. d) Symptoms of corneal edema include blurred vision, halos around lights, redness, and burning.

118. c) Hypoxia is a lack of oxygen. Higher-powered lenses are thicker, either in the center (plus lens) or at the edges (minus lens). Either way, this can create a decrease in the amount of oxygen getting to the cornea.

120. b) If a patient wearing extended wear contact lenses develops edema, try refitting with a different material or water content. A larger lens will tend to make the problem worse. You probably fit the lens on K to begin with. Cleaning solutions would not make a difference.

121. a) Vascularization, or the development of new, abnormal blood vessels in the cornea, results from a lack of oxygen (hypoxia).

122. b) The superior limbal area of the cornea (under the upper lid) is most often the spot where vascularization occurs.

123. b) Changing solutions won't affect neovascularization, which is not an allergic response to begin with. A looser, thinner, or higher water content lens would allow more oxygen to get through.

124. d) A rigid lens that does not center properly and continually rubs on the limbus may stimulate the growth of corneal blood vessels. It should ride on the central cornea, be lifted, and then drop a bit with each blink. Enzymatic cleaner will have little effect, if any.

125. b) *Pseudomonas* ulcers are more common in extended wear soft lenses. The sleeping eye is the type of warm, oxygen-poor environment in which bacteria thrive.

126. a) A corneal ulcer is not caused by sensitivity to contact lens chemicals. It is possible for a chemical keratitis to develop if solutions not meant for use directly in the eye are instilled by mistake, but that is different from an ulcer. Corneal ulcers associated with contact lens wear may be due to infection, trauma, or lack of oxygen.

127. d) Although gas-permeable contact lens wearers may develop ulcers, they usually are not related to the lens itself. Ulcers are more commonly seen with soft contact lens wear.

128. a) GPC is considered to be an allergic response of the body to the protein deposits on a contact lens (usually soft). As the deposits break down, an allergic response is triggered.

129. c) The signs and symptoms of GPC include itching, mucus, lens intolerance, and the formation of large papillae on the inner surface of the upper eyelid. (The palpebral conjunctiva lines the lids; the bulbar conjunctiva covers the sclera.)

130. c) New lenses, with an admonition to keep them meticulously clean, are in order. Heat disinfection is used rarely these days. Extended wear lenses are more likely to be associated with GPC problems due to increased opportunity for protein build-up and lens contact with the upper lid. Vasoconstrictor drops may decrease the redness but will not address the allergic component of the problem.

131. c) Symptoms usually start 2 to 3 hours after removing the lenses.

132. a) The typical slit lamp findings in OWS are diffuse apical erosions that stain deeply with fluorescein.

133. b) Spectacle blur is the phenomenon noticed by contact lens wearers when they remove their contacts and experience blurred vision with their glasses. This blur can last from several minutes to weeks.

134. d) Spectacle blur is due to corneal edema (excess fluid in the cornea because of hypoxia) and/or corneal molding (where the cornea's shape is altered by the pressure of the contact lens).

135. b) Gas-permeable contact lenses reduce the amount of noticeable spectacle blur. While corneal edema may occur with GPCLs, the edema is more diffuse (spread evenly over the corneal surface), instead of central as with PMMA lenses.

136. b) Vision that fluctuates with blinking is often associated with a loose or tight lens. The word "always" in answer d) should have been a red flag that it is incorrect.

137. b) A tight or loose lens is not the only thing that can cause vision to fluctuate with a blink. If there is excessive movement, the patient may not be looking through the optic zone. Vision through a peripheral part of the lens will not be as sharp. Fitting a lens with a larger optic zone might be part of the answer, along with reducing the movement.

138. b) Blurring after reading for long periods of time is usually due to dehydration. The patient gets so intent on reading that they forget to blink. The same thing can happen when watching TV or working on a computer. You weren't given enough information (ie, the patient's age) to decide if the patient was presbyopic or not.

139. d) See Answer 138. If the lens and cornea look good, try having the patient use rewetting drops before you go into a lot of fitting changes. The other items can cause blurring, but dehydration is the most common.

140. d) The lenses are switched. The over-refraction is of equal amounts but opposite signs, which is the big giveaway. The least myopic eye, now wearing a stronger lens, can accommodate and still see 20/20. The more myopic eye, now wearing a weaker lens, simply cannot see as well.

Chapter 19

Ophthalmic Imaging

Ledford JK.
Certified Ophthalmic Technician Exam
Review Manual, Third Edition (pp 443-451).
© 2023 Taylor & Francis Group.

> ## ABBREVIATIONS USED IN THIS CHAPTER
>
> - FA   fluorescein angiography
> - HRT   Heidelberg Retinal Tomograph
> - OCT   optical coherence tomography
> - RNFL   retinal nerve fiber layer

Fluorescein Angiography*

1. If, after absorbing energy, the molecules of a material are excited and light is emitted when they return to a ground state, this is termed:
   a) electromagnetic spectrum
   b) luminescence
   c) gamma radiation
   d) incandescence

2. If luminescence stops after the exciting light has been removed, this is termed:
   a) hypofluorescence
   b) incandescence
   c) phosphorescence
   d) fluorescence

3. Blood that has been mixed with fluorescein will glow when excited by the appropriate wavelength of light because the fluorescein then:
   a) absorbs blue light and emits yellow-green light
   b) absorbs green light and emits yellow light
   c) absorbs all light except blue
   d) reflects all light except yellow-green

4. FA is which type of test?
   a) diagnostic
   b) subjective
   c) radiation
   d) ultrasonic

5. The blue filter that stimulates the fluorescein to emit a higher wavelength is a(n):
   a) barrier filter
   b) Wratten #12 filter
   c) diffuser
   d) exciter filter

6. The barrier filter:
   a) absorbs unwanted blue (exciter) light
   b) is red
   c) is used to take the monochromatic (red-free) photo
   d) is not needed during the "late phase" of an angiogram

---

* For questions regarding the phases of an FA study, see Chapter 11: Supplemental Testing.

7. **If the FA exciter filter is worn out, one must:**
    a) stop the fluorescein study immediately
    b) inject more fluorescein
    c) simply replace the exciter filter
    d) replace both the exciter and the barrier filters

8. **One must carefully review the orders for a FA in order to determine:**
    a) which eye should be photographed in the red-free photos
    b) which eye should be photographed during the transit phase
    c) which eye should be photographed during the late phase
    d) which arm should be used when injecting the fluorescein

9. **The first step in a fluorescein dye study is:**
    a) patient education and informed consent
    b) applying a tourniquet
    c) disinfecting the patient's skin
    d) selecting the injection site

10. **The side effects or complications of fluorescein dye injection include:**
    a) yellowish skin and urine
    b) nausea and vomiting
    c) infiltration
    d) all of the above

11. **Prior to taking the control photos, one must:**
    a) dilate the pupils
    b) loosen the tourniquet
    c) start the camera's timer
    d) all of the above

12. **A photograph is taken prior to dye injection using a green filter in order to:**
    a) document any pseudofluorescence
    b) provide a clinical representation of the subject
    c) make sure the photo card has enough memory
    d) identify the patient's face

13. **The actual act of injecting the fluorescein should start when the:**
    a) intravenous needle is inserted
    b) photographer is ready
    c) tourniquet has been tightened
    d) patient gives the go-ahead

14. **Leakage from a retinal blood vessel will manifest as:**
    a) hypophosphorescence
    b) hyperphosphorescence
    c) hypofluorescence
    d) hyperfluorescence

15. **If a retinal blood vessel is occluded, this will be manifest as:**
    a) hyperincandescence
    b) hypoincandescence
    c) hyperfluorescence
    d) hypofluorescence

16.   **Even with the advent of OCT, FAs are still used. One of the most common instances for FA is:**
a) proliferative diabetic retinopathy
b) glaucoma
c) dry macular degeneration
d) retinal detachment

Corneal Topography

17.   **Which of the following may be used to generate a 3-D map of corneal curvature?**
a) hand-held Placido's disc
b) keratometer
c) corneal topography
d) pachymeter

18.   **The difference between corneal topography and tomography is that *tomography*:**
a) evaluates the corneal cap
b) is used exclusively for intraocular lens calculations
c) evaluates the corneal anterior and posterior surfaces
d) also measures axial length

19.   **Calibration of topography unit must be done for any of the following *except*:**
a) once daily when activating the instrument
b) after transporting
c) prior to every measurement
d) after someone rams it with their electric scooter

20.   **Corneal topography has implications in each of the following *except*:**
a) keratoconus
b) trichiasis
c) contact lens fitting
d) refractive surgery

21.   **When looking at a corneal topographic map, which is represented by cooler colors (ie, those closer to the blue spectrum)?**
a) central areas
b) thinner areas
c) steep areas
d) flatter areas

22.   **A "bow-tie" pattern on corneal topography represents:**
a) regular astigmatism
b) thin areas
c) irregular astigmatism
d) that corneal refractive surgery has been done

Heidelberg Retinal Tomography

23. Which of the following is used to create images with the HRT?
     a) mega-ultraviolet light
     b) magnified ultrasonic waves
     c) confocal scanning laser
     d) photon torpedoes

24. The HRT's use in evaluating glaucoma is mainly for imaging of the:
     a) corneal endothelium
     b) RNFL
     c) macula
     d) optic nerve head

25. The HRT is used mainly to evaluate glaucoma, but is also used to assess:
     a) potential acuity
     b) keratoconus
     c) dark adaptation
     d) retinopathy

26. You are performing an HRT on a patient with glaucoma who has had 4 previous scans. The analysis is displaying some areas in red. This means that:
     a) there has been disease progression
     b) the scans were inadequate
     c) the patient should not have any more scans
     d) you must discontinue the scan

Optical Coherence Tomography

27. Which of the following tests is noncontact?
     a) Schiøtz
     b) Schirmer's
     c) electroretinography
     d) OCT

28. High-resolution imaging with light is used in which of the following?
     a) HRT
     b) OCT
     c) fundus photography
     d) brightness acuity tester

29. Which of the following testing modalities can be used to image and measure the cornea and the RNFL in cross-section?
     a) teleretinal imaging
     b) OCT
     c) pachymetry
     d) FA

30. **Which of the following would *not* be evaluated using OCT?**
    a) macular edema
    b) macular degeneration
    c) cataracts
    d) glaucoma

31. **Each of the following can be evaluated using OCT *except*:**
    a) pituitary gland
    b) keratoconus
    c) partial vitreous detachment from the macula
    d) LASIK flap

32. **In order to view the ocular surface, one would use:**
    a) anterior chamber OCT
    b) anterior segment OCT
    c) hypocorneal OCT
    d) posterior chamber OCT

33. **Which of the following signal strengths indicates that a repeat scan is definitely necessary?**
    a) 5
    b) 7
    c) 8
    d) 10

34. **Black areas on the OCT scan represent:**
    a) false positives
    b) false negatives
    c) missing tissue
    d) missing data

35. **When interpreting an OCT for glaucoma, the practitioner will also take into account the patient's:**
    a) axial length
    b) scleral rigidity
    c) anterior chamber depth
    d) latest visual field test

36. **All of the following regarding "red disease" on an OCT are true *except*:**
    a) It may be caused by anything that enhances the signal.
    b) It may indicate false positives.
    c) It may occur in people with high myopia.
    d) It may result in overtreatment of glaucoma.

37. **"Green disease" on an OCT:**
    a) is backed up by visual field results
    b) shows normal when there may be a problem
    c) means everything is normal
    d) indicates that intraocular pressure is normal

Study Notes

Suggested reading in *Principles and Practice in Ophthalmic Assisting: A Comprehensive Textbook:*
Chapter 15: Ophthalmic Photography (*Fluorescein Angiography* pp 285-289)
Chapter 16: Diagnostic Imaging (*Corneal Topography* pp 298-300, *Optical Coherence Tomography* pp 300-303, *Confocal Scanning Laser Ophthalmoscopy* pp 303-304)

Explanatory Answers

1. b) Luminescence occurs when a suitable material is exposed to incidental light. This causes the electrons (orbiting atomic particles) to jump to different orbits. When the electrons later fall back into their original orbits, a photon of light is given off.

2. d) Fluorescence is a type of luminescence where the excited material glows only while stimulated with the exciting light. (If it lasts for a long time, it is called phosphorescence.)

3. a) Properly excited fluorescein absorbs light in the 465 to 490 nm wavelength range (blue light) and emits light in the 520 to 530 nm range (yellow-green light). This property holds true even when the fluorescein is mixed into the bloodstream.

4. a) Fluorescein angiography is a diagnostic test that provides information about the patient's internal vasculature.

5. d) The blue exciter filter emits the light that stimulates the fluorescein. When the dye absorbs the blue light, it is pushed to a higher wavelength and emits yellow-green light. Regarding the barrier filter, see Answer 6. A Wratten #12 filter is a yellow filter used at the slit lamp with topical fluorescein. A diffusing filter equalizes light across a field of observation.

6. a) The yellow barrier filter acts to block out the blue light of the exciter filter so that the fluorescence will be picked up in the photo. It is not used for the red-free photo but is still needed during the late phase.

7. d) The exciter and barrier filters are matched in order to maximize the fluorescent effect on film. If you mix filter types, you may get filters that overlap, resulting in less than optimum images.

8. b) The transit phase of the study starts about 10 seconds after the dye is injected and involves rapid-fire photos (every 1 to 3 seconds) for another 30 seconds or so, making it impossible to image the transit phase of both eyes. You need to know which eye to concentrate on before you start. The red-free and late phase photos are taken on both eyes.

9. a) FA involves injection of dye into the blood stream. It is imperative that the patient be advised about risks, possible complications, and side effects. A written consent *must* be obtained.

10. d) The patient should be informed that the skin and urine may be discolored for several hours after injection. Side effects of the dye can include nausea and vomiting (always have an emesis basin available). Infiltration (extravasation) occurs if the dye is injected into the tissues instead of into the vein; ice may help. Allergic reaction (including rash, itching, shortness of breath, and anaphylaxis) can also occur, so it is essential to have a properly equipped crash cart handy.

11. a) The pupils need to be well dilated prior to the control photos. (A control photo is taken with both filters in place before the fluorescein is injected.) The timer is started at the same time that the dye is pushed.

12. b) The green filter is used to create a "red-free" photo of the fundus. This filter makes the blood vessels appear black, increasing the contrast and making the vessels more visible. The optic nerve appears white. The photo provides a reference photo to compare to the angiogram.

13. b) The photographer needs to be the one to say when the injection should start. If the dye is pushed and the photographer is unaware of it, valuable photographs will be missed in the sequence. In addition, the timer on the camera is started when the dye is pushed.

14. d) Extra fluorescein will show up in areas of a leak. The prefix "hyper" = over, so there is dye over the usual amount, or hyperfluorescence.

15.   d) In the case of a blockage in a retinal blood vessel, the dye will be blocked from entering (a filling defect) and hypofluorescence will occur. (The prefix "hypo" = under, so there is dye under the usual amount.)

16.   a) In spite of the widespread use of OCT, FA remains the go-to evaluation for diabetic retinopathy, especially the proliferative type.

17.   c) The corneal topography unit evaluates light reflections off the cornea in order to create a map of the cornea's surface. These images are then compiled and evaluated by computer and used to generate a topographic representation of the cornea's curvature. The topographer is actually based on Placido's disc, which is simply a round disc with concentric circles on it through which the observer views the eye. It does not create a map. The keratometer measures the curvature of the corneal cap, and the pachymeter measures only corneal thickness.

18.   c) While topography evaluates the corneal surface, tomography evaluates both the anterior and posterior surfaces.

19.   c) The unit should be calibrated after transporting, or if it has suffered impact or thermal shock, and daily before starting. It is not necessary to calibrate prior to each measurement.

20.   b) Trichiasis is where the eyelashes grow backward and rub on the cornea; it is not evaluated with corneal topography. However, corneal topography plays an important role in diagnosing and following keratoconus patients, in complicated contact lens fittings, and in pre- and post-procedure refractive surgery evaluations.

21.   d) Cool colors (blues, purples) signify flatter areas of the cornea. Areas with a more warm color (red, orange, yellow) are steeper (HINT: you *steep warm tea*").

22.   a) A pattern like a "bow-tie" or "figure 8," where the 2 halves join at a narrow point roughly in the center of the image, represents regular corneal astigmatism. This means that the steepest and flattest meridians are 90 degrees from each other. It is not an indication of corneal thickness or that refractive surgery has been done. In irregular astigmatism, the pattern is ambiguous because the meridians are more or less than 90 degrees apart.

23.   c) The HRT uses harmless scanning laser to create images of the optic nerve and the area around it. It takes multiple scans, analyzes them and calculates an "average," then displays a 3-D image. The terms mega-ultraviolet light, magnified ultrasonic waves, and photon torpedoes are all made up. (Well, photon torpedoes *do* exist in the Star Trek universe!)

24.   d) HRT has been considered the "gold standard" for imaging the optic nerve head to detect erosion of the nerve in glaucoma, especially in early stages. While the RNFL can be imaged with HRT, this is usually done via OCT. The macula can also be imaged but is not the area of greatest interest in glaucoma.

25.   d) The HRT was designed mainly for glaucoma but is also useful to evaluate retinopathy (diabetic retinopathy, macular degeneration, etc).

26.   a) The analysis program will display red in areas where loss has occurred since the last scan. Green indicates that the area is stable.

27.   d) Of those listed, all require contact with the globe except OCT. The Schiøtz is an indentation tonometer that contacts the cornea. In Schirmer's tear testing, filter strips are placed in the inferior cul-de-sac. The ERG involves electrodes that are placed on the numbed cornea.

28.   b) The OCT uses high-resolution imaging, which involves near-infrared light. The HRT uses laser. Fundus photography may use filters but is still visible light. The brightness acuity tester does not involve imaging.

29.   b) The OCT uses high resolution with near-infrared light to image cross-sectioned "slices" of the eye, especially useful in retinal evaluations but also that of the cornea. Teleretinal imaging involves taking fundus photos that are relayed via internet to a practitioner who evaluates them remotely. Pachymetry measures the thickness of the cornea, and fluorescein angiography is a "simple" photographic technique that does not image cross-sections.

30. c) Cataracts, being a media opacity, actually interfere with OCT imaging. They are diagnosed with the slit lamp.

31. a) The OCT is a light modality and cannot penetrate opaque structures such as those that stand between the eye and the pituitary. The penetration of the OCT is also not deep enough to image the pituitary even if it was visible. The other entities are often evaluated with OCT.

32. b) The anterior segment of the eye is from the external cornea to the back of the crystalline lens. The anterior *chamber* is from the corneal endothelium (ie, inside) to the pupil; the posterior chamber is from the pupil to the back of the lens. (Remember, the posterior segment would be from the back of the lens through the vitreous and to include the retina.) "Hypocorneal" is a bogus term. So this was, actually, more of an anatomy question.

33. a) Minimum acceptable signal strength for an OCT is > 6.

34. d) The OCT displays areas of missing data as black.

35. d) Because the optic nerve fibers are damaged in a specific pattern in glaucoma, the physician will look to match areas of fiber loss to corresponding defects in the visual field.

36. a) In "red disease," the OCT "detects" disease that isn't really there. This may occur due to anything that blocks (*not* enhances) the signal such as floaters, cataracts, the pupil edge, a smudge on lens, or a blink. The appearance of all that red may induce the practitioner to treat for a disease process that isn't there or isn't as severe as the scan would suggest.

37. b) In "green disease," the RNFL scans as normal but is actually missing a problem. Missed optic nerve damage may mean that a person with damaging intraocular pressure is left untreated.

Bibliography

Asrani SG. OCT and glaucoma: artifact alert. *Rev Ophthalmol*. Published Feb 23, 2013. Accessed March 18, 2023. http://reviewofophthalmology.com/article/oct-and-glaucoma-artifact-alert

Khouri AS, Fechtner RD, Fingeret M. Heidelberg Retina Tomography. Entokey search engine. Accessed March 18, 2023. https://entokey.com/heidelberg-retina-tomography/

Optical + Biomedical Engineering Laboratory. Introduction to OCT. OBEL Website. Accessed March 18, 2023. http://obel.ee.uwa.edu.au/research/fundamentals/introduction-oct/

Podoleanu AG. Optical coherence tomography. *J Microsc*. 2012;247(3):209-219. doi:10.1111/j.1365-2818.2012.03619.x

Chapter 20

Photography and Videography*

* For questions/information about specific disorders/entities, see Chapter 16: General Medical Knowledge.

Ledford JK.
Certified Ophthalmic Technician Exam Review Manual, Third Edition (pp 453-467).
© 2023 Taylor & Francis Group.

ABBREVIATIONS USED IN THIS CHAPTER

- DSLR   digital single-lens reflex (camera)
- OD   right eye
- OS   left eye
- UWF   ultra-widefield
- WF   widefield

Photography Basics

1. **Every camera includes the following elements:**
    a) aperture, shutter, and sensor/film
    b) lens, sensor/film, and diaphragm
    c) camera body, lens, and frame counter
    d) aperture, camera body, and sensor/film

2. **A good camera lens system will:**
    a) effectively focus an image at any distance from the subject
    b) have the same focal length for all sensor/film formats
    c) be made up of only plus (convex) lenses
    d) produce sharp images on the sensor/film plane when properly focused

3. **The focal length of a camera lens is defined as:**
    a) the distance between the sensor/film and the subject
    b) the distance between the lens and the subject
    c) the distance between the lens and the sensor/film
    d) the distance between the lens and the object in focus

4. **Which of the following lenses makes the image appear larger or closer because of its longer focal length?**
    a) telephoto
    b) normal
    c) wide-angle
    d) micro lens

5. **Which of the following lenses has a variable focal length?**
    a) Soper lens
    b) macro lens
    c) zoom lens
    d) micro lens

6. **Depth of field is defined as:**
    a) the point at which the camera is focused
    b) the distance between the subject and the sensor/film
    c) the distance range within which objects are focused clearly
    d) the width of the field that will appear on the sensor/film

7. **As a general rule, the depth of field covers:**
    a) a field width equal to 1/2 of that of the human eye
    b) the entire field visible through the camera
    c) 1/2 behind and 1/2 in front of the point of focus
    d) 2/3 behind and 1/3 in front of the point of focus

8. **Which of the following modalities is the standard for transmitting and storing medical images and information?**
    a) DICOM
    b) JPEG
    c) GIF
    d) Fortran

Slit Lamp/Anterior Segment Photography*

9. **Before taking anterior segment photos with the slit lamp, one should:**
    a) wipe all lenses and mirrors with a dry tissue
    b) focus each ocular
    c) instill lubricating drops
    d) instill topical anesthetic

10. **You are taking a photo of a conjunctival nevus. Which of the following tips will help ensure a clear image?**
    a) Focus on the nevus, pull back a little, then slowly go forward until the nevus first becomes clear.
    b) Focus on the nevus, go forward a little, then slowly pull back until the nevus first becomes clear.
    c) Focus on the nevus and take the image.
    d) Focus on the nevus then move slightly left and right until the nevus is clearest.

11. **When performing slit lamp photography, a photograph of the eye using low magnification and diffuse lighting is recommended to:**
    a) judge the patient's tolerance to the flash
    b) judge the corneal reflection
    c) provide identification
    d) provide orientation

12. **Which of the following regarding use of the diffuser is *not* true?**
    a) It provides uniform illumination across the field.
    b) It increases the perception of depth.
    c) The beam should be open prior to introducing the diffuser.
    d) It eliminates some reflection.

13. **Which of the following is *not* appropriate for imaging using the diffuser?**
    a) cornea
    b) eyelid
    c) conjunctiva
    d) iris

* For questions regarding basic slit lamp use including illumination techniques, see Chapter 11 section *Proper Use of Slit Lamp*.
  In retrospect, I feel that many of the slit lamp photography and fundus photography questions in the *Certified Ophthalmic Assistant Exam Review Manual, Third Edition* were more of a COT® level; I have included some of the same questions in this section to make sure you are prepared for your exam.

14.   By convention as well as for ease of use, the illuminator in slit lamp photography is usually positioned:
   a) nasally
   b) temporally
   c) temporally for OD and nasally for OS
   d) nasally for OD and temporally for OS

15.   When imaging the cornea using direct lighting, the light should be focused so that:
   a) the light is reflected back from the iris
   b) the diffuser is in center frame
   c) the pupil is in sharp focus
   d) the background is dark

16.   When taking a slit lamp photo, if one wished to highlight the contours of an iris tumor, the illumination technique of choice would be:
   a) tangential
   b) diffuse
   c) pinpoint
   d) retroillumination

17.   If one was to take a slit lamp photograph of spoking in a cortical cataract, an effective illumination technique would be:
   a) tangential
   b) diffuse
   c) pinpoint
   d) retroillumination

18.   The higher the magnification, the more difficult it can be to get clear photos. This is due, in part to the magnification of:
   a) lashes
   b) patient movement
   c) lids
   d) tear film

Fundus Photography*

19.   In fundus photography, in order to achieve a clear image at the sensor/film plane:
   a) the reticule and subject must be in focus simultaneously
   b) the ocular(s) must be set for the subject's refractive error
   c) the diopter correction dial must be set at plus
   d) the ocular(s) must be set at zero

20.   The purpose of the reticule in fundus photography is:
   a) to compensate for the subject's refractive error
   b) to compensate for the photographer's refractive error
   c) to superimpose a measurement scale on each photograph
   d) to provide a reference point for focusing

* The IJCAHPO® flash cards have a lot of questions on phases of fluorescein angiography under this topic. I have covered these in sections of Chapter 11: Supplemental Testing.

21. **The primary component of the optical imaging system of the fundus camera is a(n):**
    a) aspheric lens that acts as an indirect ophthalmoscope
    b) astigmatic lens that acts as an indirect ophthalmoscope
    c) aspheric lens that acts as a retinoscope
    d) divergent lens that acts as a microscope

22. **In fundus photography:**
    a) the clarity of the cornea and lens do not make a difference in photo clarity
    b) the camera's internal lens system is the only consideration
    c) the patient's cornea and lens become part of the camera's optical system
    d) the dioptric power of the lens and cornea are discounted

23. **The illumination exposure system of the fundus camera includes:**
    a) both halogen and tungsten light bulbs
    b) a fixation light and flash system
    c) the view lamp and the electronic flash system
    d) a beam splitter and view lamp

24. **When aligning the fundus camera, it is best to:**
    a) have the patient look straight ahead while you look through the camera, adjusting the joy stick
    b) have the patient close both eyes so you can see the donut projected on the eyelid as you adjust camera position
    c) have the patient look straight ahead so you can see the donut projected on the cornea as you adjust camera position
    d) have the patient sit back and relax until you have the camera in position

25. **You are centering on the fundus when a light yellow crescent appears in the upper left of the viewing field. This is caused by:**
    a) illumination set too high
    b) reflection off of a cataract
    c) pathology in the fundus
    d) reflection off of the edge of the pupil

26. **In the previous scenario, you should:**
    a) reduce illumination
    b) move the camera slightly down and to the right
    c) move the camera slightly up and to the left
    d) use the dioptric compensation device

27. **Poor detail on a fundus photograph can be caused by all of the following *except*:**
    a) improper focusing
    b) hazy media
    c) retinal pathology
    d) failing to set the eyepiece accurately

28. **Inadequate dilation results in fundus photographs with:**
    a) half of the frame unexposed
    b) a general blur
    c) a gray, fuzzy quadrant
    d) streaks

29.   **Astigmatism during fundus photography may be induced by:**
      a) the patient's accommodation
      b) the photographer's accommodation
      c) the angle of the camera to the cornea
      d) use of dioptric compensation

30.   **The photographic result of uncorrected induced astigmatism is:**
      a) overexposure
      b) a bright crescent at the periphery
      c) blurring in one meridian
      d) distortion

31.   **Standard fundus imaging in diabetics involves:**
      a) imaging 7 fields
      b) taking stereo angles of 3 fields
      c) centering the macula, then imaging to right and left of macula
      d) centering the optic nerve, then imaging above and below the nerve

32.   **In diabetic fundus imaging, part of each image overlaps part of another (or several) image(s). A single, panoramic view from combining these images is known as a:**
      a) diorama
      b) triptych
      c) diabetic panorama
      d) montage

33.   **Standard fields diabetic fundus photography allow imaging of what field of view?**
      a) 25 degrees
      b) 75 degrees
      c) 360 degrees
      d) 435 degrees

34.   **Of the following disorders, WF and UWF fundus photography is *most* helpful in evaluating:**
      a) macular degeneration
      b) diabetic retinopathy
      c) glaucoma
      d) vitreous floaters

35.   **All of the following are advantages of WF and UWF *except*:**
      a) decreased distortion of color and size of lesions/findings
      b) decreased patient discomfort from exposure to flash
      c) decreased need for scleral depression
      d) photos can be sent to the patient's smartphone

36.   **The technique of imaging the same area of the retina from slightly disparate angles is known as:**
      a) panoramic retinal imaging
      b) collage imaging
      c) stereo retinal photography
      d) standard mosaic photography

37. **The purpose of stereo fundus imaging is to create:**
     a) a high-contrast image
     b) a low-contrast image
     c) a moving image
     d) a 3-D image

38. **In stereo fundus imaging the disparate images are created by:**
     a) moving the camera base horizontally
     b) tilting the camera vertically
     c) moving the camera base vertically
     d) moving the fixation target

39. **The conventional sequence of taking stereo fundus images is:**
     a) first a basic central image and then the left and right images
     b) first a basic central image and then the upper and lower images
     c) first a central red-free image, then color left and right images
     d) macula, optic nerve, periphery

40. **Match the artifact/error to the photograph (Figures 20-1A through 20-1D):**
     __ camera too close
     __ camera too far back
     __ patient blinked
     __ pupil cut

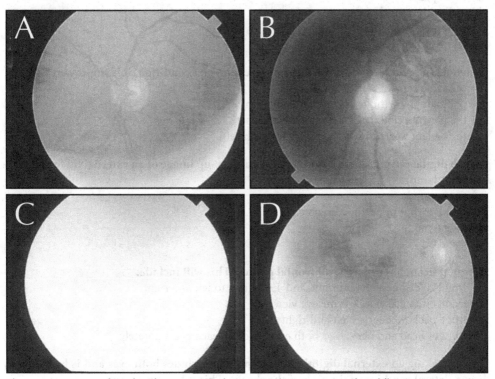

Figure 20-1. (Reproduced with permission from Eyesight Associates of Middle Georgia.)

External Photography

41. **In digital photography, the higher the number of pixels:**
     a) the less vivid the color
     b) the easier it is to copy
     c) the greater the image resolution
     d) the longer the film must be exposed

42. **When using a point-and-shoot digital camera, one must be sure to:**
     a) wait until the flash activates
     b) hold the shutter button halfway down until the image is taken
     c) hold shutter button halfway down, wait, then push button all the way down
     d) press the shutter button all the way down quickly

43. **For head and neck images and facial images, a point-and-shoot digital camera is generally sufficient. For better resolution of finer details, however, the preferred digital set-up is a:**
     a) cell phone camera
     b) digital single-lens reflex camera
     c) modified fundus camera
     d) disposable camera

44. **Which of the following is an appropriate background for external photographs?**
     a) black panel
     b) wall with enamel paint
     c) patterned wallpaper
     d) white or light blue panel

45. **When taking photos to document the progression of a condition, it is important that:**
     a) the same camera is used for each set
     b) photography settings are the same for each set
     c) the patient's clothing is the same for each set
     d) the patient wears the same jewelry for each set

46. **Which digital setting would be used to take a close-up image of an external lid lesion (ie, *without* a slit lamp)?**
     a) macro mode
     b) standard, but move the camera closer
     c) digital mode
     d) standard

47. **Your physician has ordered full frontal photos. This will include:**
     a) front, 90 degrees left and right, and 45 degrees to left and right
     b) front, bird's eye view, worm's eye view
     c) front, back, 90 degrees left and right
     d) front of head and neck, face, both eyes together, each eye separately

48. **You are taking an external digital photograph that includes both eyes and is bordered by the brows, lateral canthi, and the arch of the cheeks. This is known as a(n):**
     a) stereo view
     b) brow/cheek view
     c) double-monocular view
     d) eye frontal view

49. **Your patient has a left head turn with a left head tilt. In such a case it is important to:**
   a) take photos only in the diagnostic gazes
   b) take a photo of the patient in this "natural" position first
   c) position the patient's head so it is straight before starting
   d) position the patient's head to right turn and right tilt

50. **External photographs taken prior to strabismus surgery will include (at a minimum):**
   a) upgaze, downgaze, and primary positions
   b) a head shot, primary position, and worm's eye view
   c) 9 positions of gaze plus a head shot
   d) right gaze, left gaze, primary position, and bird's eye view

51. **An external photograph taken of both eyes using DSLR is generally at which degree of magnification?**
   a) 1/8X
   b) 1/4X
   c) 1/20X
   d) 1X

52. **To reduce the reflection of the flash in the patient's cornea (and thus on the photograph), the flash unit of choice on a DSLR is a:**
   a) bracket-mounted flash with a large reflector
   b) point source flash
   c) ring light
   d) hand-held point flash with a large reflector

53. **A patient's insurance might not reimburse the practice for external photography if the purpose of imaging is to:**
   a) document external changes over time
   b) document preoperative condition
   c) document treatment results
   d) enhance the medical record

54. **The purpose of external photos taken for insurance prior to a blepharoplasty are intended to document:**
   a) the cosmetic need for the procedure
   b) the progression of the problem
   c) the extent of the problem
   d) visual field loss

55. **A general consent for external ophthalmic photography would include all of the following *except*:**
   a) publication in print
   b) digital publication
   c) use in advertising
   d) use for education of staff

56. **Once taken, a patient's digital images are:**
   a) given to the patient
   b) part of patient's medical record and subject to privacy laws
   c) considered public domain
   d) publishable to the clinic's website

Specular Microscopy

57. **What is the average corneal endothelial cell density?**
    a) 800 per mm^2
    b) 1200 per mm^2
    c) 2500 per mm^2
    d) 4000 per mm^2

58. **Which of the following is *not* evaluated during specular microscopy?**
    a) cell density
    b) cell function
    c) cell shape
    d) cell size

59. **Videotape is frequently used in specular microscopy because:**
    a) the microscope uses such high magnification
    b) individual frames can be photographed later
    c) individual frames can be "frozen" for evaluation
    d) all of the above

60. **In addition to the quality of the cells viewed with specular microscopy, the number of cells are calculated by using:**
    a) an overlay grid
    b) a computer program
    c) template cards
    d) any of the above

61. **Specular microscopy is most likely to be ordered prior to performing:**
    a) cataract surgery
    b) intravitreal injections
    c) scleral buckle surgery
    d) laser capsulotomy

62. **At what age is the corneal endothelium the most dense?**
    a) 10 to 29 years
    b) 30 to 49 years
    c) 50 to 69 years
    d) 70 to 89 years

63. **You are looking at a specular microscopy image and note random dark "holes" in the mosaic. These are most likely:**
    a) corneal bullae
    b) corneal guttata
    c) epithelial breaks
    d) polymegathism

Video

64. **Uses of video systems in ophthalmology include all of the following *except*:**
     a) specular microscopy
     b) pachymetry
     c) documenting surgical procedures
     d) documenting eye movements (positions of gaze)

65. **The main disadvantage of video recording is:**
     a) expense of the equipment
     b) complexity of the equipment
     c) poor resolution of the image
     d) difficulty in reproducing the video

Study Notes

Suggested reading in *Principles and Practice in Ophthalmic Assisting: A Comprehensive Textbook:*
    Chapter 12: Slit Lamp Microscopy (*Methods of Illumination* pp 220-226)
    Chapter 15: Ophthalmic Photography (pp 275-296)
    Chapter 16: Diagnostic Imaging (*Specular Microscopy* pp 304-305)

Explanatory Answers

1. d) Every camera must include an aperture, camera body, and a digital sensor or film. Believe it or not, a lens is not necessary, although it will make the resulting photograph much sharper.
2. d) While a camera does not have to have a lens, most do. The function of the lens is to focus the image onto the sensor or film. Some cameras incorporate minus (concave) lenses as part of the lens system, but their additive effect is convergent (a property of plus lenses).
3. c) The focal length of a camera lens is the distance from the lens to the sensor/film plane. As in optics, this represents the distance from the lens to the focal point. In this case, the focal point falls on the sensor/film.
4. a) A telephoto lens has a longer focal length. This has the effect of bringing distant objects closer by magnifying them. A normal lens gives a 1:1 ratio (ie, images appear life-sized). A wide-angle (micro) lens has a short focal length and is used to give a wider field.
5. c) The zoom lens is adjustable, and thus has varying focal lengths. The Soper lens is a type of contact lens for keratoconus. The macro and micro lenses are not adjustable, having a fixed focal length.
6. c) Depth-of-field refers to the area in which objects are in acceptable focus.
7. d) One-third of the depth of field is usually in front of the focused subject (point of focus) and two-thirds are behind. Thus, if the depth of focus is 3 ft, objects that are within 1 ft in front of the subject will still be focused, and objects that are within 2 ft behind the subject still will be focused.
8. a) DICOM stands for Digital Imaging and Communications in Medicine. It is a protocol and format for transmitting medical files, usually photographic. JPEG stands for Joint Photographic Experts Group and is a format for compressing photo files. GIF stands for Graphics Interchange Format, which is used to create animated and still images. Fortran (a word made by combining the words formula and translation) is a programming language rarely used now except in physics.

9.   b) It is possible for the eye/lesion to look clear to you, yet the image turns out to be blurry. Insert a focusing rod* into the slit lamp. (There is a hole where it inserts; check your user's manual.) Set magnification to 16X. Turn the oculars all the way counterclockwise, then slowly turn clockwise until that first instant where the focus rod becomes clear. *Don't go past that.* Focus each ocular (yes, one at a time); this gives you a better chance of achieving "what you see is what you get." Once the oculars are focused, take a picture of the focusing rod. The photo should be clear.

10.   a) This technique will help ensure a clear image. If you are accommodating, you will have a "range" where the nevus is clear. If you take the image at the closest point (closer to the patient), the image will be blurred. When you are focusing, move forward until the nevus is clear, then back up (toward yourself) until the image just begins to blur. Then move a tiny, tiny bit closer until the nevus is *just* clear and *no farther*. Snap the image.

11.   d) Before photographing pathology, take a photo of the entire eye using diffuse lighting and lower magnification. This helps orient the viewer when photos are examined later, as well as provides documentation. (It is very difficult to identify a patient, however, from a shot of a single eye.)

12.   b) Using the diffuser decreases shadows, making it more difficult to perceive depth. If you want to highlight the elevation of a structure, you should not use the diffuser. The other statements are true.

13.   a) The cornea (and crystalline lens) will be better imaged *without* the diffuser. The other entities, which are opaque and do not have a layered structure, are well imaged using the diffuser, if desired.

14.   b) Illumination for slit lamp photos is usually directed from the temporal side. This convention helps orient the viewer, for one thing. For another, it avoids the physical limitations of the patient's nose when positioning the illuminator.

15.   d) When using direct lighting to image the cornea (for corneal dystrophy, for example) you want the background behind the area of interest to be dark. You may have to adjust the angle of the lamp and/or oculars in order to achieve this. A dilated pupil also makes it easier. What you do not want in this case is light reflecting off the iris, which would back-light the cornea (creating retroillumination). The diffuser spreads the light evenly over the entire image; it cannot be "centered."

16.   a) In tangential illumination, the light source is angled at the eye. This emphasizes the contours of structures, using shadow to show contrast. For further study, see Table 11-1 in Chapter 11.

17.   d) Retroillumination would use light reflected off of the retina to illuminate the lens from behind. This would outline the spokes of the cataract.

18.   b) The higher the magnification, the larger even very tiny movement becomes, increasing the chance for blurring.

19.   a) The reticule and subject must be in focus simultaneously. The ocular is set for the photographer's refractive error, not necessarily at zero. Unless the patient has high myopia (or external pictures are being taken with the fundus camera), the dioptric setting should be plano. FYI: *Reticule* and *reticle* are the same thing: a grid or ruler inscribed in the ocular (eyepiece) of a camera or other piece of optical equipment for focusing and measuring.

20.   d) The reticule is needed to give a reference point for focusing. It is not printed on the photograph.

21.   a) The primary component of the optical imaging system of the fundus camera is an aspheric lens that acts as an indirect ophthalmoscope. A retinoscope is used in refraction.

22.   c) The patient's optical media become part of the camera's lens system. If there is a corneal or lenticular opacity, the photographs will not be clear. The dioptric power of the eye cannot be discounted. If the patient has high myopia or hyperopia, the dioptric compensation device must be set. Some fundus cameras have a compensation device for astigmatism, as well.

23.   c) The view lamp and the electronic flash system are collectively known as the illumination exposure system. A beam splitter is part of a slit lamp camera system. Only tungsten bulbs are used. The fixation light does not play a role in exposure.

---

* A focusing rod comes with each instrument, but they are interchangeable.

24. b) Have the patient close both eyes while you align the donut on the closed lid. This is more comfortable for the patient and allows you to avoid fumbling around with the camera looking for the eye. *Note*: Many modern fundus cameras no longer focus externally, or indeed have an ocular for the photographer to view through. Instead, focusing is done on the unit's monitor.

25. d) The little yellow crescent is caused by a "pupil cut."

26. b) To compensate for a pupil cut, move the camera directly opposite from the crescent.

27. c) Retinal pathology does not cause blurred photos in and of itself.

28. b) In addition to causing pupil cuts, inadequate dilation can cause a general blur on the photographs.

29. c) In some shots needed for fundus photography (notably during diabetic fields, or to document peripheral lesions), the angle of incidence between the camera and cornea can induce astigmatism. This can cause blurring of the photograph in one meridian. Accommodation is spherical, not cylindrical.

30. c) See Answer 29.

31. a) The ETDRS study established protocol for fundus photography in diabetes as 7 fields, starting with the optic disc, then the macula, then temporal to the macula (in more or less a straight line marching across the "line" from disc to macula), then 4 more positioned superior/inferior/temporal/nasal.

32. d) A montage is a melding of images, aligning areas of overlap to give one single, large image.

33. b) Using the standard 7 field diabetic fundus photography protocol, there is a 75 degree field of view. Newer, widefield photography can capture up to 200 degrees.

34. b) Because WF and UWF are able to image a much broader area of the peripheral retina, they are especially ideal modalities to use for evaluating diabetic retinopathy and other disorders that may appear in the far periphery such as retinal vein occlusion, some pediatric retinal disorders, uveitis, and retinal detachment. While useful for macular degeneration and glaucoma, WF and UWF are *most* helpful in evaluating diabetic retinopathy.

35. a) A disadvantage of WF and UWF is that because you are taking a 2-dimensional image of a 3-dimentional object, there can be distortion of the size of lesions and other findings. Because these cameras use specific laser wavelengths for photography, colors may be distorted as well. The other statements are true. WF and UWF require only a single capture, so there is less exposure to bright lights, making them more comfortable for the patient. Dilation is not required. Because the periphery is visible in the photos, there is less need for the physician to perform scleral depression. The photos can be sent to the patient's phone, if equipped to receive them.

36. c) In stereoretinal photography, the same area is photographed twice, each photo from a slightly different angle.

37. d) The creation of a 3-dimensional image allows the viewer to appreciate depth perception, creating a more "real" image of what the area really looks like. It is useful in evaluating the relative position of retinal structures.

38. a) The 2 images for stereo are taken by moving the camera base via joy stick slightly to the left and then to the right, taking an image at each position.

39. a) By convention, a central image is taken first. Then the camera is shifted left, image taken, then the camera is shifted right and a final image taken.

40. **Matching**:
     D_ camera too close
     B_ camera too far back
     C_ patient blinked
     A_ pupil cut

41. c) In the digital world, an image is made up of pixels. In photography we usually talk of mega pixels (one mega pixel has a million pixels). The more mega pixels the camera has, the greater the resolution of the image. There is no film in a digital camera.

42. c) Due to shutter lag focus, you must hold the shutter button halfway down, wait, and then fully depress the button in order to capture the image.

43. b) The DSLR camera is the preferred set up for external photography for external photos of the eyes, especially magnified monocular photographs of lids, globe, and conjunctiva/cornea.

44. d) The ideal background is a single-colored, light-colored screen or surface without any pattern, and with low reflectivity.

45. b) When documenting a progression in a condition or treatment of same, or when taking pre- and post-op photos, all variables should be kept the same. This includes illumination, flash, background, patient position, etc. The patient should remove jewelry, hat/scarf, glasses, and (usually) makeup for medical photography involving the head/face/eyes.

46. a) Macro mode (usually indicated with a flower icon) provides the "zoom" needed for taking close images of small lesions and other findings. Moving the camera closer may cause image distortion.

47. a) A full frontal series (also called *face view*) includes frontal, left, right, and oblique (45 degree) images. A worm's eye view is taken from below (ie, "up the nose"). In contrast, a bird's eye view is taken from the top of the head down (eg, to show exophthalmos).

48. d) The view described (just above the brows, just at the malar arch, lateral canthi as the side boundaries) is the eye frontal view. The other answers are bogus.

49. b) If the patient has a head turn or tilt, you should document this with frontal photographs prior to taking other images that are in the anatomical or diagnostic poses.

50. c) External photography generally includes one head shot for orientation and documentation. A strabismus series would then involve shots showing just the 2 eyes in the 9 positions of gaze. (External photos for ptosis or plastics would include a head shot, then both eyes in primary position, upgaze, and downgaze.)

51. b) The bilateral view is usually 1/4X or 1/3X (where the image is 1/4 or 1/3 the size of the photographed subject, respectively). Full head shot is 1/8X, 1/2X to 1/1X for monocular lids, 1X or 2X (life-size or double life-size, respectively) for the globe. 1/20X was a bogus answer.

52. b) The goal is to avoid obscuring pathology with the flash reflection. The smallest reflector available should be used. A point source is better than a ring flash, especially if it is mounted on an adjustable bracket so it can be rotated.

53. d) If the only reason a photo is taken is to add information to the patient's record, their insurance may not cover the cost. What *may* be covered is documentation of a condition or treatment over time, or photos required to document a condition prior to its surgical correction.

54. c) The insurance company wants to know if the condition is "bad enough" to qualify for reimbursement (ie, by them). They are interested in function, not cosmesis. Visual field loss is not documented by photos but should correlate. (That is, if the field shows marked loss of upper field yet the lids are barely drooped, insurance might think twice about approving the procedure.)

55. c) The general consent for ophthalmic imaging includes publication for education and research, including print and digital forms where the patient's name or identification is removed or obliterated. To use the images in advertising would require a separate (and carefully worded) consent.

56. b) Photographs are considered part of the patient's medical record. So all laws, rules, and regulations regarding privacy and the release of information apply to the images, just like chart notes. The patient may request copies according to legal and clinic release regulations. Public domain means that anyone can use the image without a copyright/consent, which is not the case since the photos are part of the patient's private medical record. Nor can the clinic use images publicly without specific consent.

57. c) The "normal" range for density of the corneal endothelium is 2000 to 3200 per mm^2; average is approximately 2500 per mm^2.

58.   b) Of the characteristics listed, cell function cannot be tested via specular microscopy. Cell density (or count: average 2500 per mm² with no gaps), cell shape (each cell should be a crisp hexagon), and cell size (cells should be uniform in size) are all evaluated with the scan.

59.   d) Because of the high magnification used, even a tiny movement of the eye sends the view of the cells swooshing across the eyepiece or monitor. Video film is used to tape the viewing session, then individual frames are projected and examined later. Individual photographs can then be created from a single video frame.

60.   d) Any of the listed methods may be used. A grid may be laid over the viewing screen. The cells within the boundaries are counted, as well as the cells touching one vertical and one horizontal line of the square. This number is then multiplied by a constant. (Check the user's manual to find the constant for a particular instrument as well as the specific grid.) Some instruments provide a computer printout. Other manufacturers supply template cards that are pictures of cells. You compare the patient's display to the cards and select the best match.

61.   a) Because cataract surgery involves inserting and withdrawing instruments and material through the anterior chamber, there is a risk that cells will be lost or compromised.

62.   a) Average corneal endothelial cell density is highest in the 10- to 29-year age bracket (up to 3500 mm²). After that there is usually a steady decline to an average of 1500 to 2300 in the ninth decade.[1]

63.   b) Corneal guttata are areas where endothelial cells have been lost and show up as a dark "hole" in the natural mosaic (honeycomb pattern). They can occur as a part of natural aging, as well as from trauma and disease. Bullae and epithelial breaks would be external. Polymegathism occurs as remaining endothelial cells stretch out and move in an attempt to "cover" the area that is left empty by the lost cell(s).

64.   b) There is no need to use videotaping for pachymetry.

65.   c) Video recordings are great because they provide instant playback. However, the resolution (sharpness) of the images isn't the best, especially when a frame is paused. Compared to other pieces of ophthalmic equipment, video equipment is inexpensive and uncomplicated. Digital video is easily copied.

Reference

1.   Thomas C. Use specular microscopy to diagnose corneal disease. *Rev of Optom.* 2009;146(06). Accessed March 18, 2023. www.reviewofoptometry.com/article/use-specular-microscopy-to-diagnose-corneal-disease

Bibliography

Graziano J. Introduction to slit lamp imaging basics. American Optometric Association Website. Accessed March 18, 2023. https://www.scribd.com/document/413144096/Introduction-to-Slit-Lamp-Basics-pdf# Published 2015

Kim EL, Moshfeghi AA. Wide-field imaging of retinal diseases. *US Ophthalmic Rev.* 2015;8(2):125-131. doi:10.17925/USOR.2015.08.02.125

Mukherjee B, Nair AG. Principles and practice of external digital photography in ophthalmology. *Indian J Ophthalmol.* 2012;60(2):119-125. doi:10.4103/0301-4738.94053

Nyberg WC. External eye photography. Ophthalmic Photographers' Society Website. Accessed March 18, 2023. www.opsweb.org/page/Externaleye

Chapter 21

Equipment Maintenance and Repair*

* This topic carries little weight (1%) on the COT® exam. More questions can be found in the *Certified Ophthalmic Assistant Exam Review Manual, Third Edition*, if desired.

Ledford JK.
Certified Ophthalmic Technician Exam Review Manual, Third Edition (pp 469-474).
© 2023 Taylor & Francis Group.

ABBREVIATIONS USED IN THIS CHAPTER

- AED   automated external defibrillator
- IV   intravenous
- Rx   prescription (glasses)

---

1.   **Which of the following instruments is considered self-calibrating?**
   a) corneal topographer
   b) automated perimeter
   c) Goldmann perimeter
   d) Goldmann tonometer

2.   **The first step in cleaning any lens is to:**
   a) spray with lens cleaner
   b) wipe with a tissue
   c) gently remove surface dust
   d) fog it with your breath

3.   **A contact gonio lens should be disinfected by:**
   a) nothing; single-use lenses are now recommended
   b) water and gentle detergent
   c) commercial disinfectant wipe
   d) soaking in ether

4.   **A Goldmann tonometer should be calibrated:**
   a) daily
   b) prior to each use
   c) only by a professional
   d) every 1 to 2 months

5.   **At what settings is the Goldmann tonometer calibrated?**
   a) 0, 2, and 6
   b) 0, 2, and 4
   c) 0, 1, and 6
   d) 2, 4, and 6

6.   **The manual keratometer can be calibrated:**
   a) by reading a trial lens of known curvature
   b) only by a professional
   c) using a zeroing-out gauge
   d) using metal spheres of known curvature

7.   **The accuracy of a manual lensometer may be tested:**
   a) by reading trial lenses
   b) reading glasses of known Rx
   c) clearing the mires at Plano
   d) only by a professional

8. **Which parts of a phoropter may be wiped with alcohol?**
   a) roto-o-chart
   b) Maddox rod lenses
   c) face shield and forehead rest
   d) none of it, alcohol ruins the finish on all parts

9. **Spot-cleaning of a dirty lens in the phoropter can be done with a lint-free applicator and any of the following *except*:**
   a) alcohol
   b) ether
   c) mild abrasive cleaner
   d) commercial lens cleaner

10. **A thorough cleaning and lubrication of the phoropter should be done:**
    a) only by the practitioner
    b) only by a professional
    c) every month by the tech
    d) prior to every use

11. **You are using a projector and mirror system in a 12-foot room. What must be done in order to standardize the size of the optotypes?**
    a) the patient chair must be moved
    b) the mirrors must be appropriately tilted
    c) the projector must be moved
    d) the projector must be calibrated

12. **The slit lamp stage is not sliding smoothly. You should:**
    a) clean and lubricate the glide plate
    b) spit on it
    c) scrub it with cleanser
    d) clean it with lens cleaner

13. **Which of the following about instrument bulbs is *false*?**
    a) Retinoscopy bulbs can warp if the instrument is stored upright.
    b) In general, bulbs should not be handled with the fingers.
    c) Clean bulb contacts using a pencil eraser.
    d) Let bulbs cool before handling.

Maintain Emergency Equipment

14. **Because of potential of life-threatening emergencies, especially during procedures such as fluorescein angiogram, the office should maintain a mobile trolley containing life-saving equipment and drugs. This is known as a(n):**
    a) code blue cart
    b) code red cart
    c) automated external defibrillator
    d) crash cart

15. **All of the following need to be regularly checked on the office AED *except*:**
    a) expiration dates on electrode pads
    b) test primary and backup batteries
    c) airway attachments
    d) stock secondary supplies

16. **Which of the following regarding fire extinguishers in the clinic is *false*?**
    a) They must be easily accessed.
    b) They should be sprayed periodically to ensure functioning.
    c) There should be no major dents and no cracks.
    d) There should be no evidence of rust, corrosion, or chemical leaks.

Order and Maintain Medical and Clinical Supplies

17. **The process by which items or goods get from supplier to user is the:**
    a) mail chain
    b) supply web
    c) chain of flow
    d) supply chain

18. **A list of stocked supplies that are needed in order for the clinic to function is a(n):**
    a) inventory
    b) duty roster
    c) goods debit
    d) invoice

19. **Which of the following would *not* be considered part of "consumable" inventory?**
    a) disinfecting wipes
    b) mydriatic sunglasses
    c) Goldmann tonometer tips
    d) Tono-Pen covers

20. **Stock of consumable items must be monitored closely in order to:**
    a) identify waste and theft
    b) prevent over/under stocking
    c) monitor for out-of-date products
    d) all of the above

Study Notes

Suggested reading in *Principles and Practice in Ophthalmic Assisting: A Comprehensive Textbook:*
>   Chapter 5: Ophthalmic Equipment (pp 57-68)
>   Chapter 12: Slit Lamp Microscopy (*Maintenance and Troubleshooting* pp 219-220)

Explanatory Answers

1. b) Of the instruments listed, only the automated perimeter is self-calibrating. The corneal topographer should be calibrated daily prior to its first use, and any time after it has been jarred or transported.

2. c) You wouldn't want to "grind" any surface debris across the lens. Before wiping any lens, surface dust should be removed with an ear syringe and/or a camel's hairbrush.

3. a) With the advent of COVID-19, the American Academy of Ophthalmology recommends that any diagnostic or laser procedure requiring a contact-type lens be done using a disposable lens.[1]

4. d) The manufacturer recommends calibrating the Goldmann tonometer every month.[2] (Other sources vary, from every month to every 6 months. I'd go with the manufacturer.)

5. a) The Goldmann tonometer is calibration checked at the settings of 0, 2 (20), and 6 (60). The 2 setting is especially important as it is critical in the evaluation of glaucoma.

6. d) The manual keratometer comes with a set of stainless steel balls of a given curvature. One of these is placed in a holder (using a magnet; don't touch them with bare fingers) and read with the instrument. If not accurate, return the instrument to the manufacturer for servicing.

7. a) To make sure your manual lensometer is accurate, pull out a few trial lenses and read them. If not accurate, return the instrument to the manufacturer for servicing.

8. c) The removable face shields and the forehead rest are made of plastic/nylon, which can be wiped with alcohol. If the face shield has a "lens" in it (to protect the instrument's internal lenses), do not soak it with alcohol; this can cause the glue to loosen and the lens to fall out. *Note:* You may see roto chart also spelled Roto Chart, Rotochart, and rotochart. "Rotochart" may have started out as a Reichert trademark, but there are now generic formats with corruptions of the item's name.

9. c) Above all, you want to avoid abrading the lenses. Any of the other answers may be used. Never spray cleaner into the phoropter; apply cleaner to the applicator and gently wick or squeeze out excess.

10. b) Only a professional should disassemble, clean, and lubricate a phoropter. References vary as to how often this should be done (I've read 18 months to every 3 years). Surface cleaning, appropriate disinfection of patient contact points, and spot-cleaning of lenses can be done as needed by techs.

11. d) When the projector is to be used in a room less than 20 ft, the optotype size must be calibrated using a template that is included with the instrument. A test optotype (usually the 20/200 E) is projected and the template is held next to it. The projector tube is slid back and forth until the size of both Es is the same.

12. a) If the slit lamp isn't moving smoothly, you should clean the glide pad with a moist cloth and then lubricate it with a drop of machine oil. Alternately, it may be cleaned and lubricated with commercial spray oil, sprayed on a soft cloth and then applied to the glide plate. Hope I made you laugh with Answer b)!

13. a) Retinoscopy bulbs can warp, but this happens when the instrument is stored or habitually laid on its side. The remaining statements are true. Handling bulbs with the fingers can leave prints on the bulb, which may "burn on" once the lamp heats up. Bulbs can be very hot, so be sure to let them cool off before handling. You can clear bulb contacts of corrosion by rubbing the contact with a pencil eraser.

14. d) The mobile chest of drawers containing emergency supplies and equipment is called a crash cart. It must be regularly inspected, and items approaching end-of-use date replaced. An inventory list should be printed out and kept with the cart. Common contents include an AED, airway equipment, IV equipment, aspirin, naloxone (narcotic reversal), epinephrine, and nitroglycerin.

15. c) An AED does not provide pulmonary resuscitation. The electrode pads do expire, so check the dates regularly. Batteries should be checked to make sure they don't need replacing. Secondary supplies might include a razor, alcohol preps, toweling, gloves, and scissors. Also to be checked: a data card, if installed (this would contain a recording of each use situation).

16. b) Discharging the extinguisher is not a part of maintenance. In fact, if used even briefly, the extinguisher should be inspected and refilled. The extinguisher must be in a place that is easily accessible and not blocked or covered with anything. The canisters can explode, so a unit with major dents or cracks should be replaced, as should an extinguisher with major rust or any evidence of chemical leakage.

17. d) The "supply chain" at its most basic is the "flow of goods and services." For our purposes, it is the steps it takes to get a product/commodity to the customer. (Technically, it also includes product development, marketing, distribution, etc.)

18. a) At its most simple, inventory is a list of the supplies you must keep on hand in order for the clinic to run smoothly. This can be as basic as a paper list to more sophisticated animated programs utilizing bar codes. Inventory helps you know how much of an item to stock, because it shows your patterns of use.

19. c) Of those listed, the Goldmann tonometer tips would not be considered consumable. (There are disposable Goldmann tips now, but that was not specified in the question.) The other items are used up and discarded (or sent out the door, as in the case of the sunglasses).

20. d) Inventory of consumable items can help you identify items that are not used or rarely used. Since keeping items in stock means that clinic money is tied up and not available for anything else, you can rethink whether or not the clinic actually needs to stock an item as well as how much. When reviewing inventory, you should reconcile tallies (ie, how much you should have) with physical materials (ie, how much you do have). The inventory data should also include expiration dates where applicable.

References

1. Nguyen MT, Jung H, Taylor LE, Yee P. Coronavirus (COVID-19). Eye Wiki, Website of AAO. Modified March 22, 2021. Accessed March 18, 2023. https://eyewiki.aao.org/Coronavirus_(COVID-19)
2. Haag-Streit Diagnostics. Instructions for use. Applanation tonometer AT 900*/870. Accessed March 18, 2023. http://haag-streit.com/fileadmin/Haag-Streit_USA/Diagnostics/tonometry/download/01-IFU_AT900-7006000-04230_eng_01.pdf

Bibliography

Thulsiraj RD. Managing your eye unit's supplies. *Community Eye Health*. 2011;24(76):32-35. Accessed March 18, 2023. https://www.cehjournal.org/article/managing-your-eye-units-supplies/

Chapter 22

Medical Ethics, Legal, and Regulatory Issues*

* In no way is this book or any information in it intended to be construed as legal advice.

Ledford JK.
*Certified Ophthalmic Technician Exam
Review Manual, Third Edition* (pp 475-485).
© 2023 Taylor & Francis Group.

ABBREVIATIONS USED IN THIS CHAPTER

- AAAHC   Accreditation Association for Ambulatory Health Care
- AMA   American Medical Association
- ANSI   American National Standards Institute
- ASC   ambulatory surgical center
- CPT   Current Procedural Terminology
- E/M   evaluation and management
- EHR   electronic health record
- FCLCA   Fairness to Contact Lens Consumers Act
- FDA   Federal Drug Administration
- FTC   Federal Trade Commission
- HIPAA   Health Insurance Portability and Accountability Act
- IJCAHPO® International Joint Commission on Allied Health Personnel in Ophthalmology
- OSHA   Occupational Safety and Health Administration

Coding

1. **In medical practice, coding is used to:**
    a) identify disorders and procedures when submitting claims
    b) maintain patient privacy
    c) identify the patient
    d) set standards of care

2. **Improper coding can result in:**
    a) disputes between patients
    b) HIPAA violations
    c) OSHA violations
    d) declined reimbursements

3. **Each of the following would have a procedure code *except*:**
    a) intraocular injection
    b) chalazion
    c) corneal pachymetry
    d) Goldmann visual field test

4. **Codes used to identify the level of service a patient receives at an office visit are:**
    a) procedure codes
    b) E/M codes
    c) routine codes
    d) diagnostic codes

5. **E/M codes are used:**
    a) to indicate the type, level, and diagnosis of an eye exam
    b) only for patients who have not been seen previously
    c) throughout medicine to indicate the level of an exam
    d) only for patients who have disorders listed in the coding guide

6.   The 3 major components of E/M documentation are all of the following *except*:
     a) fair billing
     b) history
     c) physical exam
     d) medical decision making

7.   Eye codes are used along with E/M codes in order to:
     a) represent the type, level, and elements of the eye exam
     b) indicate the time spent with the patient
     c) document the level of HIPAA compliance
     d) comply with OSHA regulations

8.   Each of the following would be identified by a diagnostic code *except*:
     a) dermatochalasis
     b) coloboma of lid
     c) hyperpigmentation of lid
     d) chalazion excision

9.   Regarding procedure and diagnostic codes:
     a) any combination is acceptable
     b) informed consent must also be included
     c) there must be a direct correlation between diagnosis and procedure
     d) only modifiers may be used

10. Your patient is here today for a laser iridotomy. Their record must include:
     a) elements for a full eye exam
     b) that a verbal consent was obtained
     c) a diagnosis of narrow angles
     d) a recent fundus examination

11. Your patient is a healthy 42-year-old whose only complaint is decreased vision at near. The provider's diagnosis is presbyopia, and the patient is given a prescription for bifocals. The remainder of the exam is normal. This exam would be considered:
     a) medical
     b) routine
     c) compliant
     d) nonessential

12. Your patient is a healthy 42-year-old whose only complaint is decreased vision at near. During the exam, the provider discovers a retinal hole that needs to be treated. The exam can now be considered:
     a) routine
     b) refractive
     c) medical
     d) essential

13. Your patient is a 42-year-old with diabetes and a history of retinopathy, whose only complaint is decreased vision at near. This exam would be considered:
     a) routine
     b) preoperative
     c) presbyopic
     d) medical

14. A code that is "tacked on" to a CPT code indicating that the procedure was altered in some way is a(n):
    a) modifier
    b) extender
    c) red flag
    d) transformer

15. Which of the following statements regarding the "global period" of care for surgery done on one eye is *false*?
    a) It begins on the day of surgery.
    b) It includes having the same procedure done on the fellow eye.
    c) Its length varies according to the procedure.
    d) Within the time frame, it applies to all visits related to the procedure.

Government/Institutional Rules and Regulations

16. The FTC *Ophthalmic Practices Rules* states that:
    a) the patient must pay in full before a glasses prescription is released
    b) the practice may charge a fee for a patient's glasses prescription
    c) the patient must be given their glasses prescription
    d) the patient's glasses prescription is protected by privacy laws and may not be released

17. A patient fit with contact lenses must be provided with a prescription. This is known as the:
    a) FDA Contact Law
    b) ANSI Standards for Contacts
    c) OSHA Soft Lens Requirement
    d) Fairness to Contact Lens Consumers Act

18. Matching, one answer:
    a) AAAHC   __ governs patient privacy
    b) ANSI   __ oversees employee safety
    c) FDA   __ establishes standards for eyewear
    d) FTC   __ certification body for ASCs
    e) HIPAA   __ approves drugs and medical devices
    f) IJCAHPO®   __ enforces laws concerning consumer protection
    g) OSHA   __ oversees your certification
    h) The Joint Commission (formerly JCAHO)   __ accredits hospitals and health care organizations

Quality Assurance

19. According to one source, *this* "is judged by how well the dimensions of clinical care conform to expectations and standards."[1] To what is the author referring?
    a) quality
    b) standard of care
    c) informed consent
    d) medical ethics

20. Which of the following is *not* an example of problems in quality control?
     a) abandonment
     b) overuse
     c) underuse
     d) misuse

21. Who is responsible for quality assurance in the eye clinic?
     a) the physician/owner
     b) American Medical Association
     c) every member of the clinic team
     d) The Joint Commission

Ethical and Legal Standards

22. The branch of study that involves discerning between right and wrong is known as:
     a) morality
     b) justice
     c) integrity
     d) ethics

23. Who can take action against an eye care professional who may have breached ethical principles?
     a) patients
     b) employer
     c) colleagues
     d) all of the above

24. What type of action can be taken against an eye care professional who has breached ethical principles?
     a) civil
     b) criminal
     c) disciplinary
     d) any of the above

25. Which of the following could be considered an ethical breach?
     a) Explaining your patient's findings, by name, to a supervisor for help in determining what tests are needed.
     b) Posting your patient's findings, with a full-face photo, on an ophthalmic tech Facebook page to get others' opinion.
     c) Writing up your patient's findings as an anonymous case study without the patient's permission.
     d) Submitting photos of full-face before and after blepharoplasty photos for an article in a journal, where a photo release is in the patient's record.

26. You are attending a lecture on glaucoma treatment. The presenter shows a slide that notes they have been involved in studies involving the new eye drop featured in the lecture, but does not receive any compensation from the company. They do this in order to avoid a possible:
    a) confidentially breach
    b) proprietary infringement
    c) conflict of interest
    d) double entendre

27. As an ophthalmic tech you are permitted to do some tests and procedures but not others. These permissions and restrictions are known as:
    a) scope of practice
    b) legal parameters
    c) clinic protocol
    d) licensure

28. A 3-year-old patient needs to be dilated. You have explained the procedure and side effects to the parent, who is holding the child. You quickly put in the anesthetic, and the child starts screaming. You quickly grab the dilating drop to put it in. The child is crying, and the mother says to you, "let's not do this." You go ahead and put in the dilating drops. What are the possible consequences?
    a) a charge of malpractice
    b) a charge of negligence
    c) a charge of assault and battery
    d) a charge of breaking and entering

29. A patient with iritis has been using a steroid drop for 1 week. A new tech in your office fails to check the patient's intraocular pressure at the recheck appointment, and the physician doesn't notice the omission. The patient returns for a recheck in another week and the intraocular pressure in the eye is 36. This could be a case of:
    a) malpractice
    b) negligence
    c) ignorance of the law
    d) breach of ANSI standards

Scribing

30. The person who has been delegated to document an eye exam in real-time is called a:
    a) scribe
    b) physician's assistant
    c) chaperone
    d) nurse assistant

31. When using a scribe, the physician can devote their attention solely to the patient. This increases:
    a) exam complexity
    b) patient satisfaction
    c) billable time
    d) patient confusion

32.   **It is beyond the scribe's scope of practice to do which of the following?**
     a) find the results of a patient's lab work
     b) be thoroughly familiar with the clinic's EHR system
     c) diagnostic testing
     d) document exam findings

Confidentiality

33.   **You are having lunch in the office break room with some of your colleagues and one of them says, "I saw Jacob Pelham this morning. You know, the fellow that had a total retinal detachment last month? He just can't seem to understand that he's never going to have 20/20 vision again. It's so sad." Which of the following is *false*?**
     a) Your colleague has breached the patient's confidentiality.
     b) Your colleague could be charged with a HIPAA violation.
     c) Your colleague has committed an ethical breach.
     d) This is permissible because the comment was made in-house.

Informed Consent

34.   **You are about to perform a slit lamp exam on a patient. You place the instrument in front of the patient, who leans forward into the head rest. This is an example of:**
     a) formal consent
     b) conformed intent
     c) implied consent
     d) leniency

35.   **You are about to dilate the patient and have explained its purpose and possible side effects. Then you say to the patient, "Will that be alright?" The patient says, "Yes." This is an example of:**
     a) express consent
     b) formed consent
     c) waived consent
     d) informed intent

36.   **You are scribing for the doctor on a patient who needs a laser capsulotomy. The physician says to the patient, "This procedure uses an yttrium-aluminum-garnet laser to ablate the posterior capsule." This ineffective communication poses a(n):**
     a) breach of contract
     b) avoidance behavior
     c) lack of consent
     d) barrier to learning

37.   **Informed consent might involve any of the following by the patient *except*:**
     a) declining treatment
     b) electing an alternative
     c) asking as many questions as desired
     d) providing guaranteed results

38. **The patient is a legally emancipated minor, age 17 years, who wants a cosmetic ptosis repair. Which of the following is *true*?**
    a) A minor of this age cannot sign their own consent.
    b) The patient may sign their own consent.
    c) A minor of this age must be in the military in order to sign informed consent.
    d) A parent/guardian must co-sign the consent.

39. **You work at a teaching hospital, where residents often perform procedures under the supervision of a physician. Which of the following is *true*?**
    a) The informed consent must contain a notation that trainees will or may be participating in the patient's care.
    b) Any trainee that may be involved in the procedure must supply a copy of their license to the patient on request.
    c) Not applicable; trainees are not permitted to perform procedures.
    d) The informed consent need not specifically mention trainees, because it is a teaching facility, and everyone knows the students will participate.

40. **At some level, informed consent must include each of the following *except*:**
    a) patient education with comprehension
    b) patient involvement in the decision
    c) explanation of benefits and all risks
    d) opportunity for the patient to ask questions

Study Notes

Suggested reading in *Principles and Practice in Ophthalmic Assisting: A Comprehensive Textbook*:
    Chapter 6: Scribing and Chair-Side Assisting (pp 69-76)
    Chapter 40: Surgical Assisting (*Informed Consent* p 665)
    Chapter 41: Around the Office (*Terminology* pp 684-685)
    Chapter 43: The Basics of Coding in an Outpatient Setting (pp 695-703)
    Chapter 44: Health Care Compliance and Regulatory Issues (pp 705-714)

Explanatory Answers

1. a) Coding in the medical realm is used to identify diagnoses, as well as treatments and tests (procedures). It is used when submitting bills and claims.
2. d) If a procedure and/or diagnosis is not coded properly, insurance companies can (and will) refuse to pay. Or you may not be properly reimbursed, leading to problems in an audit if you received too much money. HIPAA applies to patient rights. OSHA is concerned about safety in the workplace.
3. b) A chalazion is a diagnosis. The other items are procedures (ie, tests or treatments).
4. b) E/M codes indicate an encounter between patient and caregiver. The encounter may be face to face or virtual. E/M codes are actually a *subset* of procedure codes, making b) the best answer.
5. c) The E/M codes are used across medicine for all patients, not just those with specific disorders, and not just in eye care. They do not include diagnostic codes.
6. a) Documentation needed to properly assign E/M codes must include notes regarding the history (our bailiwick), the actual physical exam (part us, part physician), and an indication of medical decision making (the physician's prevue, which includes diagnoses that follow from the history and exam, as well as a plan to treat or otherwise deal with the diagnoses). Fair billing is not involved in E/M coding.

7.   a) The level of an exam depends on what was done. The more complex the exam, the more exam elements must be fulfilled. If all requirements are there except one, the exam must fall to the next lower level.

8.   d) Of the items listed, all are diagnoses except for the chalazion excision, which is a procedure.

9.   c) The diagnosis and procedure codes *must* go hand-in-hand. If there are multiple diagnoses, the first one must relate to the chief complaint.

10. c) The procedure needed must be backed up by the matching diagnosis, in this case narrow angles. Informed consent for a procedure must always be written.

11. b) In the absence of any pathology or contributory disorders, this exam would be considered routine/refractive. If the provider discovers some underlying disorder that needs treatment, then the physician might order a follow-up exam to evaluate or treat that problem and *that* exam would then be medical.

12. c) In this case, a visit that started out to be a routine/refractive vision exam may be converted to a medical exam because the provider has identified ocular pathology that needs treatment.

13. d) Because the patient has been diagnosed with ocular pathology, this is considered a medical exam. (An exam on a diabetic without history of retinopathy would also be a medical exam.)

14. a) Adding a modifier to a CPT code indicates that a procedure was done but was modified in some way. An example would be a postop cataract surgery patient who comes in because of an injury to the *other* eye. The "red flag" answer is sort of a joke, because overuse of modifiers can be a red flag to Medicare, instigating an audit.

15. b) The global period starts with the specific procedure and extends for a specific amount of time. It does not include any procedure done on the other eye during the global period for the first eye. The most common example is cataract surgery.

16. c) The eyeglass prescription release rule requires that once the exam is done, the patient must be provided with a glasses prescription. It may not be withheld, for example, until the patient pays their bill.

17. d) The FCLCA was enacted in 2004. If a patient is fit with contact lenses, they must be given a prescription for them. They cannot be required to order the lenses from the fitter's practice.

18. **Matching:**
     e) governs patient privacy
     g) oversees employee safety
     b) establishes standards for eyewear
     a) certification body for ASCs
     c) approves drugs and medical devices
     d) enforces laws concerning consumer protection
     f) oversees your certification
     h) accredits hospitals and health care organizations

19. a) I liked the way this author described *quality* so well that I chose to quote him. He further states, "The Institute of Medicine describes quality care as the degree to which health services for individuals and populations increase the likelihood of desired health outcomes and are consistent with current professional knowledge."[1]

20. a) Problems in quality control are divided into 3 general areas: overuse, underuse, and misuse.

21. c) Every member of the clinic team is responsible for quality assurance, at least for areas that they oversee or work in. It takes a group effort to make sure that every item, every exam, and every procedure is done for the patient's good, and is the best you can reasonably provide. Improvement is everyone's business.

22. d) Ethics (or moral philosophy) is a branch of study that involves the determination of what is right or wrong in a given situation at a given time in a given society. Ethics involves morality, probity, and integrity.

23. d) Any of the above may seek action if they believe that an ethical breach has occurred.

24. d) Unprofessional/unethical conduct may be actionable by civil (commonly by fines/penalties, behavior modification, restitution, etc), criminal (fines, jail/prison, restitution, etc), or disciplinary (eg, revocation of credentials, reprimand, etc) action. Civil disputes are between 2 parties (private rights); criminal disputes are guided by the penal code (crime and punishment). Crimes are considered to be breaking a law that has been established by government (such as drunk driving, theft, murder). Neglect is more commonly a civil matter (such as breach of contract, property damage, defamation, malpractice); a crime (eg, embezzlement) is more likely to involve intent.

25. b) You are not permitted to post or otherwise share any information that would specifically identify that person without the patient's permission if it is outside the scope of care. Asking your supervisor for assistance, even with identifiers, is permitted. If there are no identifiers, you are permitted to write up a case study about a particular patient without that patient's permission.

26. c) A conflict of interest can exist when a person stands to profit in some way from promoting a product.

27. a) Scope of practice refers to what a person at a given level of expertise, certification/licensure, etc, is allowed and not allowed to do in the scope of their profession. It is governed by law, as well as professional bodies and clinic protocol. Certifying and licensing organizations (eg, AMA, IJCAHPO®) and clinic protocol are not permitted to run counter to the law.

28. c) In assault, the victim has reason to anticipate physical injury, while battery is the actual act that causes physical harm. Once the parent says no, you have to stop. You might try re-educating about the purpose of dilation/cycloplegia, but if parent declines, you can't put the drops in. Malpractice is a failure to follow known standards of care. Negligence is a mistake that causes unintentional harm.

29. b) Negligence is a mistake that results in unintentional harm, and this is the most likely result if the patient was injured in some way (in this scenario because of the elevated intraocular pressure). However, I'm not a lawyer! I suppose an argument could be made for malpractice on the part of the physician, since the technician works under the physician's license.

30. a) Scribing is a relatively new development in medicine. Eye care is especially adapted to it. The scribe takes charge of making notations in the patient's record while the exam is going on. (Of course, this requires that the physician verbalize their findings.)

31. b) Because the practitioner does not have to turn to the patient's record (paper or electronic) for reference and making notations, the patient becomes their sole object of focus. This usually gives the patient a sense that the physician is interested and engaged, increasing patient satisfaction. Time is actually saved.

32. c) It is beyond the scribe's scope of practice (see Answer 27) to perform any diagnostic testing, including history taking, visual acuity, and pupil evaluation. The exception would be if the person is a trained scribe/tech. A scribe may be called upon to locate lab or test results in the patient's chart. They should be completely fluent with the practice's EHR system (and may be able to navigate it better than the practitioner!).

33. d) This kind of comment, where the patient was identified by name, is an ethical and confidentiality breach and is considered a violation of the patient's rights under HIPAA. In this case, a casual conversation over lunch, there was not a need on the part of your colleague to collaborate with the rest of you regarding the patient's care. (See also Answer 25.) That makes d) the false answer.

34. c) Implied consent means that something the other person does (ie, an action by the other person) or doesn't do (ie, by remaining silent on a matter) indicates their permission and willingness for something to take place or be done. In this case, leaning forward into the instrument (and remaining silent) implies that the patient permits the slit lamp exam.

35. a) In express consent, the patient's permission is given verbally (as in this case) or in writing.

36.   d) A barrier to learning is anything that may compromise the patient's ability to understand the information presented. It may include a lack of information (eg, leaving out one of the requirements, such as explaining possible risks), poor communication (as in this example), cultural barriers, and the patient's lack of health literacy.

37.   d) No one in the medical field, in any capacity, should ever guarantee any type of results for any type of treatment or procedure.

38.   b) If legally emancipated (examples: under 18 and married, a parent, able to prove they are financially dependent, or in active military service), this patient may sign their own consent form for the procedure. Otherwise, a parent must sign for the minor (known as *informed permission*).

39.   a) The institution's informed consent must contain a statement regarding the fact, if trainees/residents will participate in and/or perform the procedure.

40.   c) Surprised? The word "all" might have tripped you up. The discussion of risks must, yes, include *the most common ones*, or those that a "reasonable person" would want to know. An example would be the risk of infection following a cosmetic procedure. It is potentially impossible to list every single possible risk. The argument might be made that informed consent would have to include mention that if the patient is allergic to eye drops used during the same procedure, they could die of anaphylactic shock. But while there is a risk there, it is so remote that most would agree that there's no need to specifically mention it.

Reference

1.   Margo CE. Quality care and practice variation: the roles of practice guidelines and public profiles. Accessed August 26, 2020. http://v2020eresoucre.cor/content/files/qualitycare_practice.htm

Bibliography

Association of American Medical Colleges. Report V. Contemporary issues in medicine: quality of care. Accessed March 18, 2023. Published August 2001. http://v2020eresource.org/content/files/quality_of_care.pdf

Study and Test-Taking Strategies

Ledford JK.
Certified Ophthalmic Technician Exam
Review Manual, Third Edition (pp 487-496).
© 2023 Taylor & Francis Group.

Setting goals seems to be a human passion. Perhaps it wasn't too long ago when you set your sights on becoming certified as an ophthalmic assistant. Now you have chosen a new goal, expanding your horizons and increasing your value to your employer and patients. Your decision also means that you must once again buckle down and study. Allow the worthiness of your major goal (becoming certified) to empower and motivate you as you take the smaller steps that move you in that direction, whether it is breaking brand new technical ground or just completing the day's reading. Having a goal when studying will give you purpose and motivation to continue and to improve.

Hitting the Books

Reading

It may be your tendency to zip through everything you read. In and of itself, fast reading is not necessarily poor reading. The key in study-reading is to comprehend what you read, regardless of your reading speed.

Here are several suggestions to help you increase your reading speed and comprehension:
1. Before you start, know why you are reading. In our case, we are seeking to learn and understand new material. We are looking for information.
2. Glance over the headings and subheadings to get a quick grasp of the main ideas before you start to read.
3. When reading the material for the first time, take it slow and easy.
4. Look up any words you don't know. Increasing your vocabulary will increase your cumulative reading speed.

There are several bad habits that will slow down your reading. You'll need to eliminate them. Here are the biggest offenders:
1. Using your finger or a pencil to track along as you read.
2. Moving your whole head as you read across the page. Instead, you should move your eyes across the page, keeping your head still.
3. Moving your lips as you read. (To find out if you do this, hold a pencil between your lips while reading. Don't bite or grip it with your teeth, just hold it gently between your lips. If the pencil waggles and falls out as you read, you're afflicted. The remedy is to put the pencil between your lips every time you read for a week or so. Concentrate on holding the pencil still. You eventually should be able to retrain yourself and kick the habit.)
4. Reading each and every word independently. Train yourself to read groups of words instead.

Here are a few pointers on careful reading:
1. Before you start, have an idea of what you're looking for. Skim the headings to see what's in store.
2. As you read, concentrate. Pay attention to what you're doing. (More on this later when we talk about studying.)
3. Relax. Try to leave your problems behind. Focus on your reading.
4. Don't panic if you didn't seem to catch on after reading the material for the first time. Don't freeze up. Read it again.
5. Take a break after 45 minutes or so of straight reading. Reward your brain and body with a nice long stretch. Your eyes need a break, too. But instead of closing them, gaze at something far off in the distance for a minute or so. This will relax the ciliary muscle and help prevent accommodative spasms.

Good reading habits can be learned. With practice (and you'll be getting plenty of that!) your reading skills gradually will improve. If you have a serious reading deficit, you should consider professional counseling.

Study Strategy

Like reading, good study habits can be learned and developed over time. If you have an interest in the topic, it's easier to study. Your study will be focused and purposeful. In the exam/certification game, your study habits can make or break you.

With a little bit of preplanning, your study time will become second nature. To avoid hit-and-miss studying, you need to plan your work and then work your plan, as the saying goes.

First, choose a place where you will study. I know you've heard this before, but here it is again: study in the same place every session. The ideal study conditions include:

1. Ample desk room—a good writing surface with enough space to spread out. If you can create a place for yourself that is off-limits to anyone else, that would be best. Then you can leave your materials there and won't have to regather everything each session.
2. Good lighting.
3. Comfortable temperature. It'll be hard to study huddled over a space heater in the basement!
4. A sturdy, comfortable chair (but not too comfortable).
5. No distractions, or at least minimal distractions. We usually think of distractions as noise. But there may be visual distractions as well. We'll talk about minimizing family interruptions later. Meanwhile, turn off the cell phone and computer notifications while you're studying.

There is another type of distraction that can be the toughest one to eliminate: drifting brain syndrome. These are internal distractions—thoughts that pop into your head unbidden as you try to study. You may be worried about paying the rent, or your daughter's football game (she's the quarterback!). The dog may have fleas and the 2-year-old may have temper tantrums. But try to put these things aside (as much as possible) when it comes to your study time. All of your problems will still be there when you've finished your assignment.

Once you've carved out your study niche, the next item on the agenda is *when* you are going to study. You need to be a good time manager since you probably are adding studying to an already crowded schedule of obligations. Trying to fit your studying between or after other activities can lead to problems.

To help decide what time is best for you, consider what part of the day you are at your best. Try to schedule at least some of your studying during that time. For "morning people" that means studying early before the day really starts. If mornings make you queasy, study at night after the kids are in bed. Either the early morning or late-night time slot will eliminate or at least minimize those family distractions we were looking at earlier.

So set a definite time you will study and commit yourself to it. Set your highest priorities and put them on your calendar. For now, studying for your exam will have to be one of those high priorities. Add other things around your study schedule as you are able.

To help carve out your study time, try to become more efficient in your other tasks. Find online hints to learn ways of saving time. Your family won't cave in if you don't squeeze your own orange juice or fix your own car. This need to study is temporary, anyway. Teach the kids how to make their own peanut butter and pickle sandwiches. (And ask them to make you one, too, while they're at it!)

How long should you study each day? That depends in part on how much time you have before the date of your exam. But you should understand that the shorter the study time, the sooner you will forget what you've learned. In fact, you may not learn much at all, having stored the information in your short-term memory. Most of it (maybe even 80%[1]) will pop back out after the test. In order to truly *learn*, you must assign meaning to the information, not merely look at words. Ways to do that are coming up shortly.

As you plan your study time, remember that to be efficient and avoid fatigue you should give yourself about a 10-minute break after each 45 minutes or so of intense study. This break time must be included as a vital part of your study schedule.

Having a schedule for study has several advantages:

1.   It puts you in control. You're never biting your pencil wondering what to do next.
2.   It decreases anxiety. You're not overwhelmed by all those areas in the criteria book because you know that each item is going to be covered.
3.   You'll work efficiently. You'll know you have a certain number of pages to cover. You won't spend time flipping through your books trying to decide what to read next.

Organizing a Study Schedule

Creating a study schedule for yourself is a matter of listing what you need to accomplish, then fitting those items into the amount of time you have. Giving yourself 6 months to get ready for the exam should be plenty of time to proceed at a relaxed but steady pace. Of course, everyone is different, and each person's situation is different. Here is a sample 6-month plan, remembering that you'll need to accomplish the work listed regardless of the time you have available.

Month 1: Download criteria booklet and application. Review requirements and obtain necessary verifications (proof of completion of formal COA® or COT® program, continuing education credits, employer's record of hours worked, etc).

Assemble study texts, using index and table of contents to find information appropriate to content areas. Make a list of the topics and corresponding page numbers/web addresses. Don't get distracted with material that's not on the test. Decide when you will study (days and times) and divide the material accordingly. Allow several weeks before the test for review.

Month 2: Submit your application. (This way you'll be ahead of schedule if there are any problems with your paperwork.) Begin working your study schedule.

Month 3: When you receive notification regarding your eligibility to take the exam, you must register for it within 90 days. Your acceptance letter includes information on how to do this. You can also access the test modality's website, where you will find information on their page set-up and other helpful tips. Continue following your study schedule.

Month 4: Continue study plan.

Month 5: Finish study plan. Register for the exam if you haven't already done so. (See the IJCAHPO® *Criteria Handbook* if you need an extension of time, have extenuating circumstances, etc.) Make arrangements for travel and accommodations, if necessary.

Month 6: Review. Eat properly and get plenty of rest. Final days of review.

Square What?

Okay. So you've chosen a time and a place. You've formulated a study schedule, which gives you a goal for each study period. Your textbooks are on your desk and you're ready to get to work. What's next?

Next is a nifty little method of study-reading called the SQ3R method.[2] The letters and number are a mnemonic for the 5 general steps for good study-reading. SQ3R stands for survey, question, read, recite, and review. Here's how you use it:

1.   Survey. Before reading, leaf through the pages you will be covering that study period. Skim the headings and subheadings, pictures, and captions for an overview. As you glance over the material, you will probably recognize some of it. This scanning process will give direction to your reading and aid in your concentration.

2.   Question. From your survey, formulate some mental questions about what you're going to read. What do you expect to learn? Turn the headings into questions. For example, suppose you notice the sub-heading "Laws of Ocular Motility." You could ask yourself: "What are these laws? How do they affect eye movements? How do they affect the way I evaluate a patient?" Also ask yourself, "What do I already know about this topic?" These questions will help you concentrate as you look for the answers. If you have trouble doing this, you may want to write down your questions for several sessions just to get the hang of it. After that you can just keep them in your head.

3.   The 3 Rs.

   a.   The first R refers to the actual reading. As you read, you will be checking for 3 items. First, you'll be looking for the answers to the questions you've just formulated during the questions stage. Second, you'll be paying attention to those "little extras"—captions, graphs, illustrations, and so forth. Third, you'll be alert to words and phrases that are boldface, italicized, or under-lined. Look up any words you don't know.

   b.   The second R stands for recite. After you have read a short portion of your assignment, stop and summarize it. Condense the material into key words and phrases that will jog your brain to remember what you just read. There are several ways to do this. First, recite orally. This gives you extra stimulation by involving your hearing, not just your vision. A second method of recitation is to go back over the material quickly and underline or mark important parts of the text. Underline only key words or phrases, not entire sections. This gives you something to refer back to when you begin to review for the test. Later, when you glance over the material and see the words you highlighted, you will remember what you read about. A third way to recite is to make notes after you read, jotting down key words and main ideas. Summarize the material in your own words. You could even make these notes on index cards, creating valuable flash cards for later study. (By all means, take advantage of IJCAHPO's® flash cards if you wish. But your personally created cards are made for specifically for *you*, emphasizing the material *you* need to retain.)

   c.   The last R of SQ3R stands for review. After you've read the entire assignment, stopping several times to recite, you should go back over all the material one more time. Look over the headings again, thinking over what each section was about. Let the marked words and phrases jog your memory.

Each day when you sit down to study, it's important to crank up and get going; don't dawdle or day-dream. Remember to take breaks and be sure to reward yourself in some way when you've finished. Watch TV or take a bubble bath. (But be cautious about rewarding yourself with food. If you do that, you'll probably find that you have gained a bit of weight by exam time. Then the self-discipline you've been using to study will have to be applied to dieting. Yuck! So if you want to reward yourself with a snack, stick to fruit and carrot sticks. You'll be doing yourself a favor!)

How to Prepare for a Test

Managing Pretest Stress

Things might have been pretty relaxed when all you had to do was read. Now that test time is close, the heat is on and you may be feeling the pressure. Actually, a moderate amount of stress is good for you. Not enough stress and you will be too carefree. Too much stress and you will freeze. So let's take an honest look at the situation.

What's at stake? This is not a do-or-die risk we're talking about. You can retake the test if you need to. Regardless of the results, you will come out alive. Maintain a realistic perspective!

Uncontrolled stress is not productive. Focused stress can help you think more clearly and sharpen your perception. Later, we'll talk about what to do if you panic during the test. But for now you need to relax so you can review productively. There are many ways you can prepare yourself for the exam and control your stress.[3]

1.   Academic preparation. Study! The other 3 are useless without this one. We'll talk about reviewing in a minute. If you've taken the test before, use the printout of missed items to strengthen weak areas.

2.   Psychological preparation. Be positive! Build yourself up. Remind yourself of the benefits of passing. I was studying for my COMT® exam during the Summer Olympics. I got a lot of encouragement in watching the competition. I knew I never would compete in an Olympics, but I had my own important job to do. I was reaching for my own gold. The athletes didn't give up, no matter what; I wouldn't either. By the same token, don't compare yourself with others. Look at the test as an opportunity rather than an adversary. Avoid self-pity by planning to reward yourself in some way when the test is over.

Pick up some new calming techniques. This might be as simple as closing your eyes and concentrating on your breath. There are lots of suggestions online. Be sure to include methods you can also use during the exam itself that don't require external objects that you won't be able to bring with you to the test site.

It might seem odd to mention this as part of your psychological readiness, but try to avoid smoking or eating when you study. You won't be allowed to do either during the exam, and that might throw you off.

Get some information about the test itself. Knowing what to expect reduces stress. How many questions are there? What topics are covered? What type of questions might be asked? How long do you have to take the test? Do you need to take pencils and paper? All these are answered for you in the criteria booklet. Talk to friends who have taken the test. If possible, visit the test site ahead of time. Then the place will be familiar.

If you have a history of panic during tests, consider getting counseling ahead of time. Also, there are some things you can do to handle panic—we'll cover them later.

3.   Physical preparation. The proper food and rest are important all the time, not just the night before the test. In the weeks before the exam, reduce sugars and increase protein and vitamins. Omega-3, anti-oxidants, and other supplements may help as well; do your research and/or consult a professional. And stay hydrated!

4.   Logistical preparation. Make early plans for getting to the test site and have a backup plan ready. Be sure to take your admission card and IDs. Don't forget your watch and any materials you may require.

Review Techniques

Study Material

Now that your reading is completed, you are armed with some formidable study aids. From the "question" part of SQ3R you have study questions. From the "recite" portion of SQ3R you have highlighted text, written notes, and flash cards. Dig out your old home study course test. (Make sure the answers are correct!) Some books (eg, *Principles and Practice in Ophthalmic Assisting: A Comprehensive Textbook*) have questions at the end of the chapter. Of course, you will plan on spending time daily with *this* book.

Ask questions at work about anything you don't understand. Talk to others who have taken the test, picking their brains for what they remember. You might want to make a new schedule to allot specific review times for specific material.

The test includes diagrams (you match the letter on the picture to the correct answer) and single best answer questions (a statement or questions followed by 4 possible answers, one of which is best; ie, multiple choice). Both of these types of questions call for recognition more than recall. If your study methods include asking yourself the tougher type of fill-in-the-blank and short answer questions, you will be even better prepared for the actual exam.

Another study aid you might consider is a formal ophthalmic technician review class. These are offered by various individuals and groups across the country, both online and in person. There are many advantages to such a course. For one, you get the benefit of being taught by someone who has already taken and passed the exam. If you attend a live conference you have a chance to rub shoulders with others who, like you, are determined to pass. Finally, you'll get handouts/downloads and other valuable material to study. The class also should help you identify your areas of strength and weakness.

Instead of a review course, you might attend a meeting that allows you to choose the topics you want or participate in some webinars. Select classes that fall into the content areas. Check IJCAHPO's® website for a list of review classes and seminars near you.

The Review Session

Successful review starts long before a mere 4 weeks prior to the exam. It's a fact of life: you have to study the material before you can review it. But since you made and followed a reading schedule months ago, you're ready to review. Way to go!

When reviewing, start with the material you feel least confident about, then move to the easier topics. Don't worry yourself over what they "might" ask. Concentrate on what they're *most likely* to ask.

Go back through your reading material, skimming what you marked. The next time you go through it, skip over what you know. Then grab a friend and recite, going over the material verbally. If you didn't make flash cards when you originally read the material, do so now. This will help you with memorization (covered in the next section).

How to Memorize[4]:

1. Repetition—practice! This is another reason why flash cards are so great. You can pull them out of your pocket while you are in the line at the grocery store and get in 5 minutes of study. Going over the material again and again really gets it into your conscious and subconscious brain. Depending on how you learn best, repetition may take the form of reading, listening (to an online lecture or reading aloud to yourself), or practice (use your book-learning in a practical way, such as performing retinoscopy).

2. Association—associate new information with something you already know. Here's one of my favorites: the edges of a minus lens bow inward, giving the lens the appearance of being *caved* in. That's how I remember that it is a con*cave* lens. Mnemonics are words or phrases (codes, really) merely intended to assist the memory. Do you remember Roy G. Biv? That silly name is used to memorize the colors in the spectrum. Each letter of the name stands for one of the hues. (Can't remember them? Go look it up!) You can make up memory tricks for yourself.

3. Stimulation—of as many senses as possible. Making your own note and flash cards serves several purposes. Your sight is stimulated by reading, touch by writing (and hearing when you recite aloud).

Fifteen to 20 minutes at a time of intense memorization is enough. Committing material to memory is more concentrated than reading, so give yourself more frequent breaks.

Study Groups

Study groups can be a great way to review the material for your exam. If there isn't anyone nearby to gather with, be sure and check out the online study groups that have sprung up. These may be as simple as an online group that messages each other as they are able, or a more organized session that meets in real time. Whether virtual or actual, group study can also help you manage stress simply by knowing that there are others going through the rigors of test preparation.

Ideally, someone who has already taken and passed the exam should function as group leader and mentor. If there is no one available to be your guide, members could take turns at being the facilitator. One person might be especially good at a particular task or subject and could conduct that review.

Use the same strategies in a group as you have for your own private study. Set a specific time and place and be sure to schedule breaks. This is a *review*, so everyone should have a good understanding of the material already. Try to stay on target, but don't forget that laughter is a great stress-reliever. Listen and learn from each other. Someone else may have a fresh perspective that will "turn the lights on" some topic you may have been struggling with. Or they may have a mnemonic or some other way of remembering that will help you. Be sure to share your discoveries, too. Use the same review materials in the group as you would alone. Another idea is to ask each group member to write several multiple-choice questions to share. Perhaps each person could do a different content area.

Remember SQ3R? Use R2 (recite) as a study aid. Have a partner scan your reading material and ask you to:

1. Explain the chapter title, headings, and subheadings
2. Define bold or italicized words and phrases
3. Answer questions based on the pictures and tables
4. Answer questions from the end of the chapter, this book, or old home-study tests.

There are several cautions about study groups, however. If someone in the group tends to panic or be anxious, they can affect the whole group. If encouragement doesn't help, you might have to ask them to refrain from making negative comments. If you are beginning to get upset yourself, it might be better to study alone.

Before You Know It ... Test Day

Actually, let's look at test day minus one. The day before your exam needs to be as laid back as possible. Eat well and get plenty of rest. Plan what you will wear tomorrow (something comfortable) so you won't be scrambling around in the morning. If you must travel to the test site and spend the night before, allow plenty of time to get there. If possible, drive by the test center so you know where it is. Ideally, go in and look at the room itself. This will help you psychologically. Review your notes for about 1 hour before going to bed. Refuse to upset yourself by thinking about all that you don't know.

Now the alarm rings, and it's test day. Get up early enough so you're not rushed. Eat a good breakfast that includes protein but avoid eating anything too heavy in the 2 hours just prior to test time. Remember your admission card, 2 valid IDs, watch, and any materials. Arrive early. If possible, choose a distraction-free seat. It's probably best not to talk to others about the test beforehand. Try to relax. Focus on being calm and confident.

How to Take a Test

Listen to the proctor. Read instructions carefully. Be sure to enter your name and number correctly.

Remember how many questions there are. In the COT® exam, there are 3 hours to answer about 200 questions. That is about 1 minute per question. Use this information to pace yourself. When your time is half up, if you haven't worked to the halfway point, go there anyway.

Read the entire question before looking at the answers. Think of an answer before you read the choices. Read each choice before marking an answer.

A multiple-choice question is actually a group of true/false questions. Try out each answer. Does it make the statement true or false? One answer will be "truer" than all the rest.

Answer the easy questions, then go back to those you're not sure of or have to figure out (you can "flag" these on the computer). You might jot a note or 2 about a tougher question to help you when you come back. When you've been through the test once and are going back to answer the harder questions, continue to pace yourself. If you feel the need for spending a while on a question, move on again and come back later. Your subconscious will be looking through your brain files for the answer while you move on. When you come back to a question, it may have "incubated" long enough and the answer will come right to you.

Multiple-choice questions often contain one answer that is obviously wrong, 1 or 2 answers that appear reasonable, and 1 or 2 correct answers. (If there are 2, one is more correct than the other). If the answer to a question is not obvious to you, eliminate any answers that you are sure are wrong. Then try to pick the best answer from those that are left.

If the question involves math, read the problem carefully. What do they want to know (lens power, cylinder axis, minus cylinder)? Estimate the answer before you start the actual calculations.

Every now and then one question will contain the answer or hints to another. Lucky you! But don't waste too much time looking back through trying to find something. Do your best to concentrate on one question at a time.

Beware of the following words: *none, most, never, always, must, only, all, some, usually, sometimes, every, many, few, often, seldom, more, equal, less, best, good, bad, worst, exactly,* and *may.* If used in the question, be sure to read *very* carefully.

Managing Panic

If you panic, stop (before you freeze). Take a brief break. Close your eyes. Talk to yourself. Remember all you did to prepare for the exam. Then breathe! Inhale for 3 seconds, hold it for 12, then exhale for 6 seconds. This helps even out your blood gas level and puts you in control. Remind yourself that you know what to do—you have a plan. Refocus on the task at hand. Concentrate on one question at a time, not on the whole test. Imagine yourself in a familiar setting, at work on a task that you know you can perform. Hold that thought, then get back to work.

Taking the Practical Exam

The testing modality will provide you with pass/fail information and how you did on specific elements of the test, but it's not official until you receive the snail mail notification from IJCAHPO®. Once you receive the good news that you've passed the written test, you realize that not only have you accomplished something great, but you get to take another test! Certification as an ophthalmic technician requires that you also pass a practical exam. The practical is given in the form of a computer simulation.

After you pass the written COT® exam, IJCAHPO® will issue you an application for the skills evaluation. After the application is approved, you will be given a link to an online tutorial and have 90 days to take the test.

The skill evaluation covers lensometry (NON-automated), automated visual fields, phoria/tropia testing, keratometry, retinoscopy and refinement (ie, refraction), and applanation tonometry. The retinoscopy/refinement and lensometry sections are offered in plus and minus cylinder. You have 1.5 hours to complete the exam. A "warning" will appear onscreen when you have 5 minutes left to finish a specific task.

A Final Word

So there you have it. You've studied, prepared, and probably even sweat a little. You can do this! Obtaining your COT® is quite an accomplishment. It's something to be proud of and maintain, both personally and professionally.

So what are you doing here? Go celebrate!

References

1. League L. Why cramming fails and study plans succeed. Q Practice Website. Updated October 21, 2019. Accessed March 18, 2023. www.qpractice.com/cramming-fails-study-plans-succeed/
2. Education Corner Website. The SQ3R strategy for reading textbooks. Accessed March 18, 2023. www.educationcorner.com/sq3r-textbook-strategy.html
3. Online Schools Center Website. 20 effective ways to calm your nerves before an exam. Accessed March 18, 2023. www.onlineschoolscenter.com/20-effective-ways-to-calm-your-nerves-before-an-exam/
4. Major C. 21 best, easy memorization techniques for students. Developing Human Brain Website. Accessed March 18, 2023. www.developinghumanbrain.org/memorization-techniques-for-students/

Bibliography

Berry M. *Help Is on the Way For: Tests*. Children's Press; 1985.

IJCAHPO. Core Criteria Handbook for Certification and Recertification. 2019 2nd ed. Accessed March 19, 2023. https://documents.jcahpo.org/documents/Certification/IJCAHPO_Core_Examination_Content_Areas.pdf

Lenz E, Shaevitz MH. *So You Want to Go Back to School*. McGraw-Hill; 1977.